THE SPARKS THAT ENDURE

Why Our Core Human Drives Survive Mental Illness

By Clovis Raymond, MD

Editor: Cynthia Constantino

Copyright © 2025 by Clovis Raymond, MD

All rights reserved. No part of this publication may be reproduced, stored in a retrieval system, or transmitted in any form or by any means—electronic, mechanical, photocopying, recording, or otherwise—without the prior written permission from **the author**, except in the case of brief quotations embodied in critical articles or reviews.

ISBN: 979-8-9935477-3-2

Library of Congress Control Number: 2026900680

Cataloging-in-Publication Data: Pending

Publication year: 2025

Edited by Cynthia Constantino
Cover and interior design by Andy Magee

Praise for The Sparks That Endure

"In The Sparks That Endure, Dr. Clovis Raymond illuminates the often-overlooked truth that core human drives—such as the need for meaning, intimacy, and self-expression—do not disappear in the face of serious mental illness. With clinical insight and deep compassion, he challenges us to see our patients not solely through the lens of pathology, but through the light of their enduring humanity. This book is a necessary addition to the evolving field of person-centered psychiatry."

—Mardoche Sidor, MD, *Quadruple Board-Certified Psychiatrist, Founder of SWEET Institute, Author of* Mindset, Mood & Memory

"Dr. Raymond, in his book, The Sparks That Endure, *brilliantly, elegantly, and humanistically demonstrates how one is more than their illness. This holistic point of view mirrors what I have witnessed for years in my therapy room. Dr. Raymond refreshingly highlights the common human needs of connection, meaning, and purpose—the 'sparks' that refuse to be extinguished despite a debilitating illness and its significance in establishing therapeutic rapport and providing treatment. This book is a must-read and I'll be recommending it highly to every clinician and non-clinician alike."*

—Dr. Andreia Harris, PhD, *Licensed Clinical Psychologist; Clinical Supervisor at Health & Hospitals Corporation (Rikers Island); Former Deputy Director of Mental Health at Rikers Island; Former Training Director in Psychology at Mount Sinai Hospital/Elmhurst Hospital Center; Former Executive Clinical Director at On-Site Psychological Services; Former Director of Psychotic Disorders Program at NY Hospital, Cornell/Westchester*

"*In both medicine and nursing education, we're taught to assess symptoms, manage conditions, and measure outcomes. But rarely are we trained to see the enduring desires—the sparks—that remain alive beneath a diagnosis. In* The Sparks That Endure, *Dr. Clovis Raymond delivers a powerful, paradigm-shifting message: that even amid serious mental illness, individuals hold onto deep and vital longings—connection, joy, purpose, creativity. As a physician and the director of a nursing institute, I see this book as essential reading for clinicians,* educators, and caregivers alike. It challenges us to treat not just the illness, but the humanity that persists within it."

—Roger Fimerlus, MD, Founder & Director, Hearts Institute Nursing School, Florida

"In a world where wellness is often reduced to quick fixes and surface solutions, The Sparks That Endure dares to go deeper. Dr. Clovis Raymond brings compassion, clarity, and hard-earned wisdom to the conversation around mental health, reminding us that healing is not about erasing struggle but reconnecting to the drives that make us feel alive. Dr. Clovis Raymond doesn't just talk about mental illness—he listens deeply to what still burns beneath it. As a radio host who hears real stories every day, I can tell you this: people want to be seen, not just diagnosed. This book does exactly that. It's powerful, human, and long overdue."

—Seema Roc, Director of Community Affairs; Radio Host

"In The Sparks That Endure, Dr. Clovis Raymond brings a wealth of insight as a professor, psychiatrist, scholar, and practitioner. His perspective is global, cross-cultural, and combines scholarly research with profound practicality."

—Dr. F. Adam Souffrant, Lead Pastor, Maranatha Evangelical Church of the Nazarene, Philadelphia, PA; Church Consultant; Member at Large, New York State Association of Protestant Chaplains

"As someone who has guided countless young people through life's pivotal transitions—from high school to higher education, from confusion to clarity—I find The Sparks That Endure to be a profound and necessary work. Dr. Clovis Raymond has captured something we often miss in both education and mental health: that the core human longings—like meaning, connection, creativity, and joy—do not disappear in illness. They persist. They endure. They guide. Whether in my role as a school counselor, a Sunday school director, or a Christian mentor, I've seen firsthand how these sparks sustain hope and ignite transformation, even in the most discouraged hearts. This book is not only a compassionate guide for professionals—it's a mirror for every one of us who believes healing is not just possible, but purposeful."

—Denet Alexandre, MA, School Guidance Counselor; Director of Christian Education; Chair, Board of Trustees, Falkenstein Library; Christian Ministry Counselor, Spring Valley, NY

"I appreciate Dr. Raymond's adroitness in peeling the nuances which envelop the indestructible sparks that feed the intricate webs of our humanity, even when affected by the most severe forms of mental disorders. Through his sympathetic *therapeutic alliance with his patients, he has uncovered their enduring determination to thrive and to generate hope. This book is an indispensable tool for mental health practitioners, researchers, scholars, and anyone who is concerned with mental health recovery."*

—Dr. Emmanuel Charles, LMSW, Former Forensic Program Administrator and Forensic Treatment Team Leader (Kirby Forensic Psychiatric Center)

Dedication

To my beloved parents, whose lives and memories continue to guide and ground me.

Your love lit the first spark.

You are forever present in every word and every purpose behind this work.

Acknowledgments

Writing this book has been both a professional journey and a deeply personal one. It is the culmination of years spent listening to the quiet, persistent voices of patients—voices that remind me daily that humanity endures, even in the depths of serious mental illness.

To my patients: you have been my greatest teachers. Your courage, resilience, and honesty have given this work its heart.

To my wife, Emmanuela: your compassion as a nurse and your unwavering support have mirrored my own path and strengthened it. You understand, perhaps better than anyone, the quiet dignity in caring for those who suffer.

To my family: your patience and love have been my grounding force through the long hours of writing and reflection.

To my brothers, sisters, and extended family—thank you for being the foundation from which I have grown. Your support, laughter, and wisdom—spoken and unspoken—echo through these pages.

To my alma mater, Universidad Central del Este, for shaping not only my knowledge, but my vocation.

To Harlem Hospital Center – Columbia University: thank you for teaching me to sit with suffering, to listen between the silences, and to witness the enduring humanity in mental illness. You shaped me into the psychiatrist I am today.

To my mentor, Dr. Zana Dobroshi: you believed in me before I believed in myself. Your faith made this work possible.

To Rockland Psychiatric Center: thank you for the daily lessons in dignity, courage, and the resilience of the human spirit.

To my colleagues and mentors in psychiatry: your insights and shared commitment to person-centered care have deeply influenced this book.

And to every caregiver, clinician, advocate, and reader who picks up this book in the hope of better understanding the people they serve—or the people they love—thank you for joining me on this journey.

This book is dedicated to the enduring spark of humanity in all of us.

About the Author

Dr. Clovis Raymond is a board-certified psychiatrist with extensive clinical experience in General and Child & Adolescent Psychiatry. He earned his medical degree from Universidad Central del Este in the Dominican Republic, where he graduated as valedictorian. He completed his residency and fellowship at Harlem Hospital Center – Columbia University, where he now serves as Assistant Clinical Professor of Psychiatry.

Dr. Raymond is Chief of Psychiatry at Rockland Psychiatric Center in New York and maintains a private practice in Bardonia. He is also a retired Major in the United States Army Reserve.

Throughout his career, Dr. Raymond has worked with individuals facing some of the most severe and stigmatized psychiatric conditions—schizophrenia, schizoaffective disorder, bipolar disorder, and related illnesses. He didn't set out to write a book; he set out to understand why, even in the most disorganized mental states, people remain tethered to certain elemental drives—money, sex, food, music, ritual, movement, and more.

His professional interests include the role of enduring preoccupations ("sparks") in patient identity, narrative psychiatry, and trauma-informed, recovery-oriented care. He is a sought-after educator and speaker in these areas.

In *The Sparks That Endure*, Dr. Raymond weaves clinical insight, patient stories, and personal reflection to argue that these persistent desires are not distractions from illness—but essential expressions of identity, agency, and meaning.

More than a physician, Dr. Raymond is a witness to suffering, resilience, and the light that refuses to go out in even the most troubled minds. This book is his testament to the enduring humanity within us all.

Table of Contents

Foreword 15
Preface 16
Introduction 19

Part I – Foundations of Desire and Survival
1. The Enduring and Unforgotten Desires of the Mind 23
2. The Neurobiology of Desire 36
3. Understanding Serious Mental Illnesses 54

Part II – The Core Sparks of the Human Spirit
4. Sex: Intimacy, Desire, and Identity in Mental Illness 63
5. Money: Security, Power, and the Preoccupation with Wealth 100
6. Food: Appetite, Nourishment, and the Emotional Meanings of Eating 113
7. Music: Rhythm, Memory, and the Language of Healing 135
8. Spirituality: Faith, Transcendence, and the Search for Meaning 156
9. Creativity: The Impulse to Make, Imagine, and Express 166
10. Movement: The Body in Regulation and Release 178
11. Rituals: Structure, Safety, and Symbolic Practice 186
12. Nature: Grounding, Calm, and Restorative Power 195
13. Humor: Laughter, Irony, and Resilience 204

Part III – The Hidden Sparks
14. Sparks in the Shadow: The Drives that Survive Mental Illness 211
15. Touch: The Forgotten Language 217
16. Storytelling: Making Meaning Amid Madness 223
17. Hope: The Improbable Light 229
18. Freedom: Autonomy in Constraint 236
19. What Lives in the Shadows Still Burns 243
20. When the Flame Goes Out: Missing Sparks 249

Part IV – Intersections and Integrations

21. The Intersection of Sparks in Recovery 255
22. Whispers Through Time: What History's Mad and Brilliant Minds Teach Us 264
23. Sparks Across Borders: Culture and the Global Expression of Human Drives 272
24. Amplifying Voices: The Power of Lived Experience 279
25. Living Beyond Sparks: A Person-Centered Path to Recovery 285
26. Future Directions: Emerging Science, Innovation, and Policy 295
27. Practical Strategies: Bringing Sparks into Therapy and Support ... 300
28. Sustaining Sparks: Final Reflections 316

Epilogue 321
Appendices 324
Glossary 361
Index 371
Endnotes 373

Symptoms may shout, but sparks whisper. And if we listen closely, they'll tell us what still matters, what still burns.

Foreword

I have had the privilege of watching Dr. Clovis Raymond grow into the thoughtful and compassionate psychiatrist he is today. From the earliest stages of his career, he demonstrated a deep reverence for the complexity of the human mind and the quiet resilience of those living with serious mental illness. In *The Sparks That Endure*, Dr. Raymond brings that same reverence to the page. This is not a book about symptoms—it is a book about survival. About the surprising and enduring drives that persist even when a person's reality has been fractured by psychosis or mood instability. It is about the humanity that remains, often in ways that are overlooked or misunderstood.

I've long admired Clovis's ability to see his patients not only through the lens of diagnosis, but through the prism of meaning. Whether exploring the role of music, money, sexuality, or spirituality in the lives of those with schizophrenia or bipolar disorder, he asks: What does this reveal about who this person still is? What desires are still alive beneath the illness?

His writing is as grounded as his clinical work—careful, clear, and profoundly humane. He offers a lens that is simultaneously neuroscientific and deeply personal, clinical, and symbolic. The result is a work that challenges both professionals and families to rethink how we understand the lived experience of mental illness.

As a psychiatrist, *The Sparks That Endure* reminds me of why I entered this field: to witness, to listen, and to hold space for the whole person—not just the disorder. As a mentor, I am proud to see Dr. Raymond bringing these values into his writing and sharing them with a broader audience.

This book is a meaningful contribution to our field. It offers tools, yes—but more importantly, it offers truth and compassion. I am honored to introduce it, and I believe it will spark insight, dialogue, and healing for all who read it.

Zana Dobroshi, MD
Board Certified Psychiatrist

Preface

Illuminating the Sparks Within Serious Mental Illness

There is a paradox at the heart of serious mental illness. Conditions like schizophrenia, schizoaffective disorder, and bipolar disorder can fracture cognition, distort perception, and destabilize the lives of those they touch. And yet, beneath even the most severe symptoms, the fundamental drives of human existence — those tied to intimacy, pleasure, creativity, connection, and meaning — persist. The pursuit of sex, money, food, music, spirituality, creativity, movement, ritual, humor, and connection to nature endures, often in altered yet recognizable forms.

Imagine a psychological landscape frequently obscured by shadow, where the vibrant hues of everyday life appear muted or extinguished. This is the lived reality for many individuals navigating the complexities of severe psychiatric illness. Diagnostic terms like schizophrenia, bipolar disorder, and major depressive disorder with psychotic features often evoke images of suffering and loss. These associations are not unfounded; the challenges are profound. But too often, that is where the narrative stops. What gets overlooked are the persistent embers of life that continue to glow within — desires, needs, and impulses that remain vital even amidst disorganization, despair, and withdrawal.

This book emerged from a sustained clinical curiosity. Over years of psychiatric practice, I repeatedly encountered patients who, despite hallucinations, delusions, or extreme mood states, remained preoccupied with elemental human concerns. At first, these preoccupations — sexual, financial, sensory, or spiritual — appeared tangential or symptomatic. But as I listened more deeply, a different picture emerged. These were not trivial distractions or pathological residues. They were essential throughlines, vital threads of continuity tethering each person to a coherent sense of self and to the world around them.

This is a book about those threads — about the sparks of life that flicker beneath the surface of even the most severe psychiatric illness. It is an exploration of how elemental human drives are experienced, modulated, and at times magnified by mental illness, and how, when intentionally recognized and nurtured, these same drives can serve as sources of strength, purpose, and connection.

To be clear: this is not a book that minimizes the gravity of serious mental illness. It does not romanticize suffering or suggest that symptoms can be transcended by sheer will or engagement with passion. Rather, it is a clinical, conceptual, and deeply human invitation to broaden our view of what recovery entails. Recovery is not merely the attenuation of hallucinations or the stabilization of mood. It is also the restoration of vitality, meaning, and personhood — the rediscovery, and sometimes the first discovery, of what makes life worth living.

In the chapters that follow, we will explore fourteen enduring domains of preoccupation that I have come to call sparks: sex, money, food, music, spirituality, creativity, movement, rituals, humor, nature, touch, storytelling, hope, and freedom. These sparks manifest in myriad ways — some familiar, others unexpected — yet they share a common quality: they illuminate the core of a person's identity, even when that identity feels fractured or obscured by illness.

We will examine these domains through the lenses of psychiatry, neuroscience, and lived experience. You will meet individuals whose stories reveal how these sparks persist and sometimes flare amid psychosis, depression, or disorganization. We will consider how these enduring preoccupations can be pathologized, misunderstood, or overlooked in traditional models of care. More importantly, we will explore how they can be recognized, respected, and cultivated as part of a person-centered approach to treatment and recovery.

This book is written for a wide audience — for clinicians seeking new tools to engage meaningfully with their patients; for families and caregivers longing to understand the person behind the diagnosis; for individuals living with mental illness who wonder whether they remain whole beneath the weight of their symptoms; and for all who wish to see psychiatric conditions not only through the lens of disorder, but through the enduring lens of humanity.

To see a spark in someone is to recognize that they are more than their illness. To nurture that spark is to participate in a form of healing that extends beyond symptom reduction into restoration and renewal. My hope is that this work contributes to a growing movement in psychiatry — one that honors not only what is broken, but what remains unbroken and bright.

Because in the end, the truest form of healing is not merely to suppress symptoms, but to see, honor, and nurture the life force that persists — always.

Join me as we explore these sparks: not as curiosities, but as vital, animating forces — as beacons of continuity, as testaments to the enduring architecture of the human mind, and as tributes to the indelible spirit it protects.

This book advocates for a strength-based, person-centered approach — one that recognizes that alongside suffering, there is also resilience, meaning-making, and a persistent longing for connection and fulfillment. The enduring sparks of life — whether manifested through relationships, rituals, or expressions of creativity and humor — are often obscured, but never erased, by illness.

As we turn to the Introduction, we will ground this exploration in the science of desire itself — tracing how the brain, body, and psyche conspire to sustain life's most enduring drives. From dopamine pathways to cultural rituals, from neurobiology to narrative, we begin our journey into the resilient circuitry of human meaning — and the sparks that endure within us all.

Introduction

What Persists When the Mind Fractures?

Modern psychiatry has long been preoccupied with classification, diagnosis, and symptom management. Within this clinical framework, individuals living with schizophrenia, schizoaffective disorder, and bipolar disorder are often understood through the lens of their dysfunction, hallucinations, delusions, disorganized speech, affective instability, and cognitive decline. Yet even as these symptoms dominate psychiatric discourse, a more fundamental question remains underexplored: What persists when so much appears to be lost?

This book proposes that certain elemental human concerns, sex, money, food, music, spirituality, creativity, movement, ritual, humor, and connection to nature, are not eradicated by serious mental illness. Rather, they endure, often reemerging in altered forms that defy traditional clinical explanation. These enduring concerns, which I refer to as sparks, offer a profound window into the preserved architecture of personhood. They are not peripheral to psychiatric care, they are central to recovery, meaning-making, and dignity.

Through years of clinical observation, I came to recognize a pattern. Patients who struggled to orient to time or place could still recall lyrics to a beloved song. Individuals who spoke in fragmented thoughts and neologisms often retained deep anxieties about money or sexual identity. Even those living with fixed delusions frequently expressed persistent rituals, aesthetic preferences, or spiritual convictions. At first glance, these expressions might seem irrational or irrelevant. But upon closer inspection, they revealed themselves as anchors—evidence of a continuing self within a disrupted mind.

Consider the patient who, despite profound paranoia and withdrawal, still requests their disability check, not solely as a financial transaction, but as a gesture of agency and predictability. Or the woman who, though nonverbal, sways gently to music that stirs her inner world. These moments are clinically significant not because they fit diagnostic criteria, but because they signal vitality. They indicate that even in the presence of severe psychiatric disturbance, core aspects of human desire, identity, and memory remain intact.

The concept of sparks challenges the reductionist view that mental illness obliterates personhood. Instead, it suggests that beneath and beyond pathology lies a substratum of human continuity. Sparks may not always be consciously articulated or outwardly functional. They may emerge as compulsions, fixations, or symbolic acts. But they persist, illuminating a terrain of experience that is often overlooked by symptom-focused care models.

This book is organized around fourteen of these enduring domains. Each will be examined through multiple lenses: clinical case examples, neuroscience and psychodynamic theory, and the lived experience of those navigating the complexities of serious mental illness. These domains are not arbitrary; they have emerged consistently across time, cultures, and diagnostic boundaries. Their recurrence suggests they are not simply epiphenomena of illness, but central components of the human condition.

By attending to these sparks, we move beyond pathology and begin to regard individuals as whole persons. This approach aligns with recovery-oriented models of care, which emphasize not only symptom management but also purpose, connection, and self-determination. It also invites a more nuanced clinical gaze, one that resists dismissing preoccupations as mere noise, and instead asks: What is being expressed here? What is striving to survive?

Throughout this book, you will encounter individuals whose psychiatric symptoms are severe, and yet, whose enduring desires shine through the fractures. Their stories illustrate that the drive to love, to create, to move, to laugh, to connect with nature or spirit, does not disappear in psychosis or mania. It may be obscured, distorted, or delayed, but it persists.

Understanding and honoring these sparks has practical implications. For clinicians, it offers new strategies for engagement and alliance-building. For families, it provides insight into the emotional logic that remains beneath erratic behavior. And for patients themselves, it affirms that they are not defined solely by disorder, but by the enduring elements of identity that continue to seek expression.

This introduction sets the foundation for what follows: a deep, sustained inquiry into how these fourteen sparks endure in the lives of those living with serious mental illness. Each chapter will explore one domain, offering a multidimensional view that integrates scientific evidence, clinical application, and human testimony.

In doing so, we aim to reframe psychiatric care, not as a response to what is broken, but as a recognition of what remains whole.

Let us begin, then, with a reconsideration of preoccupation, not as pathology alone, but as a signal. A direction. A survival instinct. A spark.

I recognize that a work like this will invite critique from multiple directions. Some will say it leans too heavily on stories and vignettes that cannot substitute for controlled studies. Others may feel it speaks too clinically, using the language of psychiatry rather than the lived language of patients and families. Still others may find the very focus on enduring passions—sex, money, food, music, and the others—too idealistic for the realities of psychosis, mania, and institutional care. Ethical concerns will also be raised, particularly around how clinicians can safely acknowledge sparks such as intimacy, touch, or financial autonomy without overstepping professional boundaries.

These critiques are valid, and I want to acknowledge them directly. This book is not a treatment manual, nor a memoir, nor a single authoritative voice. It is instead an attempt to hold together multiple truths: the neurobiology of desire, the testimony of those living with serious mental illness, and the clinical insights of those who accompany them. Sparks are not cures, and they do not negate the very real suffering of illness. Rather, they represent enduring human drives that persist even when cognition, language, and daily life are profoundly altered. To recognize them is not to romanticize illness, but to respect the depth of humanity that remains.

My hope is not that every reader agrees with every claim, but that they recognize in these pages an invitation: to notice, to honor, and to integrate the sparks that endure. If critique arises, may it serve not to silence but to deepen dialogue. I write this as one psychiatrist among many, offering observations gathered over years of practice, but also as a fellow human being who has witnessed resilience where it might least be expected. These sparks remind us that even when illness reshapes a life, the core of desire, meaning, and connection is rarely extinguished. That truth, more than any framework or theory, is what I hope endures beyond these pages.

You may not see what I see at first. But I invite you to pause at the places where desire remains, because they're more than symptoms.

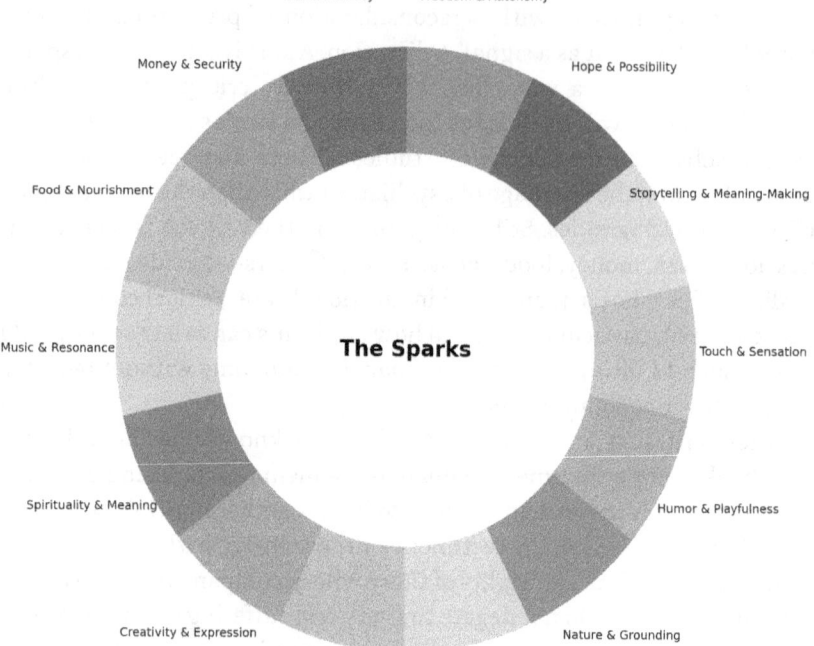

Part I – Foundations of Desire and Survival

Chapter 1:
Thee Enduring and Unforgotten Desires of the Mind: Money, Sex, Food, Music, Spirituality, Creativity, Movement, Rituals, Nature, Humor, Touch, Storytelling, Hope, and Freedom in the Lives of Individuals with Serious Mental Illness

What Persists When the Mind Fractures?

I didn't write this book because I had the answers—I wrote it because I kept seeing the same patterns, the same sparks, flickering beneath the symptoms. I wrote this chapter as a psychiatrist, but also as someone who's watched these sparks surface again and again, in places we least expect.

I remember sitting with a patient who had barely spoken for weeks. When I asked what he missed most, he quietly said, "dancing." That moment changed me. It reminded me that beneath the silence of illness, there's a person still longing for rhythm, connection, and joy.

In the depths of serious mental illness, certain desires persist—steady, recurring, and often unextinguished. These enduring interests are not merely symptoms or incidental byproducts of pathology. Rather, they are fundamental expressions of the human condition—what this volume refers to as sparks: elemental preoccupations that endure across time and diagnostic categories. These sparks offer insight into what remains resilient and meaningful within the fractured psyche.

I used to think psychosis erased personality. I was wrong. The longer I listened, the more I saw how sparks remained.

There were moments when I felt helpless. But witnessing someone come alive through food, art, or faith reminded me what healing really looks like.

This book seeks to examine those enduring desires—not simply as behavioral phenomena but as critical markers of identity, vitality, and humanity.

As a psychiatrist, I have had the privilege of working with individuals navigating the profound disruptions associated with schizophrenia, schizoaffective disorder, bipolar disorder, and other serious mental illnesses. I have witnessed how delusions dismantle familial bonds, how mood episodes destabilize entire life trajectories. And yet, consistently, I have observed a remarkable pattern: even in the presence of significant cognitive and emotional disorganization, certain preoccupations recur with striking regularity. These are not fleeting obsessions or compulsions, but deeply embedded, affectively charged themes, concerns that reflect continuity with the self rather than mere symptomatology.

Sparks represent more than interests. They are sources of meaning, engagement, and vitality, elements often obscured by clinical discourse focused exclusively on pathology. Conceptualizing sparks invites a shift in perspective: from managing dysfunction to identifying and nurturing that which persists and animates.

For people living with serious mental illness, these enduring themes may at times be distorted, exaggerated, or misdirected. Nonetheless, their presence is not inconsequential. They often signal the preservation of psychological continuity and may serve as entry points for therapeutic alliance and recovery-oriented care.

Others before me have tried to capture why certain passions refuse to fade, even under adversity. Abraham Maslow (1943) argued that higher aspirations like love, creativity, and meaning only arise once survival is secure. Yet in psychiatry, I have found otherwise: even when safety is fragile, the hunger for intimacy, music, or beauty endures. Peter Benson (2008) called these passions "sparks," describing them as the hidden strengths that guide identity and purpose. I came to see this in my patients, but also in myself. Many nights I wrote so late into the morning that my three daughters—two in eighth grade and one in tenth grade—had to wake me so they would not be late for school. Sparks persist not because life is orderly, but because they insist on expression, even in exhaustion.

Beyond Symptoms: The Relevance of Sparks in Clinical Context

Severe psychiatric disorders are frequently accompanied by apathy (a diminished capacity for interest, initiative, or responsiveness) and anhedonia (the reduced ability to experience pleasure). These negative symptoms contribute substantially to functional decline, relational withdrawal, and demoralization. However, amidst this affective flattening, sparks, whether spontaneous or elicited, can offer powerful counterweights to disengagement.

The implications are profound. Engaging with a patient's intrinsic interests, however idiosyncratic or unconventional, may offer clinicians a path forward when traditional therapeutic routes are obstructed. Even when language is limited, behavior disorganized, or affect blunted, attention to enduring interests can illuminate the path toward relational and rehabilitative progress.

Enduring Preoccupations: Intrusive or Insightful?

What we often term preoccupations in clinical language may, in fact, represent unresolved psychological content that demands recognition. Such preoccupations, whether related to sexuality, finances, food, or creative expression, can dominate thought and behavior. In clinical presentations, they may appear as delusions, compulsions, or perseverative speech. Yet to reduce them solely to pathology is to miss their symbolic and existential significance.

Indeed, these preoccupations are not randomly distributed. They cluster around core human drives: survival, intimacy, control, identity, transcendence. Whether observed in schizophrenia, bipolar disorder, personality disorders, or treatment-resistant depression, they frequently reflect universal psychological motifs distorted by illness.

Clinical Vignettes: The Spark Beneath the Symptom

Consider Jean, a man diagnosed with schizophrenia whose daily life is punctuated by auditory hallucinations and formal thought disorder. Amidst these disruptions, one element remains constant: a pronounced preoccupation with sex. His frequent masturbation and persistent sexual ideation are often dismissed as hypersexuality or disinhibition. Yet viewed differently, they may represent a fundamental expression of bodily awareness, intimacy-seeking, or identity preservation.

Or take Oscar, living with schizoaffective disorder, who grows agitated when denied a satisfying evening meal or when his modest weekly stipend is delayed. His distress is not merely a behavioral disturbance—it is a visceral response to unmet needs for nourishment and autonomy.

Robert, in his fifties, harbors an unshakeable delusion that his family is poisoning him. He inspects each meal with obsessive vigilance. Yet amid this delusional framework, he repeatedly inquires about his disability check—not merely as a financial matter, but as a reflection of agency, predictability, and control in an otherwise chaotic world.

Then there is Mary, a largely nonverbal woman with chronic schizophrenia. During a group session, a familiar song on the radio elicits a subtle but unmistakable transformation—her eyes brighten, she smiles faintly, and she begins to sway. In that moment, music bypasses the barriers of psychosis and accesses something enduring and alive.

These vignettes are not anomalies. They represent a pattern. Time and again, amidst disorganization and despair, certain preoccupations resurface: money, sex, food, and music. These are not simply remnants of premorbid functioning; they are expressions of persistent personhood.

The Concept of Sparks

Recovery in serious mental illness is neither linear nor universal—it is deeply individual and shaped by the person's environment, history, and internal resources. Within this nonlinearity, sparks emerge as signposts of retained identity and potential growth.

A spark is defined here as an enduring interest, preoccupation, or pleasure that connects an individual to their sense of self or to the broader world. These may include creative expression, spiritual practices, sensory rituals, physical activity, or even familiar routines. Though they may manifest differently across individuals and illness states, their persistence offers a window into what remains stable amidst psychiatric upheaval.

Too often, sparks are overlooked in clinical care, dismissed as fixations, obsessions, or eccentricities. Yet when reframed, they may be seen as anchors of resilience and continuity.

Crucially, sparks are not incompatible with treatment. They do not negate the need for pharmacologic or psychotherapeutic interventions. Rather, they offer complementary pathways through which recovery can be personalized and meaningfully sustained.

The Fourteen Domains of Preoccupation: Foundations of Enduring Human Experience

Even amid the perceptual distortions of schizophrenia, the mood fluctuations of bipolar disorder, or the cognitive dampening of severe depression, certain elemental human concerns emerge with remarkable persistence. These are not random or trivial, they are structured, recurrent, and often profoundly meaningful. The domains of sex, money, food, and music are frequently the most visible and recognizable. However, other equally significant domains—spirituality, creativity, movement, rituals, nature, and humor, though sometimes more subtle, are no less essential to identity and human flourishing.

Together, these fourteen categories represent archetypal human drives and expressions. They persist across cultures and clinical presentations, surfacing not as symptoms alone but as reflections of core psychological and existential needs.

For clinicians, recognizing these enduring preoccupations offers a practical and compassionate framework for patient engagement. Instead of focusing solely on symptom suppression, treatment can be reframed to include an inquiry into what persists: What continues to matter to the patient? What evokes emotion, attention, or desire, even in the depths of illness?

Each of the domains will be explored in subsequent chapters, but a brief conceptual overview is provided here to orient the reader to the scope and rationale of the framework.

Sex: The Drive Toward Intimacy and Identity

Sexuality is a foundational human drive, tightly interwoven with intimacy, identity, and bodily agency. In psychiatric disorders—particularly mood and psychotic conditions—sexual themes often become dysregulated, distorted, or amplified. Hypersexuality may emerge in manic states, while sexual content may be woven into paranoid or grandiose delusions. For some individuals, sexual preoccupations take obsessive or compulsive forms.

Rather than pathologizing these manifestations outright, a deeper analysis reveals underlying needs: the search for closeness, affirmation, or bodily recognition. Understanding sexual behavior through a biopsychosocial lens allows clinicians to explore its meaning rather than suppress its expression reflexively.

Money: Symbolism of Power, Control, and Autonomy

The preoccupation with financial matters is a recurrent theme in serious mental illness, often manifesting as compulsive spending, delusions of wealth, or extreme frugality. Money becomes more than a currency—it is a symbolic container for autonomy, survival, justice, and legacy.

In delusional systems, money may signify power, restitution, or divine reward. In depressive states, its absence may reinforce helplessness and worthlessness. Addressing financial concerns in treatment is not simply a matter of economic planning; it is an exploration of self-efficacy, trust, and identity in relation to the external world.

Food: The Terrain of Nourishment, Control, and Connection

Eating is a biological necessity, but it is also a profound social, cultural, and emotional act. In severe mental illness, food often becomes a site of struggle—whether through refusal, compulsive ingestion, or delusional distortion.

Some individuals may experience persecutory beliefs around food (e.g., fear of poisoning), while others take part in ritualized or restrictive eating patterns. Appetite disturbances are common across diagnostic categories, particularly in depressive and psychotic conditions. Understanding the meaning of food-related behaviors requires attention to both somatic and symbolic dimensions of nourishment, care, and control.

Music: Sound, Memory, and Emotional Organization

Music is perhaps the most neurologically and emotionally integrated form of human expression. It engages memory, emotion, sensory processing, and often serves as a means of self-regulation. In clinical work, music frequently surfaces in the narratives and behaviors of patients with serious mental illness—as obsessional listening, hallucinatory content, or therapeutic engagement.

Patients may use music to organize thoughts, soothe distress, or externalize affective states that are otherwise inaccessible. Far from being incidental, musical preoccupations can be leveraged to enhance engagement, access autobiographical memory, and foster a sense of agency.

Spirituality: Transcendence, Coherence, and Belonging

Spiritual beliefs and practices often remain intact—or are even heightened—during psychiatric illness. While some presentations involve religious delusions, it is essential to distinguish pathological distortions from meaningful spiritual seeking. For many patients, spirituality provides structure, hope, and a moral framework within which suffering can be understood.

Clinicians must approach spiritual content with nuance, balancing the need to assess risk e.g., in the case of command hallucinations (often voices) that tell a person to do something, through giving orders or instructions. For example, someone may hear a voice telling them to harm themselves or others. In the case of apocalyptic delusions (fixed false beliefs that the world is ending or that a catastrophic event is imminent), a person may be convinced that they are living through the end of the world, even when there is no evidence. with the potential therapeutic value of faith, ritual, and existential meaning. When respected and integrated thoughtfully, spirituality can serve as a potent source of resilience.

Creativity: The Imperative to Express and Be Witnessed

Creativity is a vehicle through which individuals externalize internal experiences. Whether through art, writing, music, or invention, creative output reflects the persistence of agency, narrative construction, and self-expression. In patients with disorganized thought or communication deficits, creative acts may serve as compensatory mechanisms for meaning-making.

Importantly, creativity in psychiatric populations is not always goal-oriented or conventionally productive. It may take repetitive, symbolic, or fragmented forms. Nevertheless, when recognized and supported, creative engagement can offer containment, visibility, and therapeutic resonance.

Movement: Embodiment and Emotional Regulation

The body often expresses what words cannot. Movement—whether as compulsive pacing, stereotyped gestures, or intentional activity—frequently serves as a means of emotional release, trauma processing, or grounding. In catatonic or psychomotor presentations, movement (or its absence) may carry diagnostic significance, but it also holds expressive and regulatory potential.

Physical engagement, including dance, exercise, or somatic therapies, may support emotional processing, interpersonal connection, and stabilization of affect. Attention to movement patterns allows clinicians to recognize embodied expressions of psychological distress or resilience.

Rituals: Repetition, Order, and Symbolic Safety

Rituals, whether cultural, religious, or idiosyncratic, provide structure in the midst of chaos. They mark time, encode meaning, and offer predictability. For individuals experiencing psychosis or mood instability, ritualized behavior may represent attempts to regain control or impose coherence on an unpredictable internal landscape.

Rather than interpreting all rituals as compulsions or symptoms of obsessive-compulsive pathology, clinicians should explore their function and meaning. In many cases, rituals are adaptive efforts to restore safety, continuity, or belonging.

Humor and Play: Resilience, Defense, and Social Connection

Humor is a sophisticated form of cognitive and emotional processing. In psychiatric contexts, it may appear incongruent, deflective, or even disorganized. Yet often, humor and play represent adaptive coping strategies that buffer against despair and foster connection.

Laughter and play are also powerful tools for building therapeutic alliance, humanizing care, and facilitating emotional processing. Far from trivial, the capacity for humor signals the preservation of perspective and relational intent, even in the midst of severe impairment.

Nature: Sensory Grounding and Existential Perspective

Connection to the natural world—through animals, landscapes, weather, or gardens—offers both sensory stimulation and existential grounding. For individuals living in clinical or institutional environments, access to nature may restore a sense of vitality, continuity, and regulation.

Nature-based interventions are increasingly recognized as legitimate components of recovery-oriented care. Even brief encounters with natural environments can reduce agitation, enhance mood, and support cognitive integration.

Each of these ten domains will be explored in greater depth throughout the book, integrating clinical vignettes, neuroscientific insights, and recovery-oriented strategies. Together, they constitute a map of enduring humanity within the experience of serious mental illness.

Touch and Sensation

The need for physical contact and sensory input. Safe, nurturing touch can soothe distress, affirm connection, and restore a sense of belonging. Even in illness, the body seeks comfort through tactile experience.

Storytelling and Meaning-Making

The human drive to shape experience into narrative. Storytelling helps integrate memories, explain suffering, and affirm identity. Through words, art, or personal accounts, people reclaim coherence in their lives.

Hope and Possibility

The forward-looking spark that sustains motivation. Hope provides resilience during despair and opens pathways to recovery, reminding us that change and renewal remain possible even in difficult circumstances.

Freedom and Autonomy

The desire to make choices and direct one's own life. Autonomy affirms dignity, supports recovery, and allows individuals to engage their sparks on their own terms, even within the constraints of illness.

The Benefits of Nurturing Sparks

Recognizing and cultivating enduring personal interests—sparks—is not a peripheral gesture of compassion; it is a core component of effective, person-centered psychiatric care. Clinical practice that attends to these sparks offers not only symptomatic relief but also enhances overall functioning, autonomy, and engagement.

The following are empirically and clinically supported domains in which nurturing sparks exerts meaningful benefit:

1. Counteracting Apathy and Anhedonia

Apathy and anhedonia, hallmark features of serious mental illness, contribute substantially to functional disability and social withdrawal. These symptoms impair intrinsic motivation and diminish the capacity to derive pleasure from formerly enjoyable activities. Re-engaging individuals through their enduring interests—like music, tactile activities, or meaningful routines—can partially restore emotional responsiveness and promote behavioral activation.

Even small interventions (e.g., enabling access to music playlists, gardening, or pet interaction) can yield noticeable improvements in affect and willingness to engage. Such efforts may precede or potentiate responsiveness to pharmacologic and psychotherapeutic treatments.

2. Enhancing Self-Esteem and Perceived Competence

Participation in meaningful, interest-driven activities reinforces a sense of agency and self-efficacy. For people living with severe psychiatric diagnoses, the internalization of stigma and repeated experiences of failure can erode self-esteem. When patients are supported in rediscovering or developing skills aligned with their sparks, they often experience a revitalization of personal competence and identity.

Clinicians and caregivers who actively acknowledge and validate these capacities play a critical role in fostering psychological growth and countering internalized helplessness.

3. Fostering Social Connection and Reducing Isolation

Many sparks are inherently relational. Whether expressed through participation in group art therapy, music-making, religious services, or recreational outings, these interests create opportunities for connection. Severe mental illness frequently isolates individuals from peers, family, and broader society; fostering shared interests offers an accessible avenue for rebuilding interpersonal bridges.

Group interventions built around shared sparks may not only reduce loneliness but also improve social cognition, perspective-taking, and affective attunement.

4. Supporting Cognitive Stimulation and Recovery

Sparks that involve cognitive engagement—like reading, storytelling, problem-solving tasks, or creative expression—offer indirect pathways to strengthen executive functioning, attention, and working memory. Neuroplasticity research underscores the importance of enrichment in cognitive recovery and adaptive functioning. Interest-driven activities can serve as ecologically valid (practically relevant) forms of cognitive rehabilitation.

Rather than framing these activities as adjunctive, they should be viewed as complementary strategies for promoting neural engagement and psychological integration.

5. Promoting Meaning and Existential Coherence

One of the most devastating consequences of chronic psychiatric illness is the erosion of a coherent narrative self. When individuals lose a sense of purpose or direction, the risk of despair increases markedly. Sparks—however modest—offer reentry points into meaning-making frameworks.

Whether it is a spiritual belief, an artistic endeavor, a caregiving role, or a connection with animals or nature, these interests often serve as existential scaffolding. They help individuals locate themselves within a personally relevant story that transcends illness.

6. Reducing the Expression of Negative Symptoms

While negative symptoms like emotional blunting and social withdrawal are notoriously treatment-resistant, structured engagement around sparks can modestly mitigate these symptoms. When individuals experience authentic interest or pleasure, even transiently, the effects can cascade into improved communication, hygiene, appetite, and affective responsiveness.

Sparks provide non-pharmacological leverage points for interrupting the inertia of negative symptom syndromes.

7. Enhancing Overall Quality of Life

Ultimately, the integration of enduring interests into psychiatric care improves subjective quality of life. When treatment extends beyond symptom control to embrace vitality, connection, and creativity, patients report greater satisfaction, autonomy, and hope. Family members and support networks also benefit when their loved one re-engages with the world in meaningful ways.

In sum, recognizing and supporting sparks should be understood not as a luxury of high-functioning patients, but as an essential element of dignified care for all individuals living with serious mental illness.

Conclusion: Sparks as Signals of Enduring Personhood

Preoccupations with sex, money, food, music, spirituality, creativity, movement, ritual, nature, and humor are not simply peripheral interests—they often define the subjective experience of individuals living with schizophrenia, bipolar disorder, and schizoaffective disorder. Far from being random distractions, these preoccupations are expressions of continuity, identity, and humanity.

When viewed through a clinical lens, a spark is a preoccupation that is both affectively charged and behaviorally persistent. It draws attention, organizes action, and resists extinguishment. In psychiatric illness, these preoccupations may at times appear intrusive, distorted, or even maladaptive. But beneath the surface, they often signify an enduring will to live, connect, and find meaning.

To overlook these signals is to risk rendering the patient invisible.

When clinicians learn to inquire about these domains—not just to catalog symptoms, but to locate meaning—they are better equipped to engage patients holistically. A concern about money may open discussions about safety and control. Sexual themes, if met with respect rather than shame, can lead to insights about intimacy and identity. Ritualized behavior may offer structure where none exists. Music may awaken memory or emotion long thought dormant.

Engaging with sparks is not a substitution for evidence-based treatment—it is a deepening of it. It is a movement toward care that is not only effective but humane.

Implications for Practice

Clinicians: Begin asking not just "What are your symptoms?" but "What do you care about, even now?" Incorporate sparks into treatment planning, therapy goals, and rehabilitation strategies.

Families and caregivers: Look for recurring patterns, interests, or rituals—even those that appear eccentric. These are likely indicators of retained identity. Families and caregivers can take simple but powerful steps: observe recurring patterns or interests, validate them without judgment, and find safe ways to encourage expression. Journaling these observations and sharing them with clinicians can turn eccentric-seeming rituals into therapeutic entry points. Above all, recognizing these sparks as signs of enduring identity can help families celebrate resilience rather than focusing only on deficits.

Systems of care: Design programming, environments, and services that make room for patient interests. Recovery is not built from symptom reduction alone, but from the restoration of meaning.

Society: Reframe the narrative of serious mental illness away from deficit and toward dignity. These individuals are not absent from the human condition; they are its clearest testament, because their struggles reveal our shared needs for connection, meaning, safety, and hope. In living with extreme vulnerability, they embody the very essence of what it means to be human: the capacity to endure, to seek sparks of vitality, and to insist on dignity even in the face of suffering.

When we attune ourselves to what endures, we are reminded that no mind is ever entirely lost. Even in disarray, the human spirit retains its sparks. These sparks do not merely survive illness—they illuminate it.

Reflection Questions

Can you recall a patient or loved one whose recurring behavior, interest, or ritual reflected a deeper spark?

How might identifying sparks influence your approach to treatment or support?

What questions could you include in clinical assessments to elicit these interests?

Have you identified your own personal sparks—those sources of meaning that remain vital even in times of adversity?

Table 1.1 — The Fourteen Sparks at a Glance

Spark	Core Drive	Clinical Relevance
Sex & Intimacy	Desire for closeness, identity, reproduction	Often silenced in care but central to recovery
Money & Security	Control, survival, autonomy	Preoccupations, delusions, or empowerment
Food & Nourishment	Sustenance, pleasure, ritual	Appetite changes, comfort, cultural roots
Music & Resonance	Rhythm, memory, expression	Regulates mood, connects identity
Spirituality & Belief	Meaning, transcendence	Anchors hope, can blur with delusions
Creativity & Expression	Making, imagining, storytelling	Enhances agency, identity, coping
Movement & Body	Regulation, vitality, embodiment	Exercise, dance, trauma release

Spark	Core Drive	Clinical Relevance
Rituals & Structure	Order, repetition, predictability	Grounding, protective, sometimes rigid
Nature & Grounding	Environment, calm, restoration	Reduces stress, supports resilience
Humor & Play	Laughter, irony, resilience	Buffers stress, fosters bonding
Touch & Sensation	Connection, safety, sensory input	Comfort or avoidance, trauma-linked
Storytelling	Identity, narrative, coherence	Meaning-making, recovery narratives
Hope	Future orientation, possibility	Essential in recovery; prevents despair
Freedom	Autonomy, choice, dignity	Balancing safety with agency

For foundational perspectives on enduring human drives and passions, see Maslow, A. H. (1943). *A theory of human motivation. Psychological Review, 50*(4), 370–396; Benson, P. L. (2008). *Sparks: How parents can help ignite the hidden strengths of teenagers.* Jossey-Bass; Csikszentmihalyi, M. (1990). *Flow: The psychology of optimal experience.* Harper & Row; Frankl, V. E. (1959/2006). *Man's search for meaning.* Beacon Press; Field, T. (2010). Touch for socioemotional and physical well-being: A review. *Developmental Review, 30*(4), 367–383; Lysaker, P. H., et al. (2007). Narrative and meaning in schizophrenia: Implications for recovery. *Psychiatry, 70*(3), 247–260.

For research on the therapeutic use of music in serious mental illness, see Gold, C., Mössler, K., Grocke, D., Heldal, T. O., Tjemsland, L., Aarre, T., ... & Rolvsjord, R. (2009). Individual music therapy for mental health care clients with low therapy motivation: Multicentre randomised controlled trial. *Psychotherapy and Psychosomatics, 78*(5), 319–327.

The term "spark" is used here in dialogue with but distinct from Benson's definition in adolescent development (Benson, 2008).

For links between hidden sparks and psychiatric recovery see: Field (2010) on touch; Lysaker et al. (2007) on narrative; Frankl (1959/2006) on hope and meaning; Frankl (1959/2006) on freedom as existential choice even in constraint.

Chapter 2

The Neurobiology of Desire: A Foundation

In the preceding chapter, we explored how fundamental human desires—what we term sparks—endure even in the midst of severe psychiatric disorders. These persistent preoccupations with sex, food, music, money, intimacy, and autonomy suggest that certain elemental drives are resilient, surfacing despite disorganized thinking, emotional dysregulation, or psychotic content. To understand why these desires survive, we must look beneath the surface of behavior and examine the brain itself—the biological foundation of motivation, craving, and emotional resonance.

Serious mental illnesses like schizophrenia, schizoaffective disorder, and bipolar disorder are not merely behavioral disruptions or failures of will. They are rooted in complex and often dysregulated neurobiological processes. These conditions alter how individuals perceive the world, regulate their emotions, construct meaning, and pursue connection. They also profoundly affect the brain's reward and motivation systems—circuits that have evolved to prioritize survival, pleasure, and social bonding.

Understanding the interplay between brain structure, neurochemistry, and enduring psychological drives allows for a more compassionate and scientifically grounded approach to care. It helps explain why preoccupations with sex, food, music, or money are not merely distractions or pathologies. They are often distorted expressions of intact biological imperatives—evidence that the person within is still seeking connection, satisfaction, and meaning, albeit in altered forms.

This persistence is not just psychological but deeply biological, connected to states researchers call flow. Mihaly Csikszentmihalyi's (1990) concept of "flow" describes the absorption and vitality people feel when fully engaged in an activity. Neurobiology shows these states activate dopamine pathways and quiet self-monitoring regions of the brain. Patients often describe flow when drawing, drumming, or walking the same path in a ward. I experienced it, too, while writing this book—losing all track of time until the sound of my daughters' footsteps pulled me back to the present.

BRAIN LABELS WITH THE 14 SPARKS

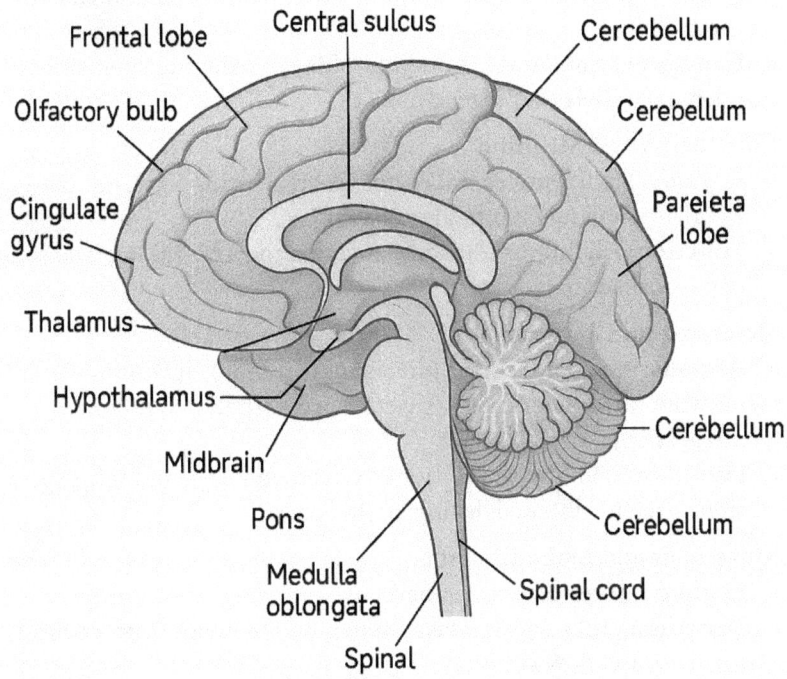

Brain Function as It Relates to the 14 Sparks

1. Sex and Intimacy
- **Regions:** Hypothalamus, amygdala, orbitofrontal cortex, ventral striatum.
- **Function:** Governs desire, attachment, reward. Oxytocin and dopamine drive intimacy and pair-bonding.

2. Money and Security
- **Regions:** Prefrontal cortex (planning, decision-making), ventral striatum (reward), anterior cingulate cortex (risk evaluation).
- **Function:** Links abstract symbols of value with survival instincts, autonomy, and social status.

3. Food and Nourishment
- **Regions:** Hypothalamus (hunger), insula (taste), orbitofrontal cortex (pleasure evaluation).

- **Function:** Integrates metabolic needs with reward learning, turning eating into both survival and comfort behavior.

4. **Music and Resonance**
   - **Regions:** Auditory cortex, hippocampus, nucleus accumbens, cerebellum.
   - **Function:** Stimulates memory, rhythm, and emotion. Dopamine release parallels that of food and sex.

5. **Spirituality and Meaning**
   - **Regions:** Medial prefrontal cortex, posterior cingulate, temporoparietal junction (default mode network).
   - **Function:** Facilitates transcendence, perspective-taking, and sense of purpose beyond the self.

6. **Creativity and Expression**
   - **Regions:** Prefrontal cortex (divergent thinking), default mode network (idea generation), parietal cortex (spatial-symbolic integration).
   - **Function:** Combines novelty, pattern recognition, and self-expression, often heightened during altered states.

7. **Movement and Embodiment**
   - **Regions:** Motor cortex, cerebellum, basal ganglia.
   - **Function:** Links body movement to mood regulation, procedural memory, and flow states.

8. **Rituals and Structure**
   - **Regions:** Basal ganglia (habit), anterior cingulate (error detection), prefrontal cortex (planning).
   - **Function:** Provides predictability, reduces anxiety, and engages dopaminergic reinforcement loops.

9. **Nature and Grounding**
   - **Regions:** Parahippocampal gyrus, anterior cingulate, insula.
   - **Function:** Exposure to green space reduces amygdala reactivity, calms stress circuits, and enhances connectedness.

10. **Humor and Playfulness**
    - **Regions:** Prefrontal cortex (cognitive incongruity), nucleus accumbens (reward), amygdala (emotional tagging).
    - **Function:** Merges surprise, relief, and joy; laughter reduces cortisol and strengthens social bonds.

11. **Touch and Sensation**
    - **Regions:** Somatosensory cortex, insula, orbitofrontal cortex.

- **Function:** Oxytocin-mediated bonding, stress reduction, and memory of safety.

12. Storytelling and Meaning-Making
- **Regions:** Default mode network, temporal lobes, hippocampus, Broca's and Wernicke's areas.
- **Function:** Shapes identity, transmits culture, builds coherence from fragmented experience.

13. Hope and Possibility
- **Regions:** Prefrontal cortex, ventral striatum, anterior cingulate.
- **Function:** Future-oriented cognition; links reward prediction with resilience and persistence.

14. Freedom and Autonomy
- **Regions:** Dorsolateral prefrontal cortex (agency), anterior insula (self-awareness), parietal cortex (sense of control in space).
- **Function:** Core to human motivation—agency drives engagement, reduces learned helplessness, and strengthens recovery.

Together, these Sparks form a **neural constellation**: the **limbic system** supplies emotional salience, the **prefrontal cortex** shapes meaning and control, the **basal ganglia and cerebellum** support habit and flow, and the **default mode network** weaves identity and narrative.

Psychological and Biological Roots of Preoccupation

Enduring preoccupations can arise from multiple intersecting factors: unresolved psychological needs, trauma, emotional deprivation, and neurodevelopmental differences. In many cases, they reflect the mind's attempt to resolve internal conflict or to reassert coherence and control. But to fully understand these fixations when it comes to serious mental illness, we must also consider the biological substrates—the neurochemical and anatomical systems that govern arousal, desire, and reward.

In this chapter, we explore the key systems of the brain involved in the regulation of desire and motivation, including:
- The dopaminergic reward system
- The limbic system, including the amygdala and hippocampus
- The prefrontal cortex and executive function

Key neurotransmitters beyond dopamine: serotonin, norepinephrine, oxytocin, and endorphins:

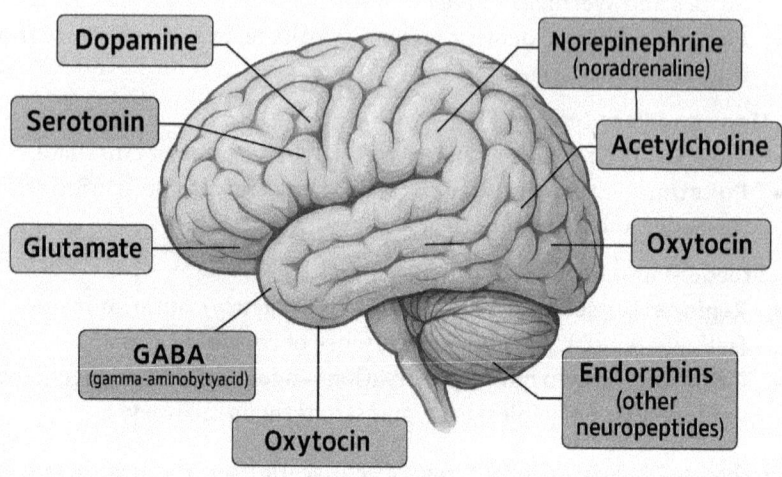

The structural and functional brain differences associated with schizophrenia, schizoaffective disorder, and bipolar disorder:

These systems shape the intensity, regulation, and direction of our fundamental drives—whether for food, sex, connection, or pleasure—and also help explain the exaggerated or distorted forms these drives may take in illness.

The Brain's Reward Circuitry and Dopaminergic Function

I didn't always see desire as something you could trace in the brain. But the science, and my patients, have shown me otherwise.

The first time I saw how dopamine lit up the brain's reward circuits, I thought, no wonder people chase what they love—even when their minds are breaking.

In residency, I once spent an entire afternoon tracing the mesolimbic dopamine pathway for a presentation. But it wasn't until I watched a patient light up when she heard her favorite song that I understood what all those neural circuits really meant. Reward is real. It's not abstract—it's alive in the body.

At the heart of the human motivation system lies the brain's reward circuitry, particularly the dopaminergic pathways. These circuits evolved to promote behaviors essential for survival—eating, reproduction, social bonding, exploration—and to reinforce them through pleasure.

Dopamine: The Neurochemical of Motivation

Often dubbed the feel-good neurotransmitter, dopamine is better understood as the chemical of anticipation, motivation, and reward prediction. It signals when something is valuable, energizing the pursuit of that goal. Whether it is food when hungry, sexual intimacy, the acquisition of money, or the pleasure of music, dopamine activation propels behavior.

When dopamine is released—particularly in the mesolimbic pathway, which connects the ventral tegmental area (VTA) to the nucleus accumbens—we experience a sense of reinforcement. The brain registers: This matters. Do it again.

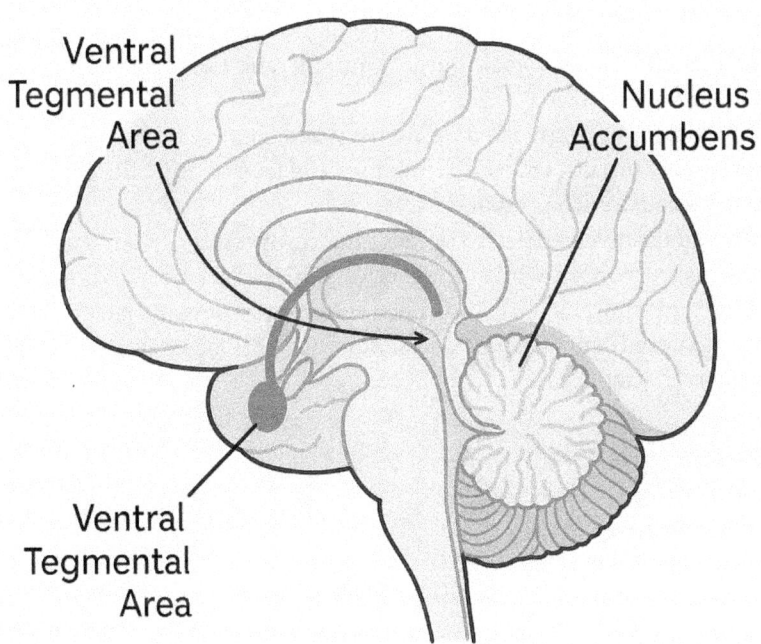

Dysregulation in Mental Illness

In people living with serious mental illness, this system can become dysregulated in two primary ways:

Excessive dopamine signaling (as in psychosis or mania) may amplify the salience of irrelevant or irrational stimuli—e.g., delusions of grandeur involving wealth or fame, compulsive sexual behavior, or exaggerated preoccupations with music.

Reduced dopaminergic activity, particularly in schizophrenia, contributes to anhedonia—a diminished ability to experience pleasure—making it harder for individuals to derive joy from sex, food, or social interactions.

In both cases, the spark remains. But its expression may become distorted, obsessive, or flattened, depending on which aspect of the dopaminergic system is disrupted.

Brain Structure and Function: Imaging the Spark

Advances in neuroimaging—including functional MRI (fMRI) and PET scans—have enabled researchers to map changes in brain anatomy and activity in people with psychiatric disorders. Several brain regions relevant to desire and motivation show consistent differences in people living with schizophrenia, schizoaffective disorder, and bipolar disorder:

Prefrontal Cortex: Often reduced in volume or function, impairing judgment, planning, and impulse control. Dysfunction here can compromise financial decision-making, goal pursuit, and the regulation of sexual or appetitive urges.

Hippocampus: Implicated in memory and contextual learning; abnormalities may disrupt emotional memory and lead to difficulty integrating past experience with present desires.

Amygdala: Involved in emotional salience; overactivity can amplify fear and threat responses, while underactivity can blunt emotional resonance.

Striatum and Nucleus Accumbens: Core components of the reward system; altered function here correlates with both obsessive pursuits and emotional flattening.

PART I – FOUNDATIONS OF DESIRE AND SURVIVAL

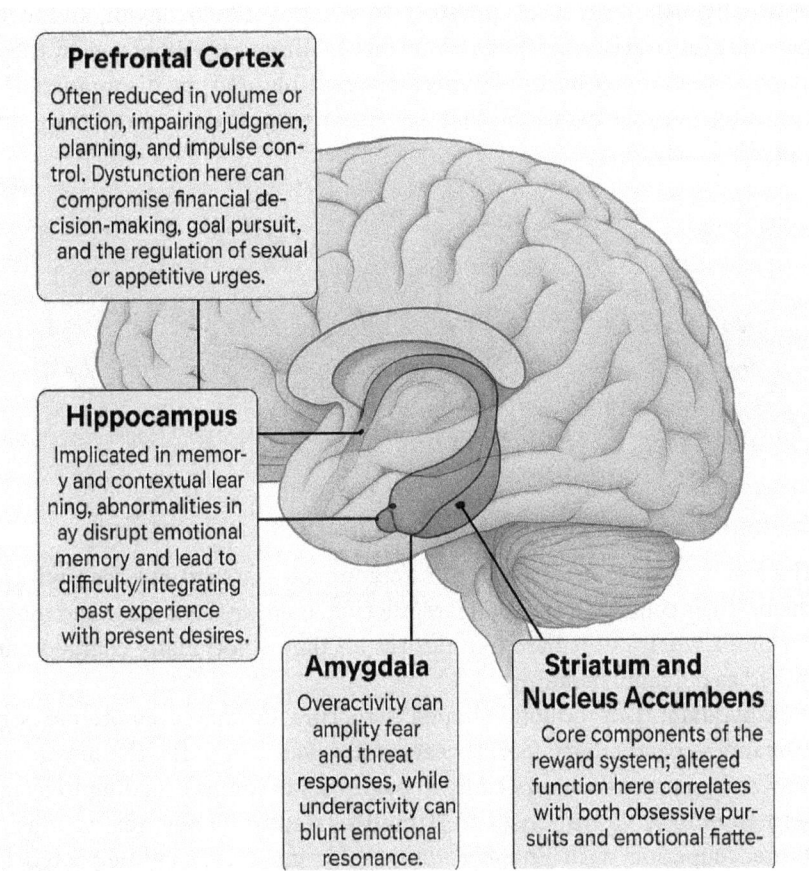

Prefrontal Cortex
Often reduced in volume or function, impairing judgmen, planning, and impulse control. Dystunction here can compromise financial decision-making, goal pursuit, and the regulation of sexual or appetitive urges.

Hippocampus
Implicated in memory and contextual lear ning, abnormalities in ay disrupt emotional memory and lead to difficulty/integrating past experience with present desires.

Amygdala
Overactivity can amplity fear and threat responses, while underactivity can blunt emotional resonance.

Striatum and Nucleus Accumbens
Core components of the reward system; altered function here correlates with both obsessive pursuits and emotional fiatte-

Importantly, these neurobiological alterations help explain why the sparks of life persist but are often experienced differently. A patient may become intensely preoccupied with wealth or sexual fulfillment not because of moral weakness, but because of disinhibited reward signaling and impaired executive regulation.

In the next section (Part 2), we will expand this foundation to examine how each brain region and neurotransmitter contributes to the expression of specific sparks—and how their dysregulation shapes the clinical realities of those living with schizophrenia, bipolar disorder, and related illnesses.

Key Brain Regions and Neurochemical Systems in the Regulation of Desire

While dopamine is central to understanding the brain's reward and motivation systems, a broader array of brain regions and neurochemicals work in concert to shape human desire. These systems, when functioning optimally, help individuals pursue pleasure, regulate behavior, and form meaningful relationships. In serious mental illness (SMI), however, these same systems may become hyperactivated, blunted, or disorganized—resulting in preoccupations that are either magnified or rendered emotionally inert.

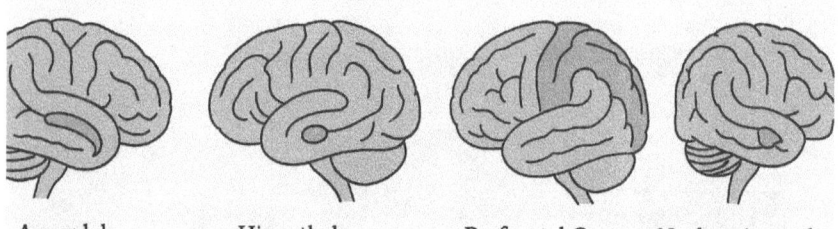

Amygdala   Hippothalamus   Prefrontal Cortex   Nucleus Accumbeı

1. The Limbic System: Emotion, Memory, and Motivation

The limbic system, a network of interconnected structures deep within the brain, is central to emotional regulation, memory encoding, and motivational salience. It is here that desires become emotionally charged and linked to personal meaning.

Amygdala: This almond-shaped structure evaluates emotional significance—particularly fear, threat, and reward. In SMIs, the amygdala may be hyperreactive (especially in psychosis or mania), leading to exaggerated emotional responses to stimuli related to money, sex, or music. A preoccupation with financial danger, for instance, may be rooted in amygdala-driven anxiety about survival or autonomy.

Hippocampus: Critical for memory consolidation, the hippocampus helps contextualize experiences. In schizophrenia, hippocampal dysfunction can lead to fragmented memory, distorting how past emotional experiences (like hunger, rejection, or sensory pleasure) inform present-day desire.

Together, the amygdala and hippocampus contribute to the affective weight of desires. When disrupted, they may intensify or blunt the emotional resonance of food, intimacy, or music, affecting the individual's pursuit and interpretation of these experiences.

2. The Hypothalamus: Homeostasis and Basic Drives

The hypothalamus serves as the brain's command center for regulating physiological drives—hunger, thirst, sleep, temperature, and sexual behavior. It monitors internal bodily states and initiates behavior aimed at restoring balance.

In SMIs, hypothalamic dysregulation can present as:
- Hyperphagia or appetite loss
- Hypersexuality or sexual disinterest
- Sleep disruption, which further dysregulates mood and impulse control

Even when higher-order thinking deteriorates, the hypothalamus continues to activate basic survival behaviors. This may explain the persistence of food and sex-related preoccupations—even when the individual appears withdrawn or disorganized.

3. The Prefrontal Cortex: Executive Function and Self-Regulation

The prefrontal cortex (PFC) is the brain's center for reasoning, decision-making, social judgment, and inhibition. It plays a critical role in:
- Evaluating long-term goals (e.g., saving money)
- Regulating impulse (e.g., delaying gratification in sex or spending)
- Navigating social interactions (e.g., courtship, collaboration)

In SMIs, PFC dysfunction undermines an individual's ability to plan, reflect, or restrain behavior. A person may want to manage finances or eat moderately but lack the neurological capacity to do so consistently. This can lead to behaviors that seem impulsive, chaotic, or irrational—but are in fact neurocognitively driven.

4. Nucleus Accumbens and the Mesolimbic Pathway: The Pleasure Center

At the heart of the dopaminergic reward system lies the nucleus accumbens, which receives input from the ventral tegmental area via the mesolimbic pathway. This circuit is critical for processing reward anticipation, reinforcement, and pleasure.

A surge of dopamine in this system reinforces behavior: the pleasure of eating, the satisfaction of sexual intimacy, the gratification of being paid, or the emotional resonance of a song.

In psychosis, this circuit may be hypersensitive, attributing excessive significance to non-rewarding stimuli (e.g., delusional beliefs or auditory hallucinations).

In negative symptom states (e.g., anhedonia), this circuit is underactive, resulting in blunted emotional response—even to typically pleasurable activities.

Understanding this circuitry helps explain why some patients relentlessly pursue exaggerated goals (e.g., wealth, food, sex), while others disengage from formerly meaningful activities.

5. Temporal Lobe: Music, Language, and Hallucinations

The temporal lobe, particularly the superior temporal gyrus, is involved in auditory processing, language comprehension, and music appreciation.

In schizophrenia, this region is often implicated in auditory hallucinations.

Abnormal activation patterns in the temporal lobe may interfere with the ability to distinguish real from imagined auditory stimuli, including music.

Emotional and cognitive responses to music may also be altered, making it either intensely meaningful or difficult to process.

Despite this, music often remains a unique bridge to emotional life in patients who are otherwise unresponsive, highlighting the temporal lobe's enduring role in connecting sound to feeling.

Part 3: Neurotransmitters Beyond Dopamine

While dopamine is central to reward prediction and motivational salience, it operates within a broader neurochemical context. Other neurotransmitters—including serotonin, norepinephrine, oxytocin, and endorphins—play essential roles in modulating desire, regulating emotional response, and influencing how enduring preoccupations are expressed or suppressed. Dysregulation of these systems in serious mental illness often contributes to the persistence, exaggeration, or inhibition of the sparks that drive human behavior.

1. Serotonin: Regulation, Impulse Control, and Mood

Serotonin (5-HT) is a key neuromodulator involved in regulating mood, impulse control, appetite, sleep, and sexual behavior. It acts as a balancing force against the more activating effects of dopamine.

Clinical Relevance:

- Low serotonin levels, commonly seen in depression and mood disorders, are associated with anhedonia, impulsivity, and diminished sexual and social interest.
- Dysregulation can result in overeating, binge behavior, hypersexuality, or compulsive spending, especially when paired with elevated dopaminergic activity.
- In schizophrenia, serotonin may play a role in altering how people see or interpret the world (perceptual distortions). Certain serotonin receptors in the brain are linked to hallucinations (seeing or hearing things that aren't there) and delusions (firmly held false beliefs).Implications for Sparks:

Serotonin dysfunction may diminish the pleasure derived from food, sex, and social intimacy—or in contrast, lead to compulsive overindulgence in these domains. When serotonin levels are destabilized, the regulation of desire becomes impaired, leading either to blunted motivation or unchecked pursuit.

2. Oxytocin: Social Bonding and Emotional Attachment

Oxytocin is a neuropeptide hormone often referred to as the "bonding hormone" or "love molecule." It is released during physical intimacy, childbirth, and social connection, and is strongly associated with trust, empathy, and attachment formation.

Clinical Relevance:

- Research indicates altered oxytocin levels in people living with schizophrenia, particularly those showing social withdrawal, paranoia, or impaired social cognition.
- In bipolar disorder, oxytocin may be dysregulated during manic or depressive episodes, impacting interpersonal relationships.

Implications for Sparks:

Deficits in oxytocin signaling can contribute to difficulties forming or maintaining intimate bonds. Even when the drive for connection exists, the neurobiological substrate for trust or emotional attunement may be compromised, leading to contrasting behaviors—e.g., longing for love while avoiding closeness.

Oxytocin is a naturally occurring neurochemical involved in bonding and trust. Therapeutically, oxytocin-based interventions (such as intranasal oxytocin sprays) are being explored as potential treatments to enhance social responsiveness and emotional regulation.

3. Norepinephrine: Arousal, Attention, and Drive

Norepinephrine (NE), also known as noradrenaline, plays a critical role in arousal, alertness, attention, and fight-or-flight responses. It helps individuals prioritize stimuli and mobilize action in response to internal or external demands.

Clinical Relevance:

- In mania, norepinephrine levels are often elevated, contributing to increased energy, impulsivity, risk-taking, and goal-directed hyperactivity.

- In depression, NE levels may be suppressed, contributing to lethargy, low motivation, and cognitive slowing.

Implications for Sparks:

High norepinephrine activity may drive compulsive behaviors like excessive spending, sexual indiscretion, or binge eating, behaviors often observed during manic episodes. In contrast, norepinephrine deficits may mute the desire to pursue once-rewarding experiences. These opposing presentations underscore the importance of arousal regulation in the expression of persistent desires.

4. Endorphins: Pain Modulation and Natural Pleasure

Endorphins are endogenous opioid peptides (the body's natural chemicals) released in response to physical exertion, emotional arousal, and pain relief. They produce sensations of euphoria and act as natural analgesics (pain killers) and mood stabilizers (feelings of well-being or euphoria).

Clinical Relevance:

- Endorphin release is often triggered by exercise, music, laughter, and sensory pleasure—key pathways for therapeutic engagement in psychiatric care.
- In some people living with SMI, diminished endorphin production may reduce stress tolerance or emotional resilience, contributing to withdrawal and disengagement.

Implications for Sparks:

Endorphins are linked to many of the sparks explored in this book: the joy of movement, the comfort of food, the catharsis of music, and the release found in laughter. Facilitating endorphin release—through rhythmic activities, creative expression, or sensory engagement—can serve as a therapeutic bridge, helping individuals reconnect with latent sources of pleasure.

Integrative Insight: The Neurochemical Tapestry of Desire

These neurotransmitters and neuromodulators do not operate in isolation. They interact dynamically across brain systems, shaping the subjective intensity, direction, and regulation of desire. In serious mental illness (SMI), these interactions are often altered, leading to desires that:
- Persist despite cognitive disruption:
  - A person with schizophrenia who struggles with disorganized thinking but still hums their favorite songs every day

- Someone with bipolar disorder experiencing severe mood swings but still craving intimate connection or seeking comfort foods
- Amplify to unmanageable proportions:
  - A manic episode where sexual drive becomes overwhelming, leading to risky behavior
  - Compulsive gambling or spending during psychosis, tied to distorted beliefs about money
  - An insatiable appetite for food despite already feeling full
- Fade into emotional numbness, yet remain neurologically encoded:
  - A person with severe depression who no longer *feels* joy from music but still turns on the radio out of habit
  - Someone with negative symptoms of schizophrenia who seems indifferent to socializing, yet whose brain circuits still respond subtly to human connection
  - A patient who reports no interest in food but physiologically still shows hunger cues and maintains routines around meals

The persistence of preoccupations—about money, sex, food, music, or connection—is thus a product of deep and resilient biological programming. Even when these desires appear irrational, exaggerated, or socially inappropriate, they often reflect disrupted but recognizable neurochemical signals.

Part 4: Synthesis and Clinical Integration

Why Neurobiology Matters for Understanding the Sparks That Endure

Having explored the key brain regions and neurochemical systems that shape human desire, we now return to a central clinical insight: the persistent preoccupations seen in serious mental illness—often regarded as pathological or irrational—are deeply rooted in core survival circuitry and neurobiological programming. These desires do not emerge ex nihilo; they are echoes of ancient neural imperatives that, even under duress, remain active.

Understanding the neurobiology of desire enables clinicians to reframe symptoms not merely as aberrations but as distorted attempts to fulfill biologically encoded needs. When patients obsess about money, food, sex, or music, they are not simply showing delusional or compulsive behavior—they are navigating the turbulent interplay of overstimulated reward systems, impaired inhibition, emotional dysregulation, and unmet physiological needs.

Persistent Drives in the Midst of Disruption

Despite the disorganization of thought and affect in schizophrenia, schizoaffective disorder, and bipolar disorder, core motivational circuits remain remarkably resilient. Indeed, in many patients, these preoccupations are the only remaining structure amidst otherwise chaotic mental states.

Examples include:

A man with schizophrenia who persistently asks about his disability check while simultaneously expressing paranoid delusions—his concern for money reflects a need for control, predictability, and agency, even in the face of cognitive fragmentation.

A woman in a manic episode who shows sexual disinhibition—her behavior is driven by intensified dopaminergic and noradrenergic activity, overriding executive control, but still grounded in the pursuit of intimacy and affirmation.

A nonverbal patient who becomes animated when exposed to familiar music—despite deficits in language and social reciprocity, her temporal lobe and limbic circuitry remain responsive to rhythm and melody, offering a route to expression.

These are not anomalies. They are reminders that, even in the presence of psychiatric illness, the architecture of human motivation remains intact, if altered.

From Pathology to Signal: A Clinical Reorientation

Traditional psychiatric models have often conceptualized persistent preoccupations as symptoms to be managed or extinguished. While safety and symptom reduction remain essential, reframing is critical:

Preoccupations are not distractions from treatment; they are portals into the patient's subjective world.

Repetitive behaviors and fixations may be expressions of unregulated survival needs or attempts at coherence, not merely pathology.

Persistent interest in a spark—like music or food—can be leveraged therapeutically as a source of grounding and motivation.

By recognizing the neurobiological basis of these behaviors, clinicians can begin to ask:
- What is this desire trying to communicate?
- How might this behavior be linked to unmet biological or emotional needs?
- Can this spark be used as a bridge for engagement, not merely suppressed?

Practical Applications in Psychiatric Care

Understanding the neurobiology of enduring preoccupations informs a range of clinical strategies:

- Psychoeducation: Explaining to patients and families that these desires are neurologically encoded may reduce shame and improve cooperation with treatment.
- Motivational interviewing: Exploring the significance of a spark (e.g., the importance of music or money to a patient) can serve as a foundation for rapport and goal-setting.
- Recovery-oriented interventions: Integrating sparks into rehabilitation plans—like music therapy, structured financial literacy programs, or sensory integration techniques—can enhance engagement and emotional connection.
- Medication management: Appreciating the roles of serotonin, dopamine, and norepinephrine allows for more tailored psychopharmacological approaches that consider both symptom control and affective vitality.

Ultimately, neurobiological insight must not become an end in itself, but a tool to deepen empathy, improve care, and restore dignity.

Conclusion: The Brain Remembers the Spark

Even when language falters, cognition declines, or emotion becomes dysregulated, the brain often holds on to what matters most. Embedded within the reward system, encoded in emotional memory, and propelled by ancient drives, the sparks of life—pleasure, safety, connection, purpose—do not vanish. They endure.

This endurance is not merely clinically significant; it is profoundly humanizing. Understanding the neurobiology of desire affirms that people living with serious mental illness are not broken beyond recognition. Rather, they are engaged in a different kind of survival—a struggle to meet basic needs with altered tools, within altered states. And even in that struggle, meaning persists.

The brain's systems for reward, motivation, and emotional regulation—the mesolimbic dopamine pathway, prefrontal cortex, amygdala, hypothalamus, and more—play pivotal roles in how individuals pursue connection, pleasure, autonomy, and self-expression. Yet these circuits never operate in isolation. Psychological forces shaped by life history, trauma, cognitive processing, and identity influence how those drives are felt, expressed, or muted.

This interplay of biology and psychology explains why symptoms such as anhedonia, disorganization, impulsivity, or mood instability can obscure the enduring sparks of life—or distort them in ways that are pathologized rather than understood. Treatment, therefore, must reach beyond symptom management. It must address both the biological substrate and the personal narrative, through pharmacological, psychotherapeutic, and social interventions that restore not only functioning but also meaning.

Healing, then, is not simply the reduction of pathology. True healing is a return to the sparks—the enduring desires that persist beneath illness. Whether it is a song that stirs memory, a favorite meal that anchors identity, or a fleeting moment of connection that affirms existence, these are signs of life. They remind us that beneath disorder lies the intact self, striving still.

As we now turn to Chapter 3, the focus shifts from systems and circuits to lived experience. We explore how schizophrenia, schizoaffective disorder, bipolar disorder, and related illnesses both shape—and are shaped by—these deep human preoccupations. The goal is not merely to define illness, but to illuminate the enduring humanity within it.

Table 2.1 — Key Neurotransmitters in Desire

Neurotransmitter	Function	Spark Relevance
Dopamine	Reward, motivation	Sex, money, food, music
Serotonin	Mood regulation, satiety	Food, rituals, spirituality
Oxytocin	Bonding, trust	Sex, touch, intimacy
Endorphins	Pain relief, euphoria	Movement, humor, music
Norepinephrine	Arousal, focus	Creativity, freedom
GABA	Calming, inhibition	Rituals, nature, spirituality

For continuity with the broader sparks framework, see Maslow, A. H. (1943). *A theory of human motivation. Psychological Review, 50*(4), 370–396; Benson, P. L. (2008). *Sparks: How parents can help ignite the hidden strengths of teenagers.* Jossey-Bass.

Csikszentmihalyi, M. (1990). *Flow: The psychology of optimal experience.* Harper & Row.

Berridge, K. C., & Robinson, T. E. (2016). Liking, wanting, and the incentive-sensitization theory of addiction. *American Psychologist, 71*(8), 670–679.

For neuroimaging findings in serious mental illness, see: Harrison, P. J. (1999). The neuropathology of schizophrenia: A critical review of the data and their interpretation. *Brain, 122*(4), 593–624; Glahn, D. C., et al. (2005). Beyond hypofrontality: A quantitative meta-analysis of functional neuroimaging studies of working memory in schizophrenia. *Human Brain Mapping, 25*(1), 60–69.

Feifel, D., & Shilling, P. D. (2010). Potential of oxytocin in the treatment of schizophrenia. CNS Drugs, 24(8), 615–628.

Chapter 3:
Understanding the Illnesses

Building on the neurobiological and psychological insights explored in Chapter 2, we now turn our focus to the clinical manifestations of serious mental illnesses and their impact on enduring human desires. While the previous chapter highlighted the interconnectedness of brain function and subjective experience, it is crucial to recognize that these underlying mechanisms express themselves in highly individualized ways—particularly when it comes to diagnoses like schizophrenia, schizoaffective disorder, and bipolar disorder.

When we speak of serious mental illness , we often refer to diagnoses like schizophrenia, schizoaffective disorder, and bipolar disorder. These conditions are marked not only by psychiatric symptoms but by the magnitude of their impact on day-to-day functioning. They disrupt cognition, mood, perception, and interpersonal relationships. Beyond clinical definitions, SMIs reflect altered modes of engagement with the world—ways of being that often disrupt connection, purpose, and identity.

This book is not about diagnostic labels but about lived experience. Serious mental illness can dismantle routines, fracture relationships, and obscure the sense of self. Yet, even amidst this disruption, the capacity to connect with fundamental human desires endures.

Schizophrenia, schizoaffective disorder, and bipolar disorder each present unique constellations of symptoms and cognitive features that shape how individuals experience and express their desires. This chapter examines the diagnostic features, prevalence, and psychosocial impact of these conditions, while reinforcing the persistence of foundational human drives like intimacy, nourishment, autonomy, and emotional expression.

Defining Serious Mental Illness

According to the National Institute of Mental Health, an SMI is defined as a "mental, behavioral, or emotional disorder resulting in serious functional impairment, which substantially interferes with or limits one or more major life activities." This category includes conditions like schizophrenia, bipolar I disorder, and severe major depressive disorder.

SMIs often:

- Disrupt education and employment
- Lead to social isolation and impaired relationships
- Require repeated hospitalization
- Increase vulnerability to homelessness and legal entanglements
- Carry significant societal stigma

Despite these challenges, people living with SMI retain their identities, dreams, and desires.

I've seen how these illnesses fracture identity—but also how parts of the self stubbornly remain.

Historical Context and Diagnostic Evolution

The conceptualization of SMIs has evolved considerably over time. From the asylums of the 19th century to the neurobiological advances of the 21st, our understanding has shifted from moral and spiritual explanations to biopsychosocial frameworks. Early classification systems by Kraepelin, psychoanalytic models of the mid-20th century, and contemporary DSM-based criteria all reflect ongoing efforts to capture the complexity of these illnesses.

The current DSM-5-TR offers structured criteria based on symptom clusters, duration, and functional impact. While invaluable for diagnosis and treatment planning, these frameworks should not eclipse the rich inner life and enduring desires of those living with SMI.

Key Conditions

Schizophrenia Spectrum Disorders: This group includes schizophrenia, schizoaffective disorder, and schizophreniform disorder. Core features include positive symptoms (e.g., hallucinations, delusions), negative symptoms (e.g., flat affect, anhedonia), disorganized thinking, and cognitive deficits. These symptoms profoundly affect an individual's interaction with basic drives like pleasure, connection, and autonomy.

Schizoaffective Disorder: Characterized by a combination of schizophrenia symptoms and mood episodes, this condition represents a complex interface between thought and affect. The variability of mood symptoms shapes the individual's capacity to pursue desires related to intimacy and nourishment, whether through food, comfort, or care from others and self-direction.

Bipolar Disorder: Defined by mood dysregulation ranging from manic or hypomanic episodes to severe depression, manic states may heighten libido and impulsivity, while depressive episodes can diminish interest and motivation. Yet, during euthymic periods, times when mood is stable and neither depressed nor manic, individuals often regain access to their core desires.

Major Depressive Disorder with Psychotic Features: This condition combines severe depressive symptoms with delusions or hallucinations. Profound impairments in motivation and pleasure often occur, yet the longing for connection and comfort often remains, even if muted.

Other Serious Mental Illnesses

Beyond schizophrenia, schizoaffective disorder, and bipolar disorder, several other psychiatric conditions may also qualify as serious mental illnesses due to their profound impact on daily functioning and quality of life. These include severe forms of obsessive-compulsive disorder (OCD), post-traumatic stress disorder (PTSD), major neurocognitive disorders with psychotic features (like dementia), certain personality disorders (notably borderline or antisocial personality disorder when associated with functional decline), and co-occurring conditions involving developmental or intellectual disabilities.

Though the symptomatology may differ, the disruption to autonomy, relationships, identity, and emotional expression can be equally profound. For instance, intrusive thoughts and compulsions in OCD can overwhelm one's ability to experience joy or spontaneity. Trauma-related hypervigilance or emotional numbing in PTSD may blunt interpersonal connection, diminish trust, and interfere with pleasure or intimacy. In dementia with psychosis, the erosion of memory and reality testing can distort formerly pleasurable rituals or meaningful connections—yet flashes of music, familiar tastes, or spiritual practices often remain accessible. In developmental and intellectual disabilities complicated by psychiatric illness, expressive modalities like movement, art, or routine can become vital sparks for self-regulation and communication.

Each of these conditions calls for a tailored, compassionate approach that recognizes not only symptom burden but also the individualized ways in which core human drives persist. Even when language falters, or behavior becomes erratic, the underlying longing for connection, structure, identity, and meaning remains—waiting for the right channel through which to be recognized and affirmed.

Substance Use and Co-Occurring Disorders

Substance use disorders frequently co-occur with serious mental illnesses and can significantly complicate both diagnosis and treatment. The interaction between substance use and the core human drives—particularly those related to sex, money, and food—is often synergistic and bidirectional. Substances may be used to modulate mood, enhance pleasure, or escape distressing symptoms, but they can also exacerbate impulsivity, distort perceptions, and impair judgment.

For example, stimulant use may intensify hypersexuality or trigger grandiose financial delusions, while alcohol or cannabis may contribute to disinhibition, poor nutritional choices, and heightened emotional reactivity. In many cases, substance use becomes entangled with psychotic symptoms, blurring the lines between voluntary behavior and illness-driven compulsion. Moreover, the neurobiological pathways involved in addiction overlap significantly with those implicated in reward processing, motivation, and desire—areas already dysregulated in SMI.

Clinically, it is critical to recognize how substance use may not simply be a maladaptive coping strategy but also a distorted attempt to fulfill fundamental human needs—pleasure, connection, agency—that remain active beneath the illness. Integrated treatment models that address both psychiatric and substance use disorders are essential for supporting individuals in reclaiming healthier, more adaptive ways of engaging with the enduring sparks of life.

Genetic Predisposition

The genetic contribution to SMIs is substantial, implicating heritable factors that increase vulnerability. Although no single gene determines illness, polygenic risk involving multiple gene-environment interactions shapes susceptibility. Individuals with a family history of SMI are at elevated risk.

Genetic predisposition influences neurotransmitter levels, brain structure and connectivity, and sensitivity to environmental stressors. These inherited traits affect how individuals experience and regulate core desires. For example, variations in genes related to dopamine and serotonin systems may impact reward sensitivity, thereby altering engagement with food, sex, music, and financial autonomy.

Psychological Impact

Cognitive impairments, affective dysregulation, and disorganized thought processes often characterize SMIs. However, despite these challenges, individuals continue to long for connection, comfort, and meaning.

Psychotherapeutic interventions aim to support these residual strengths. Social skills training enhances relationship-building; cognitive behavioral strategies address impulsivity and emotional dysregulation. These efforts can restore access to fundamental aspects of life that support dignity and purpose.

The Interplay of Neurobiology and Psychology

The neurobiological and psychological aspects of SMIs are inextricably linked. Biological changes in the brain can contribute to psychological symptoms, which in turn affect how individuals engage with the enduring sparks of life. For example, anhedonia—often rooted in altered brain function—can diminish the psychological experience of pleasure from food or music.

Similarly, effective pharmacological interventions that regulate mood may enhance capacity for intimacy or restore the enjoyment of everyday activities. Recognition of this interplay underscores the need for integrated treatment approaches that address both biological mechanisms and subjective experiences. By doing so, clinicians can more effectively support individuals in re-engaging with those fundamental human drives—connection, pleasure, autonomy—that define a meaningful life.

Cultural Influences on Desire in Psychosis

While neurobiology provides a framework for understanding the persistence of desires in severe mental illness, it is equally important to consider how cultural contexts influence the expression of these drives. Culture shapes how people experience and prioritize desires like money, food, sex, and music.

For example, in many societies, money is closely linked to identity, status, and survival. A patient with schizophrenia who believes they are wealthy may be reflecting a deeply ingrained cultural value placed on financial success. Their delusions may not be random but an amplification of societal pressures that equate success with worth.

Similarly, sexuality is often culturally regulated. Patients who experience hypersexuality or sexual delusions in mania or psychosis may be expressing, in distorted forms, the cultural significance they attach to sexual conquest, beauty, or attraction. Cultural factors like gender roles or religious beliefs about sexuality can further complicate how these desires are experienced and acted upon in psychotic states.

In food obsession, many societies equate food with comfort, social connection, and identity. Patients may hoard food or obsess over meal choices because of social norms that elevate food to a symbol of self-care or family bonding. These behaviors can reflect a deeper need for belonging and nourishment, both physically and emotionally.

Lastly, music is universal but also culturally specific. Certain genres or types of music can evoke powerful emotional responses. Patients with psychosis may gravitate toward specific types of music, not just as a source of pleasure, but as a means of grounding in a world where their perceptions are fragmented. This could be a form of reclaiming emotional stability or identity in a culture where music is a central part of the social fabric.

Spectrum of Severity

Serious mental illnesses do not present in uniform ways; rather, they exist along a continuum of severity. Some individuals experience persistent and debilitating symptoms that require intensive, ongoing care, while others may achieve periods of relative stability with appropriate pharmacological and psychosocial interventions. The extent to which these conditions interfere with an individual's capacity to engage with foundational human drives—like intimacy, nourishment, autonomy, creativity, or spiritual practice—varies greatly from one person to another.

Importantly, the presence of serious symptoms does not negate the enduring presence of human needs. Even amid severe functional impairment, individuals may continue to seek, experience, or respond to moments of joy, comfort, and meaning. The expression of these desires may be altered, delayed, or less accessible, but they are rarely extinguished.

The Importance of a Holistic Perspective

Reducing serious mental illness to a set of diagnostic criteria risks missing the broader picture of human experience. A truly holistic understanding requires attention not only to clinical symptoms but also to the sociocultural, economic, and relational contexts that shape an individual's life. While biological and psychological models offer crucial insight into etiology and treatment, they must be complemented by recognition of each person's values, aspirations, and enduring capacities.

The Value of Person-First Language

Central to this holistic approach is the use of person-first language, which affirms the individual's humanity beyond the scope of their diagnosis.

Terms like "person with schizophrenia" or "individual living with bipolar disorder" underscore that identity is multifaceted and not defined by illness alone.

Language shapes perception. By choosing words that reflect respect and dignity, we reinforce a framework of care that prioritizes autonomy, agency, and hope. This linguistic shift is more than semantic—it is a clinical and ethical imperative that aligns with the values of recovery-oriented care and reaffirms our commitment to honoring the enduring human spirit.

Conclusion

Understanding the intricate ways in which schizophrenia, schizoaffective disorder, and bipolar disorder shape the experience and expression of fundamental human desires requires moving beyond simplistic generalizations. The interplay of psychotic symptoms, mood disturbances, negative symptoms, cognitive impairments, medication effects, and sociocultural factors create a highly individualized landscape for each person. This complexity demands that we adopt truly person-centered treatment approaches that go beyond symptom management to recognize and support the persistent human yearnings that often remain intact beneath the surface.

This chapter has provided an essential foundation for appreciating the scope and impact of serious mental illnesses. Yet it has also emphasized the enduring relevance of core human experiences—those "sparks of life" that can flicker even in the midst of profound psychiatric disruption. As we move forward, each chapter will examine one of these sparks in depth: sex, money, food, music, spirituality, creativity, movement, ritual, nature, and humor. We will explore how these vital forces intersect with mental illness, how they survive, and how they can be nurtured.

To truly understand serious mental illness, we must cultivate not only knowledge but humility. We must be willing to listen—to what patients grieve, what they yearn for, and what they return to time and again. Individuals living with SMI are not passive recipients of care; they are bearers of meaning. They carry with them fragments of memory, desire, and identity that defy erasure.

This book does not minimize the severity of mental illness, nor does it romanticize suffering. Rather, it affirms that within even the most disorganized mind lies something indelible—an ember that flickers, a rhythm that persists, a spark that refuses to go out.

Let us begin there. Let us remain attentive not only to what is impaired, but to what is preserved—and what might be reignited.

Reflection Questions

1. How has your understanding of serious mental illness evolved after reading this chapter?
2. Can you recall a moment when a patient or loved one demonstrated a "spark"—something that endured despite their condition?
3. How might shifting from a deficit-based model to a strength-based model change your clinical or personal approach?
4. What sparks in your own life help you stay connected during times of distress?

In the chapters that follow, we will examine each of the ten enduring sparks in depth—beginning with sex, money, food, and music—to explore how they manifest, distort, and sustain life in those navigating the deepest psychological challenges.

Table 3.1 — Impact of Illness on Sparks

Illness	Common Spark Disruptions	Protective Sparks
Schizophrenia	Delusions of money/sex, disrupted intimacy	Music, rituals, spirituality
Schizoaffective Disorder	Mania-driven spending/creativity, disorganized rituals	Hope, storytelling
Bipolar Disorder	Hypersexuality, excessive spending, disrupted sleep rituals	Creativity, humor, spirituality

1. Insel, T. R. (2010). Rethinking schizophrenia. *Nature*, 468(7321), 187–193; Owen, M. J., Sawa, A., & Mortensen, P. B. (2016). Schizophrenia. *Lancet*, 388(10039), 86–97. (Overview of disruption across cognition, mood, perception, function.)
2. National Institute of Mental Health (NIMH). Serious Mental Illness (SMI) definition. (NIMH describes SMI as a mental, behavioral, or emotional disorder resulting in serious functional impairment that substantially interferes with one or more major life activities.)
3. American Psychiatric Association. (2022). *Diagnostic and Statistical Manual of Mental Disorders* (5th ed., text rev.; DSM-5-TR). American Psychiatric Publishing. (Diagnostic criteria, duration, functional impact.)
4. Kraepelin, E. (1919/1971). *Dementia Praecox and Paraphrenia*. (Classic nosology); Shorter, E. (1997). *A History of Psychiatry*. (Historical

evolution); Engel, G. L. (1977). The need for a biopsychosocial model. *Science*, 196(4286), 129–136. (Model shift.)

5. Drake, R. E., O'Neal, E. L., & Wallach, M. A. (2008). A systematic review of psychosocial research on co-occurring disorders. *J Subst Abuse Treat*, 34(1), 123–138; Mueser, K. T., Noordsy, D. L., Drake, R. E., & Fox, L. (2003). *Integrated Treatment for Dual Disorders*. (Integrated SUD–SMI care.)
6. Sullivan, P. F., Daly, M. J., & O'Donovan, M. (2012). Genetic architectures of psychiatric disorders. *Nat Rev Genet*, 13(8), 537–551; Ripke, S., et al. (2014). Biological insights from 108 schizophrenia-associated loci. *Nature*, 511(7510), 421–427. (Polygenic risk & biology.)
7. Green, M. F. (1996). What are the functional consequences of neurocognitive deficits in schizophrenia? *Am J Psychiatry*, 153(3), 321–330; Fioravanti, M., et al. (2005). Meta-analysis of cognitive deficits in schizophrenia. *Neurosci Biobehav Rev*, 29(2), 217–233. (Cognition & function.)
8. Kleinman, A. (1980). *Patients and Healers in the Context of Culture*. (Explanatory models); Luhrmann, T. M., et al. (2015). Differences in voice-hearing experiences across cultures. *Br J Psychiatry*, 206(1), 41–44. (Cultural shaping of symptoms/meaning.)
9. American Psychological Association. (2020). *Publication Manual* (7th ed.). (Person-first language guidance); SAMHSA. (2012). *Recovery and Recovery Support*. (Recovery-oriented principles.)
10. Anthony, W. A. (1993). Recovery from mental illness: The guiding vision of the mental health system. *Psychosocial Rehabilitation Journal*, 16(4), 11–23; Slade, M. (2009). *Personal Recovery and Mental Illness*. (Person-centered, strength-based care.)

Part II – The Core Sparks of the Human Spirit

Chapter 4:
Sex: Intimacy, Desire, and Identity in the Midst of Mental Illness

I've observed how the struggle for intimacy, often deeply impacted by illness, can paradoxically become a driving force for patients seeking connection.

I recall a young patient, Sarah, battling severe schizophrenia. For months, she was withdrawn, preoccupied by delusions, and deeply isolated. One afternoon, during a quiet moment, she hesitantly brought up a past relationship, a wistful memory of physical intimacy before her illness took place. "I wonder if I'll ever feel...that alive again," she murmured. It reminded me that even amidst profound illness, the human need for connection and self-worth, often expressed through intimacy, endures.

Sex is one of the most elemental human drives. It pulses beneath culture, cognition, and condition. In people living with severe mental illness, it rarely disappears. In fact, it often intensifies—becoming a fixation, a source of shame, a symbol, a currency, or a coping mechanism.

The clinical temptation is to frame this solely as hypersexuality, disinhibition, or risky behavior. But if we look closer, sex reveals itself as a multidimensional spark, an enduring signal of aliveness, identity, longing, and relational hunger.

When most people hear the word "schizophrenia," they picture fragmented thoughts, disordered speech, and an eerie detachment from reality. What they often miss are the deeply human needs that survive beneath the symptoms. Among them is sexual desire—a force as old as life itself. Even when the mind is clouded by delusions or battered by hallucinations, the yearning for intimacy, touch, and love often remains intact.

I have seen patients, their thinking disorganized and their realities distorted, still blush when speaking of a crush—reminders that desire does not vanish in psychosis but simply takes new forms. They still ache for the closeness of a hand held tightly, a stubborn signal of selfhood that illness cannot fully erase. Sexuality is among the most intimate and powerful human experiences. It binds us to one another, anchors us in identity, and offers connection that transcends words. In serious mental illness, sexuality may appear distorted, exaggerated, or muted—but it does not vanish.

Despite cognitive disorganization, affective instability, or psychotic thought, desire persists. Even when behavior is erratic or speech nonsensical, the pull toward closeness—toward sexual or romantic union—remains. Sometimes it emerges in troubling ways. Other times it flickers quietly: in longing looks, shy flirtations, or secret dreams.

Sex isn't merely a symptom or side effect. It is a signal—of yearning, of memory, of being alive.

For many people living with severe mental illnesses, sexuality is not just about pleasure. It becomes a constant preoccupation—an emotional need, a psychological defense, and often, a way to cope. It may function as an attempt to assert control when everything else feels lost. For some, the craving for sex becomes a pathway to reclaim agency, validate worth, or numb emotional pain.

This can lead to internal conflict. When sex becomes all-consuming, it's no longer solely about connection. It becomes entangled with fear, obsession, and self-soothing, resulting in compulsive behavior or shame-ridden cycles that feel impossible to escape.

A pervasive and damaging misconception is that people living with schizophrenia, schizoaffective disorder, or bipolar disorder are somehow devoid of desire. This dehumanizing view erases a core truth: the yearning for love, intimacy, and belonging remains a vital and enduring force, even amidst disorganized thought or emotional volatility.

Let's take a closer look at the persistence of sexual desire in serious mental illness—how it manifests, how it is misunderstood, and how we, as clinicians, can better recognize its significance. We examine how sex may be amplified or distorted by illness and how personal boundaries, identity, and social norms intersect with experiences of hypersexuality, sexual delusions, or trauma.

In the heart of psychosis, where language breaks down and time distorts, something pulses beneath the chaos—the spark of desire. Sex, one of the oldest drives in the human brain, often endures even when altered by illness: animated, erratic, tender, and tenacious. As psychiatrists, we are trained to detect dysfunction, but we must also acknowledge an essential truth: sex—in its many forms, whether chaotic, delusional, or hopeful—is not just pathology. It is a sign of life. In this chapter, we explore sex in schizophrenia, bipolar disorder, and schizoaffective disorder—not merely as symptomatology, but as a window into the inner lives of people too often reduced to diagnoses. We begin with biology, but we move into stories: love letters to strangers, imagined marriages to celebrities, small flirtations behind locked doors, and the struggle to preserve dignity in systems that fear sexual expression.

What we find is not dysfunction, but humanity.

The Neurobiology of Sexual Desire: Circuits That Survive Illness

Brain Areas and Sexual Desire: Neurobiology in Mental Illness

Brain Area / System	Primary Function in Sexuality	Clinical Impact in Serious Mental Illness
Dopaminergic Reward System (VTA→ Nucleus Accumbens → Prefrontal Cortex)	Craving, motivation, pleasure anticipation, reinforcement of sexual behavior	Schizophnenia: aberrant sallence; distortied significencce of sexual cues
Hypothalamus (MPOA, PVN, HPG Axis)	Hormone regulation (testosterone), arousal, orgasm, autonomic sexual responses	
Limbic System (Amygdala, Hippocamp- Anferior Cingulate Cortex)	Emotional regulation and attachment, yet strong emotions (love, lealousy, longing continue despite illness	
Oxytocin & Vasopressin Systems (Hypothalamus → Posterior Pituitary)	Pair bonding, trust, emotional closness, long-term attachment	
Serotonin Pathways	Hormonal bonding remains; emerging research suggests oxytocin therapy	Even with cognitive decline or psychosis, sexual desire persists in altered or distorted forms
Evolutionary Survival Circuits (ancient	Drive to species survival, ensure of desire across stress/illness	Even with cognitive decline or psychosis sexual desire persists in altered or distorfms

Sexual desire is not simply an impulse or emotion—it is a neurobiological phenomenon rooted in complex circuits of the brain. Long before desire takes shape in thought or action, it originates in the coordinated activity of neurotransmitters, hormones, and deeply embedded survival mechanisms.

At its core, sexual desire is regulated by interconnected systems involving dopaminergic reward pathways, limbic structures, hypothalamic regulation, and hormonal feedback loops. These systems—primitive yet remarkably resilient—can remain active even when higher-order cognitive functions are impaired by psychiatric illness.

Brain Areas and Sexual Desire: Neurobiology in Mental Illness

Brain Area / System	Primary Function in Sexuality	Clinical Impact in Serious Mental Illness
Dopaminergic Reward System (VTA → Nucleus Accumbens → Prefrontal Cortex)	Craving, motivation, pleasure anticipation, reinforcement of sexual behavior	**Schizophrenia:** aberrant salience, distorted significance of sexual cues
		Bipolar Mania: hyperdopaminergic activity → impulsivity, hypersexuality
Hypothalamus (MPOA, PVN, HPG Axis)	Hormone regulation (testosterone, estrogen), arousal, orgasm, autonomic sexual responses	Medication and stress can blunt function, but libido and sexual thoughts often persist even in restrictive environments.
Limbic System (Amygdala, Hippocampus, Anterior Cingulate Cortex)	Emotional tone of sexual experience, memory, bonding, sexual identity	Impaired regulation and attachment, yet strong emotions (love, jealousy, longing) continue despite illness.
Oxytocin & Vasopressin Systems (Hypothalamus → Posterior Pituitary)	Pair bonding, trust, emotional closeness, long-term attachment	Hormonal bonding remains; emerging research suggests oxytocin therapy may improve intimacy and social cognition in schizophrenia/bipolar disorder.
Serotonin Pathways	Modulation of mood, inhibition of sexual drive	In depression: suppressed libido, withdrawal, anhedonia → frustration, isolation, relationship strain
Evolutionary Survival Circuits (ancient subcortical networks)	Drive for species survival, resilience of desire across stress/illness	Even with cognitive decline or psychosis, sexual desire persists in altered or distorted forms.

1. The Dopaminergic Reward System: Craving and Motivation

The mesolimbic dopamine pathway, extending from the ventral tegmental area (VTA) to the nucleus accumbens, plays a central role in the experience of desire. This circuit is responsible for the anticipation of pleasure, motivation to seek reward, and reinforcement of behaviors that promote survival—including sex.

In people living with schizophrenia, bipolar disorder, or schizoaffective disorder, this reward system often remains hyperactive or dysregulated. In mania, for instance, dopaminergic overactivity is associated with impulsivity, risk-taking, and hypersexuality. In schizophrenia, aberrant salience attribution—the misfiring of dopamine signals—can cause individuals to assign excessive meaning or significance to sexual stimuli, even in delusional ways.

Yet even amid these distortions, the underlying signal—the drive toward connection—persists.

2. Hypothalamus: Command Center of Sexual Function

The hypothalamus is the central node for sexual behavior in the brain. It regulates the release of sex hormones (like testosterone and estrogen) through the hypothalamic-pituitary-gonadal (HPG) axis, and it governs autonomic sexual responses like arousal and orgasm.

Key regions like the medial preoptic area (MPOA) and the paraventricular nucleus (PVN) integrate sensory, hormonal, and emotional information to drive sexual behavior.

In schizophrenia and mood disorders, hypothalamic functioning may be disrupted by medication, stress, or chronic illness—but the fundamental architecture remains intact. Even in institutional settings where libido is dulled or repressed, spontaneous sexual thoughts, fantasies, and behaviors still emerge.

3. Limbic System: Emotion and Attachment

The amygdala, hippocampus, and anterior cingulate cortex link desire with emotion, memory, and bonding. These structures encode the affective tone of sexual experiences and help shape sexual identity.

Patients with psychotic disorders may have impairments in emotional regulation or attachment, yet they often continue to experience powerful sexual emotions—love, jealousy, longing, and rejection. These feelings are not delusions; they are human echoes, filtered through altered perception.

4. Oxytocin and Vasopressin: Neurohormones of Bonding

Oxytocin and vasopressin, released during sexual intimacy and physical touch, facilitate emotional closeness and pair bonding. These hormones modulate limbic circuits and reinforce feelings of trust and safety.

While often under-researched in psychiatric populations, emerging studies suggest that people living with schizophrenia or bipolar disorder may still respond to oxytocin, particularly in social and sexual contexts. Some have proposed oxytocin as a potential therapeutic agent to enhance social cognition and intimacy in these populations.

5. The Resilience of Desire

Even when executive functioning deteriorates, when insight is lost, or when cognition fragments—sexual desire can endure. This is because desire originates not only in the neocortex but in ancient, evolutionarily conserved systems designed to ensure species survival.

The persistence of sexual desire in severe mental illness is a testament to its biological resilience. It may be altered, disinhibited, or repressed, but rarely extinguished.

Serotonin and Depression: Suppressing Sexual Desire

On the flip side, in depressive episodes, serotonin dysregulation can lead to a significant decrease in sexual desire. Depressive states often bring a loss of interest in intimacy, sometimes due to overwhelming feelings of worthlessness or anhedonia (inability to experience pleasure). This can result in sexual withdrawal, where patients lose the ability to form meaningful sexual connections or even care about sex altogether. For some patients, this can contribute to feelings of frustration or isolation, especially if they are in relationships where their partner's sexual needs are unmet.

This neurobiological lens reinforces a central premise of this book: that enduring human drives—like sexuality—are not erased by illness but are often misunderstood.

Sexuality and the Human Drive

From an evolutionary standpoint, sexual desire is hardwired into our neurobiology as described above. But sexuality is more than biology; it is also psychological and social. It reflects how we see ourselves, how we seek closeness, and how we interpret pleasure, power, and shame.

Even in the midst of serious mental illness, sexuality often remains active—sometimes amplified, sometimes blunted, and sometimes misdirected. Patients may continue to long for intimacy, connection, or validation. Others may experience distressing intrusions (unwanted sexual thoughts or urges), impulsivity (difficulty controlling sudden sexual impulses), or a loss of agency (feeling unable to make free choices) related to sexual behavior.

The Impact of Illness on Intimacy and Relationships

Serious mental illness affects not only cognition and behavior but also the most tender aspects of human experience, intimacy, attachment, and sexual expression. These are often overlooked in psychiatric settings, yet they remain essential to personhood and recovery. This section explores how psychiatric disorders interfere with sexual functioning, distort intimate relationships, and yet still reveal enduring needs for connection and love.

1. Sexuality in Psychosis: Distorted but Not Erased

In psychotic states, sexual content often becomes intertwined with delusions and hallucinations. Some patients believe they are married to a celebrity, impregnated by a spirit, or seduced telepathically. Others report divine or demonic sexual experiences—astral intimacy, unseen lovers, or voices of desire.

These are not mere oddities or clinical symptoms to be dismissed. They are human longings refracted through fractured minds—distorted signals of unmet needs for touch, closeness, comfort, and safety. Sexual delusions often reflect deeper emotional truths: vulnerability, desire, trauma, or shame.

One patient with schizoaffective disorder spent hours speaking of her celebrity husband. Her entire psychotic world was organized around this fantasy. When the voices mocked her, she said he comforted her. When hospitalized, she protested, claiming we were violating her marital rights by keeping her from him. It was delusional—but it was also stabilizing, because the belief anchored her in a consistent relationship, provided reassurance when voices tormented her, and offered a framework through which she could make sense of her experiences.

Beyond clinical observations, the longing for closeness remains deeply human.

One peer advocate described how intimacy, "even in restricted settings, became a spark of identity."

His reflection underscores that intimacy is not erased by illness, but reshaped into the need for connection, dignity, and belonging.
Patients with schizophrenia or schizoaffective disorder may experience a range of sexual delusions:
- Believing they are erotically powerful or divinely chosen
- Fearing rape via technological manipulation
- Sensing their genitals are being controlled or invaded
- Believing others are secretly in love with them (erotomania)

These experiences can be terrifying, humiliating, or even dangerous. But they are not random—they reflect the emotional landscape of the person: fear, desire, identity, and memory. Understanding their symbolic meaning allows clinicians to treat the person, not just suppress the symptom.

2. How Mental Illness Affects Libido and Sexual Function

Many psychiatric conditions—especially schizophrenia, bipolar disorder, and depression—have direct biological and psychological effects on sexual functioning. These include:

Schizophrenia and Negative Symptoms:

Avolition (lack of motivation) and anhedonia (loss of pleasure) can dull libido and reduce interest in sexual intimacy. Social withdrawal and flat affect may further interfere with the initiation or reciprocation of romantic overtures.

Depression:

Often associated with a sharp decline in sexual interest, difficulties with arousal and orgasm, and feelings of worthlessness or guilt that undermine intimacy.

Anxiety Disorders:

Co-occurring anxiety, especially social or performance anxiety, can inhibit sexual arousal, lead to avoidance of intimacy, and interfere with relaxation needed for pleasure. Obsessive-compulsive disorder may cause intrusive thoughts or compulsions about sex, making intimacy fraught with guilt and fear.

Cognitive Impairments:

Impaired executive functioning and social cognition in serious mental illness can affect an individual's ability to navigate consent, recognize boundaries, read social cues, and communicate sexual needs clearly.

Yet despite these challenges, the need for connection remains. People still yearn to be loved, to feel attractive, to experience intimacy, even if the path there is complicated by symptoms or stigma.

3. Bipolar Disorder and the Instability of Desire

In bipolar disorder, shifts in libido often mirror the cycles of mood.

During mania or hypomania, dopamine levels can become elevated, leading to heightened sexual desire and sometimes hypersexuality. The intense need to pursue pleasure, combined with a lack of inhibitions, can drive individuals to take part in risky sexual behaviors, like having multiple sexual partners, engaging in unsafe sex, or experiencing sexual impulsivity that can be out of character during periods of emotional stability.

Dopamine dysregulation, especially hyperactivity in mesolimbic pathways, is strongly implicated in psychosis. But dopamine is also a key component of sexual arousal and pleasure. This biological overlap helps explain why hypersexuality may emerge during manic episodes, or why even floridly psychotic individuals may maintain preoccupations with sex. The desire is still "lit"—but it may burn without boundary.

On the pharmacological side, many antipsychotic medications antagonize dopamine receptors, especially D2, leading to decreased libido, erectile dysfunction, and anorgasmia. For patients already struggling with motivation and social withdrawal, this blunting of sexual expression can compound despair.

Still, despite these neurochemical disruptions and side effects, many patients—through fantasy, ritual, conversation, or behavior, find ways to preserve a sexual self.

These behaviors are often labeled hypersexuality, and indeed they may involve serious risks. But they are not always driven by mere impulse. They may also represent desperate attempts to feel powerful, loved, or alive.

One patient sought multiple partners during mania. It wasn't just about sex—it was about being seen. Adored. Validated. Mania, for her, was a fleeting moment where she felt desirable, worthy, in control.

Sexual desire does not vanish with psychosis. Instead, it often adapts—shaped by medication side effects, cognitive distortions, and social withdrawal. Studies have shown that people living with schizophrenia continue to experience sexual urges, fantasies, and even romantic longing, despite profound illness.

During Depression:

If dopamine ignites desire, serotonin can suppress it, especially when it comes to depression.

In major depressive episodes, serotonergic dysregulation contributes to:
- Anhedonia: the loss of pleasure, including sexual enjoyment
- Low libido: a marked disinterest in intimacy or physical connection
- Sexual dysfunction: including difficulties with arousal, lubrication, and orgasm

Depression doesn't just mute sexual drive—it can erase the capacity to care about sex at all. Feelings of worthlessness, guilt, and self-disgust may sever the emotional ties needed for intimacy. For partnered individuals, this can create rifts in relationships, leaving both parties isolated.

To compound this, selective serotonin reuptake inhibitors (SSRIs)—a first-line treatment for depression—are well known to cause sexual side effects in a significant proportion of users. These include delayed orgasm, erectile dysfunction, reduced vaginal lubrication, and blunted desire. While effective for mood, they may inadvertently inhibit one of the very aspects of life patients most miss: closeness.

For some, the loss of sexual connection becomes yet another grief within the landscape of depression.

For many living with serious mental illness, alternating poles of desire and detachment create instability in relationships. These abrupt swings—from craving closeness to pulling away—can leave partners feeling whiplashed, and often lead to emotional regret, broken trust, and stigma. James, with schizoaffective disorder, alternated between passionate declarations of love during manic phases and distant detachment when psychotic symptoms intensified. His partner described feeling "on a roller coaster I never agreed to ride."

4. Schizophrenia, Erotomania, and Delusional Intimacy

Psychotic illnesses are particularly associated with erotomanic delusions—where individuals believe someone (often of higher status) is secretly in love with them. These beliefs can drive inappropriate, obsessive, or even illegal behaviors. But beneath the surface lies a deeper emotional truth: a desperate need for connection and validation.

Other common patterns include:
- Delusions of sexual persecution
- Grandiose beliefs of sexual importance
- Misinterpreting neutral interactions as flirtation
- Disorganized sexual scripts performed repetitively

One man with schizophrenia repeated sexually charged phrases full of bravado and innuendo. He had never had a partner. For him, the sexual script was performative—a thread of identity in a life that felt otherwise disintegrated.

5. The Importance of Recognition and Support

Suppressing or ignoring sexuality in people with serious mental illness does not eliminate it. It only drives it underground—into shame, fantasy, or danger.

Healthy sexual expression can be a source of joy, agency, and dignity. Clinical support should include:
- Open, shame-free discussions about sexuality
- Assessment of sexual side effects of medication
- Psychoeducation about consent and healthy relationships
- Trauma-informed therapy to address past abuse or sexual confusion
- Couples counseling or relationship coaching, when appropriate

When clinicians address sexual health as part of holistic care, patients gain tools to better understand their desires and regulate their behaviors—often reducing distress, improving relationships, and strengthening identity.

Despite these disruptions, sexuality remains central to identity. Even when blunted or dysregulated, it offers clues to what the person values, yearns for, or remembers as meaningful.

Holding Space for the Sexual Self

Neurotransmitters don't simply regulate illness, they regulate identity. When clinicians overlook how dopamine or serotonin influence sexuality, they risk treating symptoms at the expense of personhood.

Patients are not just managing mania or depression—they are navigating what it means to be desired, to want, to lose, or to reclaim sexual connection. Supporting this exploration is not ancillary to psychiatric care; it is central to recovery.

Psychiatry's Complicated Relationship with Sexuality

Psychiatry has long had an uneasy relationship with sexuality. Historically, desire—especially when expressed outside societal norms—has been pathologized rather than understood. For generations, patients who voiced sexual feelings or sought intimate connection were met not with curiosity or compassion, but with suspicion, dismissal, or clinical labels.

Sexual expression in psychiatric patients is often framed in terms of risk: hypersexuality, inappropriateness, disinhibition, boundary violation. These terms can be useful for identifying patterns of harm or distress—but too often, they become tools of control, silencing the complexity of what sexuality truly means to the individual.

Conversations about intimacy, attraction, or bodily pleasure are frequently sidestepped. When medications blunt sexual drive, the effect is rarely discussed with the patient. When desire persists or intensifies—perhaps as a side effect of mania or as a resistance to institutional repression, it is seen as a behavioral problem, rather than a meaningful part of one's inner life.

Yet for many people living with schizophrenia, bipolar disorder, or schizoaffective disorder, sexual identity and expression remain some of the most enduring ties to personhood. A man who cannot hold a job may still crave a partner. A woman whose thoughts are clouded by delusions may still care deeply about how she looks, how she's touched, and how she's loved.

Sexuality, especially when it comes to illness, often serves as a form of continuity. Amidst fractured thought, flattened affect, or shifting moods, the wish to be seen, desired, or held can tether someone to the world in ways few other things can.

When psychiatry avoids or suppresses these conversations, it does not extinguish the desire. It only drives it underground, into fantasy, into delusion, or into shame. Patients begin to express their needs in ways that are more difficult to contain: intrusive sexual comments, inappropriate touching, or elaborate erotic delusions. These are not merely signs of illness, they are symptoms of neglect. The absence of open, affirming dialogue about sexuality leaves individuals to navigate a fundamental human experience in isolation.

Clinicians often fear that acknowledging sexuality in patients with serious mental illness will open the door to inappropriate behavior, manipulation, or risk. But the opposite is more often true. When patients are given the space to explore their sexual identities with dignity and structure, when desire is not treated as pathology but as part of their humanity, the therapeutic alliance strengthens. Shame softens. Control transforms into choice.

To move forward, psychiatry must reckon with its historical discomfort. We must replace silence with dialogue, surveillance with curiosity, and suppression with support. If we are to treat the whole person, we must be willing to honor their whole experience—including the parts that still long to touch and be touched, even in the midst of madness.

The Universal Drive: Sex and Intimacy as a Biological and Psychological Imperative

Sex and intimacy are not merely reproductive instincts or fleeting pleasures—they are fundamental human drives, deeply intertwined with our physical, emotional, and psychological well-being. The longing to be desired, to be held, to feel chosen—these are not superficial wants. They are core to our sense of identity, self-worth, and belonging.

From a biological standpoint, sexual desire arises from neurochemical and hormonal systems finely tuned for bonding and survival. But beyond biology lies something even more powerful: the emotional imperative for connection. According to attachment theory, our earliest need as human beings is to form secure, dependable bonds. As we grow, these bonds evolve into complex relationships where touch, intimacy, and mutual desire play essential roles in affirming our place in the world.

For individuals navigating the isolating terrain of serious mental illness, these needs do not disappear. In fact, they may intensify. While symptoms, stigma, and side effects often pose barriers to forming and maintaining relationships, the drive for intimacy can remain a deeply motivating force—a spark that cuts through disorganization, depression, or delusion.

The desire to be seen, desired, and loved is not extinguished by illness. It is one of the most enduring truths of what it means to be human. Sex and intimacy contribute to:

- Self-worth and self-esteem: Feeling desired or connected reinforces a sense of value and identity.
- Emotional regulation: Physical closeness can calm distress and foster a sense of safety.
- Healing and recovery: Supportive intimate relationships can anchor individuals during episodes of instability and help sustain recovery efforts.

Yet, for those living with schizophrenia, bipolar disorder, or schizoaffective disorder, these experiences often come with added layers of complexity. The illness itself may disrupt perception, mood, and social functioning. Medications that stabilize thought and emotion may simultaneously blunt libido or cause sexual dysfunction. And society—fearful of sexuality in people with mental illness—frequently pathologizes, ignores, or suppresses expressions of sexual desire.

Despite these challenges, many individuals still yearn for, and are capable of, meaningful intimate relationships. These relationships may look different—slower to build, more vulnerable to miscommunication, or requiring support from clinicians—but they are no less real. No less healing. No less human.

Sexuality is not a symptom to be managed, but a signal of vitality. When supported with care, respect, and understanding, it can become a source of dignity, resilience, and joy.

Fulfilling sexual and emotional lives are not only possible for people living with serious mental illness—they are essential. When we honor the full humanity of those we serve, including their desires and capacity for love, we help restore what the illness has tried to take away.

The Persistence of Sexual Desire: The Unquenchable Flame

In the throes of acute psychosis, many core functions of the mind unravel—reality testing fractures, language disorganizes, memory disintegrates, and affect (the outward expression of emotion) may either flatten into numbness or erupt unpredictably, with sudden outbursts of laughter, anger, or tears. Yet, amid this psychic collapse, sexual desire often persists. Sometimes, it even intensifies. One patient may be mute, unable to recognize their own name—yet speaks fluently about being pregnant with a divine child. Another, floridly psychotic and cognitively disorganized, may make frequent sexual comments or advances toward staff. These expressions may seem inappropriate, even disturbing, but they are not senseless. They are signals.

Why does sexual content endure, even when so much else dissolves?

Because sex is not merely about pleasure. It is about connection, control, identity, and vitality. In the middle of mental disintegration, sexual desire can become a lifeline to the body—a last remaining tether to the self. It may serve as an attempt to assert personhood, claim autonomy, or reconnect with sensation when everything else feels dictated by external forces.

Even disorganized or delusional sexual behavior often reflects unmet needs—to be seen, to be touched, to be known, to matter.

Sexual desire is not erased by schizophrenia, bipolar disorder, or schizoaffective disorder. It is a fundamental biological drive, interwoven with our sense of self, emotional well-being, and capacity for intimacy. While illness may distort how that desire is experienced or expressed, the underlying urge remains.

To deny this reality is to deny a basic dimension of humanity.

In clinical settings, this desire often emerges as part of the symptomatology:

- Hypersexuality during manic or psychotic states
- Sexual delusions involving celebrity marriages, spiritual unions, or persecution
- Impulsive behaviors that blur boundaries and disrupt care

These behaviors may appear chaotic, but they are rarely random. They often represent distorted attempts to cope, to connect, or to communicate. For some patients, sexuality becomes an obsessive focus, a psychological stronghold in an otherwise eroded identity. For others, desire is numbed or buried beneath medication side effects, stigma, and social withdrawal.

In schizophrenia, schizoaffective disorder, and bipolar disorder, neurobiological disruptions affecting impulse control, emotional regulation, and executive functioning can make it difficult for individuals to navigate sexual thoughts and behaviors appropriately. Sexuality can become exaggerated, delusional, or dangerously disconnected from context. Yet its presence, however altered, confirms the resilience of this core human drive.

Sex is not just a spark of pleasure, it is a spark of identity, longing, and the will to feel alive.

Acknowledging the persistence of sexual desire in severe mental illness is not an endorsement of disinhibited behavior. Rather, it is an invitation to understand its origins, to respond with compassion rather than control, and to support individuals in integrating this aspect of self in healthy, affirming ways.

The Other Side: Shame, Withdrawal, and Violation

Not all sexual experiences when it comes to serious mental illness are vivid or exaggerated. For many, sexuality is marked not by intensity, but by absence, aversion, and silence.

Some individuals retreat from sexual expression altogether—driven not by disinterest, but by fear, trauma, medication side effects, or profound internalized shame. For them, sex becomes dangerous—not as an act, but as a concept.

A man who once joked about hookups now flinches at the brush of a hand. A woman who once loved dancing hides under layers of oversized clothing. Libido doesn't disappear—it retreats. It waits for safety. It waits to be invited back.

For many patients, past abuse—whether in institutions, foster care, or the street—has left deep wounds. Others feel their bodies no longer belong to them. They may describe their bodies as "foreign," "violated," or "surveilled." Psychotic symptoms can reinforce these feelings, as patients sense that they are being watched, judged, or invaded.

This kind of sexual withdrawal is not always immediately visible. It can manifest as flat affect, avoidance of eye contact, refusal of medical exams, or persistent rejection of interpersonal closeness. Beneath the surface lies pain—often unspoken, often misunderstood.

On the other end of the spectrum are patients who become vulnerable to exploitation. Individuals who are manic, cognitively impaired, or homeless may exchange sex for survival, for a place to sleep, a cigarette, protection, or a fleeting sense of being wanted.

These encounters are too often labeled as promiscuity or poor judgment. But when viewed through a trauma-informed lens, they are better understood as acts of negotiation, survival, and emotional desperation. The body becomes currency in a world that offers them few other resources.

These aren't just choices; they're strategies. And they are almost always misunderstood.

For clinicians, this side of sexuality demands just as much attention—if not more—than hypersexuality or delusions. The absence of sexual expression does not mean the absence of need. Often, it reflects that the environment has not yet felt safe enough for those needs to be expressed.

The Clinical Imperative: Creating Space for the Silenced

It is essential that mental health professionals routinely and sensitively inquire about sexuality, intimacy, and relationship concerns. Too often, these topics are avoided—out of discomfort, perceived irrelevance, or fear of "opening Pandora's box."

But silence does not protect patients. It isolates them.

By integrating questions about sexual history, experiences, and identity into psychiatric assessments, clinicians can:
- Normalize discussion of sexual concerns
- Identify past trauma or current exploitation
- Understand how symptoms and side effects impact sexual self-concept
- Build trust through acknowledgment of the whole person

A few simple questions, asked with care and without judgment—can reopen doors long shut:
- "Has your condition affected how you feel about intimacy or touch?"
- "Have medications impacted your sexual experiences?"
- "Do you feel safe in your relationships?"

These questions invite honesty, build therapeutic alliance, and affirm that sexuality is part of recovery—not a distraction from it.

Gender, Identity, and Bodily Autonomy

For many individuals living with severe mental illness, questions of gender identity, sexual orientation, and bodily autonomy are not peripheral, they are central. These questions may arise quietly over time or emerge suddenly during episodes of mania or psychosis. And while some clinicians may be quick to pathologize these explorations, the reality is far more complex.

In some cases, gender fluidity or identity questioning during acute episodes is indeed part of the psychiatric symptomatology, connected to grandiosity, delusional beliefs, or disorganized thinking. But in other cases, these moments reflect long-suppressed truths—insights that surface only when the mind is untethered from social conformity or internal repression.

The challenge for clinicians is to discern without dismissing. To validate without idealizing. To listen without labeling.

Identity exploration is not always destabilizing. Sometimes, it is liberating. For individuals whose self-concept has long been constrained by trauma, stigma, or silence, serious mental illness may paradoxically open a window to authentic self-recognition. What surfaces may be confusing or fragmented, but it is often real.

At the same time, body image distortion, dysphoria, and sexual confusion are common in those with schizophrenia, bipolar disorder, and related conditions. Many patients express discomfort with their physical form, not only due to gender identity issues, but also as a result of:

- Antipsychotic-induced weight gain
- Sedation and fatigue
- Sexual side effects like erectile dysfunction or anorgasmia
- Feelings of being surveilled, controlled, or violated
- Trauma and bodily dissociation

In these contexts, the body becomes both a battleground and a barometer, a place where symptoms, medications, memories, and meaning all converge.

People with serious mental illness often live in bodies that feel changed, constrained, or colonized, by illness, by systems, by side effects. Restoring bodily autonomy and affirming identity must be part of recovery, not a luxury after stabilization.

Honoring the Spark of Sexual and Gender Identity

To honor the enduring spark of identity means making space for nuance, fluidity, and agency. It means approaching each patient's self-expression with curiosity rather than correction, and helping individuals reclaim ownership over their body and their desires—on their terms.

This includes:
- Creating affirming environments for LGBTQ+ patients
- Addressing dysphoria or discomfort without immediately pathologizing it
- Validating identity exploration while ensuring safety and grounding
- Helping patients interpret bodily changes caused by medications or illness

- Promoting dignity in physical care, including during exams, hygiene, and sexual health discussions

The body is not just a site of pathology—it is a source of pleasure, identity, resilience, and rebellion. In psychiatric care, we must learn to treat it as such.

Challenges and Complexities in Forming and Maintaining Intimate Relationships

Navigating intimacy is complex for everyone. But for individuals living with serious mental illness, the challenges of forming and sustaining meaningful relationships are often compounded by factors that stretch far beyond ordinary relational struggles.

While the desire for connection, love, and intimacy remains deeply intact, the path toward realizing those desires can be obstructed—by symptoms, stigma, side effects, trauma, and systemic limitations. Romantic and sexual partnerships often require vulnerability, emotional reciprocity, consistency, and communication—capacities that may be compromised or rendered unpredictable by psychiatric illness.

The result is a painful paradox: the longing for closeness remains, but the very symptoms of illness may erode the foundations on which intimacy rests.

Below, we explore the specific barriers that people living with schizophrenia, bipolar disorder, schizoaffective disorder, and related conditions often face when attempting to take part in intimate relationships.

Key Barriers to Intimacy in Serious Mental Illness

1. Affective and Cognitive Symptoms

Flat affect, emotional blunting, or mood instability can make emotional connection difficult. Partners may feel confused or rejected by inconsistent or muted emotional responses.

Cognitive impairments, including poor attention, disorganized thinking, or difficulty with abstract reasoning, can hinder meaningful communication and the ability to interpret social cues, resolve conflict, or offer empathy.

2. Distrust and Paranoia

In disorders like schizophrenia, paranoid delusions can disrupt the ability to trust a partner or sustain closeness. Even benign behaviors may be misinterpreted as threatening or deceptive.

The fear of being watched, manipulated, or harmed may lead to social withdrawal, preventing the development of intimate bonds altogether.

3. Disorganized or Erratic Behavior

Manic episodes may lead to impulsive decisions, including infidelity, oversharing, or intense declarations of love that shift rapidly into disinterest or hostility.

Disorganized speech or behavior can be difficult for partners to understand or respond to, leading to miscommunication and emotional fatigue.

4. Hypersexuality or Sexual Disinhibition

During manic or psychotic states, increased libido and reduced inhibition may result in risky sexual behaviors, boundary violations, or strained monogamous commitments.

These behaviors, while often symptoms of illness, can leave lasting emotional scars on relationships, particularly if they occur repeatedly.

5. Emotional Dysregulation and Rejection Sensitivity

Individuals may overreact to perceived rejection or misinterpret a partner's neutral behavior as criticism or abandonment.

This emotional volatility can destabilize even strong relationships, especially in the absence of insight or therapeutic support.

6. Medication Side Effects: A Physical and Emotional Disconnect

The impact of psychotropic medications on sexual function is a significant, often underreported, and routinely underestimated issue in psychiatric care. While these medications are essential for managing the symptoms of severe mental illnesses, their sexual side effects can undermine a person's vitality, identity, and quality of life.

These effects, often considered secondary or irrelevant, strike at the core of human dignity. They affect how people experience their bodies, how they relate to others, and whether they continue with treatment.

For someone already struggling to feel human, losing the capacity for sexual pleasure can feel like losing the last thread of connection to joy.

Clinicians must approach this not as a side conversation but as a core element of informed care. Open, nonjudgmental communication about these effects, and the exploration of alternative medications or mitigation strategies, can help preserve this vital spark of connection, pleasure, and identity.

How Medications Affect Sexual Function

A. Selective Serotonin Reuptake Inhibitors (SSRIs) & Serotonin-Norepinephrine Reuptake Inhibitors (SNRIs)

Commonly prescribed for depression, anxiety, and mood stabilization, these medications increase serotonin availability, but serotonin, especially when elevated at certain receptor subtypes, can inhibit sexual desire and function.

Common effects include:
- Decreased libido
- Delayed or absent orgasm
- Erectile dysfunction
- Reduced genital sensitivity

Patients often describe these effects as emotionally flattening or alienating, compounding already-present feelings of inadequacy or detachment. For someone trying to rebuild relationships or reclaim intimacy, these changes can feel devastating.

B. Antipsychotics (First- and Second-Generation)

Both typical and atypical antipsychotics can have profound sexual side effects due to their influence on dopamine blockade and prolactin elevation.

Mechanisms include:
- Hyperprolactinemia → decreased libido, erectile dysfunction, menstrual irregularities, galactorrhea
- Anticholinergic effects → vaginal dryness, difficulty achieving erection
- Sedation → diminished arousal and desire

A man who gains 60 pounds on antipsychotics may stop dating. A woman who can no longer orgasm may feel emotionally numb. These losses don't just erode pleasure—they undermine identity.

These side effects are rarely volunteered by patients, yet they are among the most distressing and influential in treatment adherence.

C. Mood Stabilizers

Medications like lithium and certain anticonvulsants (e.g., valproate, carbamazepine) can indirectly reduce sexual function through:
- Weight gain
- Fatigue
- Cognitive dulling

Though less commonly discussed than SSRIs or antipsychotics, these effects can still suppress libido, reduce romantic interest, and compound emotional withdrawal—especially in patients with bipolar disorder.

The Cycle of Discomfort and Silence

When patients experience these side effects but are not asked about them—or feel too ashamed to bring them up—a cycle of disengagement begins:
- The body no longer responds the way it once did.
- Shame, confusion, and relational strain increase.
- The patient loses interest in intimacy or stops medication altogether.

This silence is particularly harmful for patients already struggling with communication barriers, social anxiety, or paranoid symptoms. Even the idea of disclosing something so personal may feel impossible.

Clinical Responsibilities and Shared Decision-Making

Sexual agency should not be collateral damage in our pursuit of symptom control.

Clinicians must:
- Proactively ask about sexual function in every comprehensive assessment
- Validate the emotional and relational impact of side effects
- Discuss the possibility of medication adjustments, augmentations, or drug holidays when safe
- Offer psychoeducation on how medications affect the body—not as an afterthought, but as a core component of treatment planning

Patients deserve honesty. They deserve options. They deserve partnership—not just prescriptions.

7. Stigma and Social Isolation

Beyond the symptoms of mental illness and the side effects of medication lies another, quieter force, one that often goes unspoken but cuts just as deeply: stigma.

The pervasive societal stigma surrounding severe mental illness sends a clear, devastating message: You are broken. You are dangerous. You are unlovable. Over time, many individuals begin to internalize these beliefs, leading to profound feelings of shame, low self-worth, and emotional isolation.

"Why would anyone want to be with me?" is a question not rooted in delusion but in the painful echo of cultural rejection.

Internalized stigma can severely limit a person's willingness—or even perceived right—to pursue love, intimacy, or sexual expression. Many begin to believe that they are undeserving of connection, that their bodies are contaminated by illness, or that any attempt at romance would be met with rejection.

These beliefs are reinforced not only by social attitudes but also by the lived experiences of many individuals, as shown in the following examples:
- Partners who recoil upon learning of a diagnosis
- Families who discourage dating or intimacy
- Institutions that punish or suppress sexual expression
- Media portrayals that depict people with mental illness as unstable, dangerous, or asexual

All of this contributes to a cycle of self-silencing, where individuals begin to avoid relationships—not because they lack desire, but because they feel fundamentally unworthy.

This internalized shame also affects sexuality. Many patients feel too embarrassed to explore or express their desires. They may dissociate from their bodies, experience performance anxiety, or suppress libido entirely out of fear of judgment.

Mental illness does not erase the capacity for love—it obscures it behind a wall of fear and false beliefs.

I used to hesitate before asking about sex. Now, I see it as essential, because silence around desire breeds shame.

A young man with schizophrenia once asked me, "Do you think someone could ever love me?" He wasn't asking about sex—he was asking if intimacy was still possible for someone with a fractured mind. I didn't have an easy answer. But I knew that the fact he could still hope meant something vital was intact.

8. Body Image Concerns

For individuals living with serious mental illness, the body is often a site of conflict—a physical space shaped not only by illness but also by treatment side effects, trauma, and shame. While the desire for intimacy persists, the way one feels in and about their body can profoundly influence how (or whether) that desire is expressed.

Many psychiatric medications, especially antipsychotics and mood stabilizers, come with visible side effects: significant weight gain, acne, gynecomastia, hair thinning, sedation, or movement disorders like tremors or rigidity. These changes are not just cosmetic—they alter how patients see themselves, and how they believe others see them.

A patient may say, "I don't feel attractive anymore," or, "I used to go out—now I don't want anyone to look at me."

For some, these physical changes create a sense of being different, undesirable, or damaged. This can lead to:
- Avoidance of dating or physical intimacy
- Reluctance to be seen naked or touched
- Hypervigilance about appearance
- Shame during sexual encounters
- A belief that their body has betrayed them

Even when partners are affirming, patients may continue to carry a distorted self-image, shaped by years of internalized stigma and reinforced by visible side effects. For those who have experienced trauma or psychosis involving the body—like sexual delusions or tactile hallucinations—this disconnection can be even more profound.

In addition to weight gain, movement disorders (e.g., tardive dyskinesia, akathisia) can also erode confidence. Uncontrolled movements may be interpreted by others as instability or agitation, further stigmatizing the individual and reducing their comfort in social or intimate settings.

Healing the Relationship with the Body

Clinicians can take the following approaches to address body image in ways that are affirming and recovery-oriented:
- Validate concerns rather than dismissing them as "just side effects."
- Offer choices around medications when possible, including weight-neutral or prolactin-sparing options.
- Incorporate psychoeducation about the physical impact of medications, paired with strategies for physical wellness that are collaborative and stigma-free.
- Encourage therapeutic work around body image and self-concept, especially in patients with trauma histories or dissociative symptoms.

The body may change, but the right to feel at home in it does not disappear. The goal is not perfection—it's reconnection.

For clinicians, it is crucial to recognize that intimacy is not just about desire—it is about confidence. When patients feel unattractive, invisible, or repulsive, they withdraw from connection, even when they long for it. Supporting patients in reclaiming comfort with their bodies is an essential part of helping them reclaim intimacy.

9. Trauma, Taboo, and Identity

Sexual trauma is heartbreakingly common among individuals living with serious mental illness. Histories of early childhood abuse, coercion during periods of homelessness or incarceration, and exploitation in clinical or institutional settings leave deep psychological imprints—often shaping how individuals experience sexuality, intimacy, and identity throughout their lives.

For some, trauma leads to withdrawal or aversion—a retreat from all forms of physical touch or desire. Others may take part in reenactment—compulsive or provocative sexual behaviors that echo past harm. These expressions may seem contradictory, but at their core, they stem from the same unmet need: safety, consent, and meaningful connection.

Sex is not just about drive—it is also about history.

Many people living with schizophrenia, bipolar disorder, and schizoaffective disorder carry not only the burden of illness but also the scars of sexual betrayal, objectification, or confusion. In the wake of trauma, the boundaries between intimacy and danger, consent and coercion, desire and fear, often blur.

A patient may appear hypersexual or sexually provocative. But beneath that behavior could lie:

- A bid for control in a life marked by helplessness
- An effort to preemptively shape interactions they fear will become exploitative
- A learned survival strategy in unsafe environments

They may not be seeking pleasure—they may be trying to control the terms of harm they believe is inevitable.

Clinicians must learn to interpret behavior in context, not just in form. Trauma-informed care requires that we understand what sexual behavior means to the patient, not just how it looks on the surface.

The Institutional Silencing of Sexuality

Within hospitals, group homes, or forensic settings, patients' sexuality is often ignored, repressed, or pathologized. Institutional policies designed to "protect" can become mechanisms of erasure, infantilizing patients and denying them agency over their bodies and desires.

This is especially true for:

- Women, whose sexuality is often dismissed as inappropriate or pathological
- LGBTQ+ individuals, whose identities may be minimized, misinterpreted, or labeled delusional

- Transgender patients, who are frequently misgendered or denied access to gender-affirming care

I've worked with transgender patients whose entire sense of self was dismissed as psychosis. Their longing for love, for touch, for gendered recognition was reduced to symptomatology.

Yet even in these restrictive environments, sexuality finds a way to surface. Patients pass notes. They hold hands beneath cafeteria tables. They write poems, make eye contact, share brief moments of recognition and warmth. Romantic dramas unfold quietly in every unit—evidence that even under surveillance, the human longing for intimacy persists.

To ignore this is to ignore the patient's full humanity.

Reclaiming the Sexual Self Through Safety and Support

For survivors of trauma, healing requires more than abstaining from sexual behavior or extinguishing risk. It requires:
- Restoring choice over one's body
- Creating environments where safety is the norm, not the exception
- Validating the role of sexuality in self-concept and recovery
- Supporting healthy boundaries and communication around consent
- Honoring identity without assuming pathology

Clinicians must hold space for contradiction: that a person can be both terrified of touch and deeply longing for it, both dysregulated in behavior and wise in motive.

Trauma does not destroy the spark of sexuality—it reshapes it. And in the process of healing, that spark can become a source not just of pain, but of power.

10. Financial and Functional Instability

Limited income, housing insecurity, or lack of transportation may prevent individuals from participating in the social rituals that often lead to relationships, dating, going out, or spending private time with a partner.

Dependency on caregivers or staff for daily needs may also make intimacy feel impossible or inappropriate.

Dating, Disclosure, and the Search for Connection

For individuals living with severe mental illness, the terrain of dating and romantic connection is often emotionally charged and socially precarious. The desire for intimacy and partnership remains deeply human and alive, yet pursuing it may involve navigating a maze of stigma, vulnerability, and relational instability.

The Vulnerability of Disclosure

Deciding when, how, and whether to disclose a psychiatric diagnosis in a dating context can be fraught with anxiety. The fear of being judged, rejected, or misunderstood weighs heavily, especially in a culture that often equates mental illness with danger, instability, or dependency.

Some individuals choose to disclose early, believing honesty is essential. Others delay, hoping to establish trust before revealing a part of themselves that may be misinterpreted. Neither path is easy.

"If I tell them too soon, they'll leave. If I wait, they'll feel betrayed."
—A patient with schizoaffective disorder

The emotional toll of this decision-making process can be profound. For many, the potential for judgment or discrimination becomes a deterrent to dating altogether—reinforcing isolation and internalized stigma.

Lack of Understanding and Support from Others

Even well-meaning family members or friends can inadvertently discourage romantic relationships. Lacking a nuanced understanding of mental illness, they may:

- Offer overprotective or dismissive advice: "Focus on getting better first."
- Question a partner's intentions or capacity: "What if they take advantage of you?"
- Express fears about sexuality, safety, or parenting

These reactions, though rooted in care, can amplify the individual's own doubts about their desirability, competence, or rights to love and be loved.

Limited Opportunities for Social Connection

Social isolation is a common and painful reality for many people with serious mental illness. Psychiatric symptoms, transportation barriers, poverty, or institutional living can make participation in social life difficult.

Dating apps may feel overwhelming or unsafe.

Local events or group settings may be unwelcoming or stigmatizing.

Inclusive, judgment-free spaces to meet others, like community centers, peer-led groups, or therapeutic social clubs, are often scarce or inaccessible.

Consider the availability of inclusive social opportunities. If social infrastructure is lacking, individuals may never reach the threshold where meaningful relationships can even begin.

The Challenge of Episodic Illness in Relationships

Many serious mental illnesses—especially bipolar disorder, schizoaffective disorder, and recurrent psychotic disorders—are episodic in nature. Periods of relative stability may be followed by acute episodes of mania, depression, or psychosis.

This rhythm can be destabilizing in a relationship, even in one rooted in care and love. Partners may feel helpless, confused, or frightened during acute episodes. The ill individual may feel guilt, embarrassment, or fear of abandonment after recovery. Symptoms like irritability, withdrawal, paranoia, or hypersexuality can strain trust and intimacy.

Yet these challenges, while real, are not insurmountable.

With education, support, and open communication, couples can learn to navigate these fluctuations—not perfectly, but with resilience.

Clinicians can play a critical role by:
- Providing psychoeducation to both partners about the illness and its management
- Encouraging honest, nonjudgmental conversations about needs and boundaries
- Supporting the development of relational coping plans for times of crisis
- Helping patients feel empowered—not burdensome—in their relationships

Ethical Tensions and Clinical Care: Consent, Vulnerability, and Sexual Rights

Supporting sexual expression in people living with serious mental illness raises some of the most complex questions clinicians face. Issues of safety, capacity, dignity, and human rights converge in ways that defy simple answers. The following subsections explore these tensions in greater depth, highlighting practical dilemmas and ethical considerations for clinical care.

What does it mean to support sexual expression in someone who is floridly psychotic? How do we balance safety, consent, dignity, and human rights in psychiatric care?

These are some of the most ethically complex and emotionally charged questions clinicians face—particularly when caring for people living with serious mental illness. There are no simple answers.

Sexual Expression and Inpatient Constraints

In inpatient settings, sexual activity is often prohibited or tightly controlled—justified by concerns about consent, liability, and risk of exploitation. Staff may intervene at the first sign of a romantic relationship, fearing boundary violations, manipulation, or legal exposure.

Yet, in the community, people living with mental illness live unsupervised. Many, especially those who are homeless, cognitively impaired, or isolated, face significant risk of sexual exploitation, coercion, or abuse—often with no clinical oversight or protection. The disconnect between institutional restriction and community vulnerability creates an ethical tension that demands deeper reflection.

Consent Capacity: A Clinical and Moral Dilemma

One of the most ethically fraught tasks in psychiatric practice is assessing capacity to consent to sexual activity. Consider the complexity:
- Can a person in a manic episode, fueled by impulsivity and grandiosity, give informed sexual consent?
- Can someone with fixed delusions about divine marriage or telepathic lovers meaningfully distinguish fantasy from reality in a sexual encounter?

These are not abstract hypotheticals—they are daily clinical realities. Informed sexual consent requires the ability to:
- Understand the nature and risks of the act
- Appreciate the implications for self and other
- Make a voluntary and autonomous decision

Psychotic symptoms, cognitive impairments, and emotional desperation may undermine this capacity. Yet, we must guard against over-pathologizing. A consensual romantic relationship between two stable people living with mental illness should not automatically be deemed unsafe or inappropriate.

Vulnerability and the Risk of Exploitation

Individuals with serious mental illnesses may be more vulnerable to exploitation for several reasons:
- Cognitive impairments may hinder the ability to understand complex interpersonal dynamics or assess risk.
- Psychotic symptoms may distort perceptions of trust, intimacy, and danger.
- A deep longing for affection and connection can make someone more susceptible to manipulation.

- Power imbalances, especially in relationships involving caregivers, staff, or financially dependent roles, can limit autonomy and the ability to assert boundaries.

These vulnerabilities call for education, monitoring, and support—not shame, avoidance, or control.

Blurring of Boundaries in Illness

Mental illness can blur the boundaries between:
- Desire and compulsion
- Consent and submission
- Autonomy and coercion

Some patients may appear hypersexual, not out of genuine desire, but out of trauma reenactment, confusion, or attempts to control anticipated harm. Others may be withdrawn, averse, or disembodied, not because they lack desire, but because they've never been taught what safety feels like in their own skin.

The challenge for clinicians is to move beyond surface behavior and into its meaning: What does this act express? What need does it serve? What risks does it pose?

A Clinical and Ethical Imperative

Protecting the autonomy and safety of people living with serious mental illness in sexual situations is not a contradiction; it is a dual obligation. Clinicians must:
- Assess consent capacity carefully, contextually, and without judgment
- Promote sexual education tailored to cognitive and emotional levels

Normalize conversations about sexuality, moving beyond symptom checklists to include relational questions:
- "Do you feel connected to anyone?"
- "Have you ever felt safe in intimacy?"
- "What does desire mean to you?"
- Validate sexual identity and expression where appropriate.
- Monitor and address power dynamics, especially in controlled environments.

Key Factors That Increase Sexual Vulnerability
- Cognitive Impairments: Difficulty understanding complex information or making sound decisions.
- Psychotic Symptoms: Delusions or hallucinations that distort the nature of relationships and consent.

- Desire for Connection: A powerful longing for intimacy may override judgment or lead to idealizing unsafe dynamics.
- Power Imbalances: Situations where the individual is dependent on someone for housing, care, or protection can compromise consent.

Toward an Ethic of Sexual Dignity

We must advocate for a trauma-informed, dignity-centered approach to sexuality in mental health care. This includes:
- Recognizing when to intervene and when to allow for intimacy
- Supporting education, expression, and safe connection
- Developing policies that reflect ethical complexity, not blanket restriction
- Honoring that sexual identity and agency are part of recovery—not threats to it

Mental illness may complicate sexuality, but it does not eliminate the right to desire, to choose, or to love.

Hope Within the Complexity

Despite the barriers, many people living with severe mental illness form and sustain deeply loving, emotionally rich partnerships. These relationships may look different, slower to develop, more attuned to pacing and communication, but they are no less valid, no less passionate, no less healing.

What matters most is not perfection, but presence, patience, and mutual recognition of humanity between the patient and the care team. Mental illness may complicate dating, but it does not preclude love. The spark for connection still burns, even in difficult terrain. It simply needs room to grow.

Recognizing the Possibility Despite the Barriers

Despite these challenges, many people living with serious mental illness do form deeply meaningful relationships—romantic, sexual, and emotional. These partnerships may require different pacing, more support, or creative adaptations, but they are no less real, committed, or loving. What makes these relationships possible is often:
- Honest communication and psychoeducation
- Partners who are informed, patient, and nonjudgmental
- Supportive clinicians who validate the importance of intimacy
- Therapeutic environments that include sexuality and relationships as part of treatment planning

To deny someone's potential for love because of their diagnosis is to deny their humanity. Clinicians have a responsibility not just to treat symptoms, but to nurture hope—for connection, for partnership, for intimacy that heals rather than harms.

The Importance of Sexual Health Education and Support

For individuals living with serious mental illnesses, sexual health is often an unspoken but vital dimension of care. Too often, clinicians avoid the topic, institutions suppress it, and society either pathologizes or ignores it. Yet the need for intimacy, affection, and sexual expression remains enduring.

Comprehensive sexual health education must be:
- Accessible: Delivered in language that is clear and digestible, tailored to cognitive capacities, and sensitive to learning needs.
- Sensitive: Grounded in empathy and respect, avoiding judgment, shame, or moralizing.
- Comprehensive: Covering anatomy, sexual response, contraception, safe sex, STIs, consent, boundaries, healthy relationships, and recognizing abuse.
- Affirming: Validating individuals' right to desire, to explore, to set boundaries, and to define their sexual and romantic identities.
- Destigmatizing: Actively challenging shame and internalized stigma around sexuality, pleasure, and desire.

Sexual health is not a luxury—it is a fundamental component of identity, recovery, and well-being.

Therapeutic and Clinical Interventions

A holistic approach to sexual health and intimacy should be woven into routine psychiatric care. This includes:

1. Clinical Practice: Listening Without Judgment
- Shift from control to curiosity: What need is this behavior expressing?
- Create space for patients to discuss shame, pleasure, fantasy, or confusion without fear of being pathologized.
- Normalize the presence of sexuality in session.

2. Medication and Symptom Management
- Discuss sexual side effects openly.
- Collaborate with prescribers to adjust treatment when possible.
- Acknowledge and validate the emotional toll of sexual dysfunction.

3. *Individual and Group Therapy*
   - Use cognitive-behavioral therapy (CBT), sex therapy, or trauma-informed approaches to address unhealthy patterns, rebuild self-esteem, and explore intimacy.
   - Offer group therapy focused on relationship dynamics and social skills.
   - Use visual aids, repetition, and simple language to enhance learning.

4. *Peer and Community Support*
   - Facilitate peer-led groups on sexuality and relationships.
   - Encourage connection through creative or shared interests (art, music, writing, pets).
   - Promote online and community-based platforms for socialization and dating.

5. *Family and Couples Therapy*
   - Educate partners on the impact of illness on intimacy.
   - Support families in having open conversations about sexuality and mental health.
   - Help couples improve communication, build trust, and resolve conflict.

6. *Advocacy and Systems-Level Change*
   - Advocate for inclusive policies in institutions that respect sexual expression.
   - Challenge infantilizing practices that strip patients of sexual agency.
   - Promote sexual rights in mental health discourse and public health policy.

Clinical Role and Responsibility

Mental health professionals must embrace their responsibility to address sexuality, intimacy, and relationships as integral aspects of care. This includes:
- Proactively initiating discussions
- Conducting comprehensive sexual and relational assessments
- Offering accurate, shame-free education
- Collaborating across disciplines (gynecology, urology, sex therapy)
- Advocating for environments that honor rather than suppress sexual identity

A patient's sexual narrative is often a key to understanding their deepest hopes and fears. Ignoring it leaves that story untold.

Love, Longing, and the Right to Desire

Sex is not always about the act itself. It is about being seen, being wanted, being chosen.

Many patients describe a profound yearning for companionship, even amidst chaos. Some keep photos of former lovers tucked in their wallets. Others fall in love in hospitals or group homes—brief connections that offer warmth in otherwise sterile environments. These romances may be fragile. They may raise ethical questions. But they are real. They matter.

To deny this longing is to deny their humanity.

I've worked with patients who, even amid deep psychosis, still spoke of love and longing with striking clarity.

Despite the burdens of illness, the side effects of medication, and the stigma of diagnosis, the desire to love and be loved endures. And with the right support, it can be safely nurtured—not extinguished.

We must remember: People with serious mental illness are not less sexual, less deserving, or less capable of meaningful connection. They are simply more often denied the space to explore, express, and define their sexuality on their own terms.

Let us offer that space with tenderness, honesty, and hope.

Stories That Illuminate the Spark

Thomas: The Hope for a Hand to Hold

Thomas was a tall, soft-spoken man in his late twenties, diagnosed with schizophrenia in early adulthood. His speech often veered into fragmented, surreal territory, and on most days, he appeared lost in conversation with voices only he could hear.

Yet one afternoon, during a quiet moment in the inpatient unit, Thomas leaned across the table and asked with childlike earnestness, "Do you think...I could have a girlfriend someday?"

There was no delusion in the question, no hallucinated lover, no elaborate fantasy, just a clear, hopeful yearning for human connection. He spoke of wanting someone to sit with him, to watch movies, to hold his hand when the voices became too loud.

In that moment, the illness that had often obscured his identity peeled back, revealing something deeply universal: the desire to be loved. Thomas was not just a patient. He was a man still reaching for tenderness.

Yocasta: The Imagined Marriage That Soothed the Silence

Yocasta, a woman in her early forties, had lived with chronic schizophrenia for most of her adult life. She often believed she was secretly married to a famous musician—a man she had never met, whose songs played endlessly on the radio in her mind.

She described their "secret life" together with fierce devotion: imagined vacations, candlelit dinners, and late-night talks only she could hear. To an outsider, it might sound bizarre or sad. But when I listened closely, I realized something else.

Yocasta's delusion was also a survival strategy. Her imagined marriage softened the isolation imposed by her illness. Beneath the psychosis was an unmistakable longing—to be chosen, to be loved, to belong.

Even in delusion, her spark endured. Her fantasy offered structure, comfort, and a kind of emotional dignity in a world that often denied her both.

Sarah: Navigating Desire in Bipolar Disorder

Sarah, a young woman with bipolar disorder, described the emotional whiplash of dating with a condition that could swing her from exuberance to exhaustion. Mood swings made consistency hard. Medication dulled her libido.

She often feared that disclosing her diagnosis would scare partners away. When relationships ended, she blamed herself—her body, her moods, her "too much-ness."

Her story is one of bravery: learning to disclose on her own terms, to ask for understanding without apology, and to find a partner who met her with empathy instead of fear. For Sarah, intimacy became possible not when symptoms disappeared, but when she could show up authentically.

David: Paranoia and the Long Road to Trust

David, a middle-aged man with schizophrenia, struggled with persistent paranoia that made intimacy feel dangerous. He longed for companionship but couldn't shake the fear that others were plotting against him.

Simple acts—like someone asking for his number or brushing his arm—could trigger spiraling thoughts.

But David kept trying. He began attending a support group. He started naming his fears instead of hiding them. He practiced eye contact, sharing coffee, receiving touch. For David, building intimacy wasn't a leap—it was a series of slow, steady steps toward safety.

Maria: Depression and the Struggle to Feel Worthy

Maria, a woman in her fifties with recurrent major depressive disorder, described how her illness dulled not only her energy but her belief that she was deserving of affection.

"I don't want anyone to see me like this," she would say. "I don't even want to touch myself."

She avoided dating, convinced that no one would want someone "so broken." And yet, beneath the despair, she admitted: "Sometimes I just want someone to hold me. Just to be held."

Maria's healing began with therapy focused not on rekindling libido, but on restoring worth. Her spark was never extinguished—it was buried under shame. Uncovering it was the work of trust, time, and kindness.

Carlos: From Provocation to Presence

Carlos, a 32-year-old man with schizoaffective disorder, often spoke about his "sexual electricity." He believed he was destined to father a nation. He flirted with staff, crossed boundaries with other patients, and made repeated calls to ex-partners.

Rather than restrict him or medicate the behavior away, his clinician asked, "What does this electricity mean to you?"

Carlos paused and said, "When people want me, I feel real. I forget the voices. I feel like myself."

Therapy didn't aim to extinguish his spark—but to understand it. They worked on safe ways to express intimacy, recognize boundaries, and channel his energy into connection rather than chaos. Slowly, his behavior shifted. Not because he was silenced, but because he was seen.

Beneath the Illness, the Human Remains

These stories are not just case notes. They are reminders: that schizophrenia, bipolar disorder, depression, and schizoaffective illness may alter perception, but they do not destroy the yearning to love and be loved. The spark persists—sometimes quiet, sometimes wild, sometimes wrapped in delusion, but always human.

To honor that spark is not to romanticize illness; it is to reclaim the humanity too often lost beneath diagnosis.

Love, desire, intimacy—these are not luxuries. They are lifelines. And for every Thomas, Yocasta, Sarah, David, Maria, or Carlos, they may just be the most enduring sign of the self that illness could never fully erase.

Conclusion

The desire for intimacy, sexual expression, and meaningful connection is not erased by serious mental illness—it persists. Beneath the layers of psychosis, mood instability, or cognitive disruption, there remains a longing to be close, to be desired, to be known. This desire may be altered in form, fragmented in expression, or complicated by trauma and symptoms, but it is fundamentally human.

In the clinical world, it can be tempting to focus solely on what is broken: hallucinations, disorganization, delusions. But if we listen more closely, we find that the architecture of longing remains intact beneath the illness. Sexual desire in schizophrenia or bipolar disorder is not a disruption to be managed—it is a profound reminder that even in the most altered states of mind, the human heart keeps reaching outward.

For many individuals, sexuality becomes a symbol—not just of pleasure, but of connection, of worth, of identity. In a mind frayed by illness, sexual desire can act as a tether back to the world, a quiet reminder that the self, however disorganized, still yearns. Still imagines. Still touches. Still loves.

Sometimes, the fire doesn't consume. Sometimes, it simply glows—quietly, defiantly—in the corner of a forgotten room.

Sex is often the first spark judged, and the last to be understood. In serious mental illness, it can appear messy, risky, or unsafe. But it can also be healing, affirming, and life-giving. Our task as clinicians is not to extinguish this spark, but to contain it, understand it, and support the person in reclaiming it.

This means:

- Listening without judgment
- Asking not just about symptoms, but about desires
- Creating space for honest conversation
- Addressing medication side effects, trauma, and self-image
- Offering education, therapy, and support
- Honoring boundaries while affirming rights
- Seeing sexuality not as a risk to manage but a life force to nurture

Sexuality is not a distraction from psychiatric care—it's central to it. It is a barometer of dignity, vitality, and belonging. Even in the depths of illness, the body remembers its hunger for touch and closeness. To honor that spark is not unprofessional; it is profoundly humane.

This chapter affirms that with appropriate support, education, and empathy, people living with severe mental illness can experience healthy, meaningful, and fulfilling sexual and romantic lives. These connections are not luxuries; they are part of recovery, part of being alive.

To acknowledge and support this spark is to say to our patients: "You matter—not just as a diagnosis to be stabilized, but as a person to be seen, touched, and loved."

The fire may flicker. It may distort. But it endures.

And in honoring it, we do not just treat illness—we restore humanity.

Table 4.1 — Sexuality in Clinical Care

Barrier	Impact	Recovery-Oriented Approach
Stigma/taboo	Silence, shame	Open, respectful conversations
Medication side effects	Loss of desire, dysfunction	Adjust meds, normalize discussion
Trauma history	Fear, avoidance	Trauma-informed care

Seeman, M. V. (2011). Sexuality and schizophrenia. *World Psychiatry*, 10(3), 210–214.

Goodwin, F. K., & Jamison, K. R. (2007). *Manic-Depressive Illness: Bipolar Disorders and Recurrent Depression* (2nd ed.). Oxford University Press.

Pfaus, J. G. (2009). Pathways of sexual desire. *J Sex Med*, 6(6), 1506–1533.

Brown, E. C., Tas, C., & Brüne, M. (2014). Potential therapeutic use of oxytocin in schizophrenia. *CNS Drugs*, 28(8), 713–724.

Kennedy, S. H., Rizvi, S., Fulton, K., & Rasmussen, J. (2008). A double-blind comparison of sexual functioning, antidepressant efficacy, and tolerability between bupropion XL and venlafaxine XR. *J Clin Psychopharmacol*, 28(3), 329–333.

Wright, E. R., Wright, D. E., Perry, B. L., Foote-Ardah, C. E. (2007). Stigma and the sexual lives of people with mental illness. *Schizophrenia Bulletin*, 33(3), 587–596.

Serretti, A., & Chiesa, A. (2011). Sexual side effects of pharmacological treatment of psychiatric diseases. *Clin Pharmacol Ther*, 89(1), 142–147.

Mauritz, M. W., & van Meijel, B. (2013). Sexual revictimization in people with severe mental illness: a literature review. *Trauma, Violence, & Abuse*, 14(4), 305–322.

Bartlett, P., & Sandland, R. (2020). *Mental Health Law: Policy and Practice* (6th ed.). Oxford University Press. (Discussion of institutional constraints and patient rights.)

Anthony, W. A. (1993). Recovery from mental illness: The guiding vision of the mental health service system. *Psychosocial Rehabilitation Journal*, 16(4), 11–23.

Chapter 5
Money: Autonomy, Survival, and Power

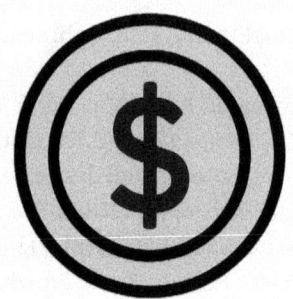

Introduction

Money is not merely currency, it is narrative, identity, survival, and, for many living with severe mental illness, a symbol of the control they often lack in other areas of life. In clinical settings, preoccupations with money are frequently dismissed as symptoms, grandiosity, delusion, irresponsibility. But to view them only through a pathological lens is to miss their deeper meaning. When understood as a spark, money emerges as a profound theme, revealing urgent needs for security, self worth, and autonomy in a world that routinely disempowers.

Despite disordered thought or emotional turmoil, many people living with schizophrenia, schizoaffective disorder, or bipolar disorder continue to hold vivid dreams about wealth. These are not just fantasies, they are lifelines. In the midst of psychosis, money becomes more than a means of exchange. It becomes a form of symbolic power, a promise of safety, agency, and relevance.

For some, money represents protection, a shield against instability. For others, it is a way to regain dignity, to prove they matter, to claim a stake in a world that often sidelines them. Obsession with wealth rarely stems from greed. More often, it arises from deprivation, of control, of respect, of choice. In this context, the fantasy of abundance becomes a coping mechanism.

You may see it clinically, the patient convinced they have a hidden inheritance, or the one who hoards coins as if stockpiling for a siege. You may see it in mania, when spending becomes compulsive and uninhibited. Or in depression, when financial fears spiral into hopelessness. These behaviors are not random, they are emotionally anchored, shaped by both illness and a deep seated need for agency.

In a culture where financial independence is equated with personal value, the struggle to manage money takes on existential weight. Money, in these contexts, is not just about transactions, it is about autonomy. About having a choice. About being someone, not just someone's patient.

In this chapter, we explore the landscape of money and mental illness. We examine how psychosis and mood disorders distort financial perception, but also how the desire for economic control reflects something enduring and human. We consider real life implications, how poverty and financial dependence affect self worth, how spending patterns may reflect attempts to reclaim control, and how clinicians can engage these concerns with empathy and insight.

Because beneath every discussion of money in psychiatric care lies a more fundamental question, what does it mean to be in control of your own life?

The Brain and Money, Reward, Motivation, and the Neuroeconomics of Mental Illness

The human desire for money is not merely cultural or symbolic, it is neurobiological. Financial reward activates many of the same brain systems that respond to food, sex, or social connection. Chief among these is the mesolimbic dopamine pathway, which we explored in Chapter 2. This circuit, linking the ventral tegmental area, VTA, to the nucleus accumbens and prefrontal cortex, is the brain's core reward engine. It lights up in response to the anticipation of pleasure, including the pursuit and acquisition of money.

Neuroeconomics, the study of how the brain evaluates value, makes decisions, and responds to risk, shows that money is encoded in the brain not only as a means of survival, but as a powerful symbol of reward, agency, and possibility. In people living with serious mental illnesses like schizophrenia and bipolar disorder, this system is often dysregulated, which can lead to distorted behaviors and beliefs around money.

The prefrontal cortex, responsible for judgment, foresight, and impulse control, plays a key role in managing financial decisions. In mania, this regulatory center is compromised. The result, disinhibited spending, risk taking, and an exaggerated sense of financial invincibility. Patients may embark on reckless shopping sprees, invest in implausible schemes, or give away large sums of money. The high becomes more about the pursuit than the payoff.

In schizophrenia and schizoaffective disorder, delusions of wealth are common. Patients may believe they are heirs to fortunes, lottery winners, or financial saviors. These beliefs often stem from dysfunction in salience attribution, a process governed in part by the striatum and dopaminergic signaling. Here, the brain assigns excessive significance to neutral cues, a receipt, a bank number, or a wallet, transforming them into tokens of imagined wealth or cosmic destiny.

Neuroimaging studies show that the same reward circuits activated in healthy individuals by the promise of money are hyperactive or misdirected in those with psychosis. When these circuits fire without proper modulation, the result is not just desire, it is conviction. Money becomes not just something wanted, but something owed, fated, or divinely granted.

Even pharmacology can enter the equation. Dopamine agonists, used in Parkinson's disease and, occasionally, in psychiatric augmentation, have been linked to compulsive gambling, risky financial decisions, and hyper focused monetary behaviors. These effects reveal how delicate the balance of brain chemistry is in governing financial self control.

Yet, neurobiology does not tell the whole story. Behind every delusion of wealth is a story, of longing, of humiliation, of a desire to matter. Behind compulsive spending is a craving for agency, identity, or relief from emptiness. The circuits may be misfiring, but the symbolic power of money remains potent. For many patients, financial fantasies are not symptoms alone, they are myths of survival.

Understanding the neuroeconomics of mental illness invites us to see not only the brain's dysfunction, but the person's meaning making. It asks us to look not only at what is broken, but at what is desired. Beyond biology, money is a story, one that patients use to explain power, worth, and hope.

Delusions of Wealth, Power, and Control

Delusions involving money are frequently grandiose or persecutory, for example,
- "I invented the internet and Google owes me."
- "I have a frozen offshore account."
- "They are monitoring my debit card."

These are not just symptoms, they are efforts to reclaim dignity and control in environments that strip both away. Even persecutory delusions can reflect real trauma, economic marginalization, systemic surveillance, and profound powerlessness.

Mania, Shopping Sprees, and the High of Spending

In manic states, money becomes kinetic. Patients max out cards, give money away, or start grandiose business plans. There is a sensuality to spending, a thrill, a click, a flash of control. But the aftermath is often devastating, debt, legal issues, shame. Spending during mania is not just impulsive, it reflects a deeper need for agency, expression, and esteem. Therapy must validate the emotions behind the behavior while building safer outlets for those needs.

Compulsive Spending, Hoarding, and Financial Chaos

Financial behaviors may manifest in extremes, including:
- Compulsive spending, shopping sprees, gift giving, reckless investments
- Hoarding, coins hidden in shoes, stashes of receipts labeled for emergencies
- Gambling, fueled by delusions or distorted risk perception

These behaviors are rarely about greed. They are responses to instability, fear, trauma, and the longing for control.

The Impact of Mental Illness on Financial Autonomy

Cognitive impairments impact budgeting and planning. Negative symptoms, for example avolition, reduce motivation for employment. Paranoia fosters mistrust of financial institutions. Grandiosity drives delusional entrepreneurship. Real world impact includes eviction, poverty, and reliance on dehumanizing systems.

Delusions involving money are a double edged sword in the treatment of people living with psychosis. On one hand, these beliefs can impede engagement, with patients resisting medication or therapy, convinced their financial destiny will resolve their suffering. On the other hand, these very delusions can be therapeutic entry points. They often express a yearning for security, autonomy, and self worth, universal needs intensified by the disorientation of illness.

Rather than dismissing these beliefs outright, clinicians can gently explore the emotional meaning behind them. For instance, a therapist might ask how wealth represents control or identity, using that dialogue to help the patient find more grounded ways of asserting agency. Empathy, without reinforcement of the delusion, can deepen therapeutic rapport and open space for healing.

One patient once told me that having money would make him a real person. That moment reframed everything I thought I knew.

Illness Specific Financial Impacts

Schizophrenia and Schizoaffective Disorder
- Grandiose wealth beliefs that drive risky spending or legal entanglements
- Paranoia about surveillance that fosters cash hoarding and avoidance of banks or benefits
- Executive dysfunction that undermines budgeting, bill paying, and employment persistence
- Avolition leading to disengagement from financial responsibilities

Bipolar Disorder

- Manic impulsivity with unrestrained spending or gifting, often charged with a sense of destiny or purpose
- Risky investments and grandiose ventures during elevated mood states
- Depressive inertia that leads to unpaid bills, avoidance, and shame

Stigma, Employment Barriers, and Economic Marginalization

Stigma impacts access to work, housing, and healthcare, for example,
- Employers may avoid hiring people with mental illness
- Housing providers may reject tenants based on diagnosis
- Healthcare may overlook physical needs because of psychiatric labels

These barriers reinforce poverty and prevent engagement with sparks such as food, music, and connection. Supported employment and housing programs can restore dignity and enable recovery.

The Symbolic Language of Money

In therapy, money often becomes metaphor, for example,

"I am rich" equals "I matter."

- Hoarding equals "I am still in control."
- Budgeting equals "I can shape my future."

Helpful clinical questions include,
- What does money represent in your story?
- How would having money change your life?

Financial Exploitation and Structural Vulnerabilities

People with serious mental illness are vulnerable to scams, theft, and manipulation because of:
- Cognitive deficits
- Social isolation
- A desperate need for connection

Protective structures like conservatorships must be paired with dignity preserving interventions. Autonomy should be nurtured, not erased.

Interventions, From Risk Reduction to Empowerment

Treatment should integrate,
- Medication to stabilize mood and modulate impulsivity
- Cognitive behavioral therapy to reframe money beliefs
- Financial education tailored to cognitive level
- Supported employment and peer mentoring

Support should aim to preserve agency, not only to control risk.

Clinical Reflections and Vignettes

- Richard, schizophrenia, convinced of inheritance, planned global ventures as a form of hope
- Martha, believed a millionaire would fund her publishing dreams, symbolic validation
- Denise, spent twenty thousand dollars in a manic week, later integrated into a recovery plan

These are not just fantasies. They are expressions of longing, grief, and self worth.

The Impact of Illness on Financial Matters

Serious mental illness often reshapes a person's relationship with money in profound ways. Symptoms such as cognitive disorganization, impaired concentration, and fluctuating motivation can undermine the ability to budget, pay bills on time, or maintain steady employment. Hospitalizations may interrupt income, while stigma and systemic barriers limit access to work opportunities and financial independence. Even when money is available, the energy and executive function required to manage it may be compromised. For many, this instability compounds a sense of dependency, eroding self esteem and intensifying feelings of being less than. At the same time, financial precarity is not simply logistical, it is existential. Without money, choices narrow. Autonomy is restricted. Recovery itself is jeopardized when basic needs like housing, food, and security cannot be consistently met.

Money Delusions, Barriers and Bridges in Therapy

Delusional beliefs about money are common in psychotic illnesses. Some patients are convinced they are secretly wealthy or destined for riches. Others fear that forces are stealing their funds or conspiring to bankrupt them. These delusions can act as barriers to therapy, making it difficult to discuss budgeting or financial planning when the very foundation of money's meaning feels distorted. Yet they can also serve as bridges. A patient who insists he is a millionaire may be expressing a yearning for freedom, recognition, or dignity. Another who believes her money is being stolen may be voicing a deeper sense of vulnerability and lack of safety. By listening for the symbolic meaning behind the delusion, clinicians can connect with the patient's underlying concerns, control, security, hope, and gently reframe the conversation toward reality based strategies.

Mania, Spending Sprees, and the Allure of Wealth

In manic states, money becomes kinetic, spent freely, invested recklessly, or given away impulsively. Patients may max out credit cards, start businesses overnight, or gamble away life savings. These behaviors carry real world consequences, but they are deeply tied to emotion and meaning. In mania, money often equals identity:

- "I deserve this," self worth
- "I must act now," urgency and invincibility
- "I am changing the world," inflated purpose

Helping patients recover from these episodes involves more than financial literacy. It requires deeper emotional work. What were they reaching for, what losses were they defending against, and what needs were they trying to meet, esteem, freedom, connection. Addressing these themes supports healthier, sustainable paths to feel powerful, connected, and alive.

Compulsive Spending, Gambling, and Financial Chaos

In serious mental illness, money does not only linger in thought, it often explodes into behavior. Financial decisions can become an emotional language, acting out distress, hope, or desperation through currency and credit. During manic episodes, individuals may order dozens of packages online, buy gifts for strangers, or invest in dubious ventures with borrowed money. Some gamble with a sense of invincibility, convinced they are destined to win. Others, caught in paranoid psychosis, may withdraw all funds, certain they are being watched or manipulated.

For those relying on fixed incomes, Social Security, disability payments, or informal labor, these behaviors carry severe consequences. A single episode can trigger eviction, utility shutoffs, or the return of hunger and dependence. These are not foolish acts. They are emotional storms, moments where inner instability bursts into economic risk. Beneath them lies shame, rarely spoken but deeply felt, as patients struggle to reconcile intentions with aftermath.

Hoarding and the Hidden Treasures

Money related distress does not always present as spending. Sometimes, it emerges as saving, rigid, obsessive, symbolic. Many patients hoard coins, old receipts, expired debit cards, or stacks of unopened benefit letters. The items are not always practical, but they are potent. They represent lost opportunities, fragile hopes, or attempts to preserve a thread of continuity in a life frequently disrupted.

One man lined his shoes with rolls of nickels, just in case the world ends. A woman slept beside plastic bags of dollar bills, each labeled in careful handwriting, for my kids, for my escape, for emergencies. These are not just survival strategies. They are personal archives. Each bag, coin, and scrap of paper tells a story of trauma, displacement, and abandonment. They mark places where trust broke down, between patient and family, patient and system, patient and self. To discard these objects might feel like discarding one's history. To guard them is to protect whatever dignity remains.

The Underlying Desire for Security and Autonomy

Even when financial behaviors appear irrational or driven by symptoms, they often reflect a deeper human desire for security and autonomy. The patient with grandiose spending may be seeking power or importance. The individual hoarding small amounts out of paranoia is likely trying to create a sense of safety and control in a world that feels unpredictable. The desire to manage funds, even in small amounts, speaks to a fundamental need for independence and self determination.

Money as a Source of Power and Identity

Money is not only a means to survival, it is also a symbol of status and identity. For people living with severe mental illness, cultural values around money are often internalized in ways that exacerbate struggle. Stigma surrounding poverty and mental illness can make individuals feel invisible or worthless. As a result, the desire for money becomes more than a practical necessity. It represents social validation and a potential means of regaining dignity.

In psychotic disorders, patients may fixate on money as a way to regain a sense of normalcy or to prove worth to others. A patient may believe that acquiring a significant amount of money will resolve all problems, from health to isolation. This can be reinforced by delusions of grandeur in which the individual believes that they are meant for greatness or power.

The Crushing Weight of Financial Strain and Poverty

The connection between financial stability and mental health is deeply interwoven and often cyclical. Managing money can be a daily struggle because of cognitive symptoms, executive dysfunction, or social challenges. At the same time, chronic financial stress can worsen psychiatric symptoms, fueling anxiety, deepening depression, and triggering paranoia or hopelessness.

Every unpaid bill or denied benefit becomes more than a bureaucratic hassle, it is a threat to survival. The fear of eviction, running out of food, or losing access to vital medications is not abstract. It is urgent and ever present. These stressors are more than external hardships, they penetrate deeply into emotional and psychological life, dimming the spark of autonomy and hope. Addressing financial insecurity is therefore central to psychiatric care and recovery.

Poverty as a Daily Reality

Many people living with schizophrenia, bipolar disorder, or schizoaffective disorder live in persistent poverty. They often depend on a patchwork of public supports, Social Security Disability, SNAP, Section 8 housing vouchers, Medicaid. These benefits offer critical lifelines, but they also come with surveillance, conditionality, and uncertainty. In this landscape, money is survival, safety, and dignity.

Common worries include,
- What if my benefits stop,
- How will I eat if I am discharged,
- Why can I not control my own money,

These concerns are often rooted in lived experience. Financial exploitation, administrative errors, sudden benefit cuts, or unexplained changes in payee arrangements are all too common. Mistrust is not always a symptom, it can be a survival strategy.

Financial Exploitation, A Hidden Epidemic

People with serious mental illness are particularly vulnerable to financial abuse and exploitation. Cognitive impairments, impulsivity, and attentional difficulties make it harder to detect scams or resist coercion. Without support, individuals can fall into debt, overdraw accounts, or become targets for manipulation.

Social isolation reduces a protective network. There may be no one to consult about suspicious calls or to help decipher a medical bill. Loneliness increases susceptibility to predatory lending and coercive family dynamics.

Guardianship and conservatorship can safeguard individuals who are unable to manage their affairs, yet these arrangements can also undermine autonomy. At their best, they protect from harm. At their worst, they become systems of control where financial decisions are made without transparency or respect for the individual's voice. The ethical task is to pair protection with dignity and self determination.

Medications, Disability, and the Price of Treatment

For many individuals with serious mental illness, the economics of treatment are as daunting as the symptoms. Disability benefits often provide only a modest monthly stipend, forcing patients to choose between medication, housing, and basic necessities. Insurance coverage may not extend to the most effective or tolerable medications, leaving patients with either suboptimal treatment or significant out of pocket expenses. Navigating formularies, prior authorizations, and pharmacy shortages requires persistence and executive function that illness itself may compromise.

When Survival Has a Copay

Money is not only a symbolic spark, it is a gatekeeper. Medication, therapy, and transportation can be out of reach for those on fixed incomes. The act of surviving becomes a financial burden. Efforts to work, even part time, can put benefits at risk. Patients face painful trade offs, earn a few dollars and lose Medicaid coverage, or stay unemployed to preserve access to care. The systems designed to promote independence can entrench dependency.

The Spark of Dignity, Financial Independence as Recovery

Despite these challenges, the drive for financial autonomy persists. Patients want to manage their money, earn income, and live with dignity. Clinicians and advocates should recognize this not as a symptom to pathologize, but as a spark to support. Financial literacy programs, supported decision making, and trauma informed benefits navigation can restore a sense of control.

The Emotional and Practical Weight of Money

The relationship between financial well being and mental health is cyclical and complex. Cognitive impairments, fluctuating mood states, and medication side effects can compromise money management. Simultaneously, the stress and instability caused by financial insecurity, fear of eviction, inability to afford medications, or persistent food insecurity, can exacerbate depression, anxiety, and psychosis. Money in this context is existential. It represents safety, control, and identity.

Treatment Implications, From Shame to Empowerment

Integrate financial support into care,
- Connect patients to disability benefits and housing supports
- Offer psychoeducation on how illness affects financial behavior
- Teach budgeting, banking basics, and scam avoidance
- Normalize financial shame and explore it as a clinical theme

Therapeutic interventions can include,
- Medication to regulate impulsive or delusional spending
- Cognitive behavioral therapy to examine and reframe beliefs
- Family support to establish healthy boundaries and collaboration
- Financial counseling to promote autonomy and reduce risk

The Ethics of Financial Control

Clinicians must balance autonomy and harm prevention. Conservatorships and payeeships can stabilize finances while eroding dignity. Recovery oriented care emphasizes partnership by using prepaid cards with spending limits, co developed budget plans, and peer mentors for financial coaching.

Dreams, Delusions, and the Symbolism of Money

Psychotic symptoms commonly include money related themes. Grandiose delusions may feature wealth fantasies, while paranoid content may include fears of theft or surveillance. These beliefs reflect deeper human desires, power, safety, recognition, and redemption. Delusions should be explored for meaning. Behind them often lies an unmet need or unresolved fear.

Real Lives, Real Struggles, Patient Vignettes

- James, schizoaffective disorder, wrestling with benefits and stigma while longing for work

- Lisa, an older adult with depression and anxiety who was scammed amid isolation
- Michael, a young man with psychosis who found dignity through supported employment
- Denise, a woman with bipolar disorder who spent a large sum during mania and later rebuilt with supported budgeting

The Role of Social Programs and Financial Literacy

Support programs, often the first line of defense, include SSDI, SSI, Section 8, and utility assistance. They are crucial lifelines yet bureaucratically complex.

Financial literacy initiatives should be tailored to cognitive needs, use simplified materials and repetition, and teach budgeting, banking, and fraud prevention.

Sustained support can come from case managers, social workers, peer mentors, and representative payees who include the patient in decisions.

The Persistent Shadow of Financial Dreams in Psychosis

Money delusions can persist even during remission. Psychosis alters reality but not the desire for control and dignity. Dreams of sudden wealth, paranoia about theft, or hallucinations involving money are common and reveal fears and aspirations, security, validation, a reachable future, fear of poverty, and anxiety about losing autonomy. Understanding these dreams guides treatment, not to silence them, but to translate them into needs for safety, recognition, dignity, and hope.

Conclusion

Achieving a greater degree of financial stability for people living with serious mental illness requires comprehensive support, accessible financial education, opportunities for employment, and safeguards against exploitation. This work is not merely economic. It is fundamental to recovery, to a sense of independence, and to nurturing the spark of autonomy that supports a life worth living. Money in this context is symbolic, emotional, and sacred. When we treat financial preoccupations not as symptoms to manage but as messages to understand, we build bridges, not only budgets. Behind every dollar there is often a dream, and every dream, no matter how distorted, offers a clue to what matters most.

Table 5.1, Money, Healthy versus Shadow Expressions

Expression	Healthy	Shadow
Money use	Independence, budgeting	Spending sprees, hoarding
Symbolism	Autonomy, survival	Grandiose delusions
Clinical role	Employment, security	Exploitation, financial stress

References

Anthony, W. A. (1993). *Recovery from mental illness: The guiding vision of the mental health service system. Psychosocial Rehabilitation Journal, 16*(4), 11–23.

Beck, A. T., & Alford, B. A. (2009). *Depression: Causes and treatment* (2nd ed.). University of Pennsylvania Press.

Davidson, L., Tondora, J., O'Connell, M., Lawless, M. S., & Rowe, M. (2009). *A practical guide to recovery-oriented practice: Tools for transforming mental health care.* Oxford University Press.

Green, M. F., Kern, R. S., Braff, D. L., & Mintz, J. (2000). Neurocognitive deficits and functional outcome in schizophrenia: Are we measuring the "right stuff"? *Schizophrenia Bulletin, 26*(1), 119–136.

Kahneman, D., & Tversky, A. (1979). Prospect theory: An analysis of decision under risk. *Econometrica, 47*(2), 263–291.

Keefe, R. S. E., Harvey, P. D., Goldberg, T. E., Hazlett, E. A., McClure, M. M., & Meltzer, H. Y. (2006). The neurocognitive effects of antipsychotic medications in patients with chronic schizophrenia: A two-year randomized trial. *Archives of General Psychiatry, 63*(6), 633–640.

Lal, S., & Chow, J. (2014). Can employment be a spark for recovery? A conceptual model based on the individual placement and support approach. *Psychiatric Rehabilitation Journal, 37*(2), 94–101.

Medalia, A., & Revheim, N. (2002). Dealing with cognitive dysfunction associated with psychiatric disabilities: A handbook for families and professionals. *New York State Office of Mental Health.*

Panas, L. J., & Davis, L. W. (2020). Financial decision-making capacity in severe mental illness: Implications for recovery and autonomy. *Psychiatric Services, 71*(7), 731–738.

Saperstein, A. M., & Medalia, A. (2016). Cognitive remediation for psychiatric disorders: Current status and future directions. *World Psychiatry, 15*(3), 233–245.

World Health Organization. (2013). *Mental health action plan 2013–2020.* World Health Organization.

Chapter 6:
Food: Nourishment, Pleasure, Comfort, Routine, Control, Communion

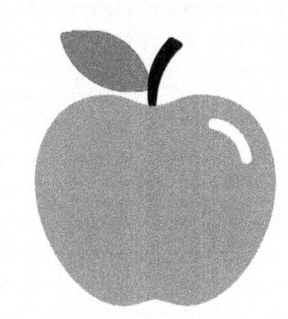

Introduction

Food is never just about calories. It is ritual, reward, identity, and memory. For individuals living with severe mental illness, food often becomes a central preoccupation—not merely as a biological need, but as a complex emotional and symbolic spark. Whether through restriction, bingeing, hoarding, ritualized eating, or spiritual fasting, the way someone interacts with food often tells a story—of what they've endured, what they fear, and what they hope to reclaim.

Food is more than sustenance—it's a way of coping, controlling, and sometimes surviving. It can bring comfort or offer control when everything else feels uncertain. In the throes of emotional distress, eating may become a way to soothe anxiety, escape pain, or create structure. For others, not eating may be a form of self-punishment or a desperate bid to regain agency.

The connection between mental illness and food is deeply layered. Individuals with schizophrenia, schizoaffective disorder, and bipolar disorder often struggle with patterns of eating that reflect internal chaos, trauma histories, or responses to psychotropic medications. These patterns may include compulsive eating, food aversions, or erratic mealtimes shaped by disorganized thought. Food behaviors can signal attempts to assert control, to feel grounded, or to express distress.

For many, food remains one of the last rituals of continuity. A familiar snack can become sacred. The precise folding of a sandwich or hoarding of a favorite candy bar may seem irrational but is often deeply meaningful. These behaviors can hold stories of scarcity, shame, comfort, or cultural identity.

Eating is also one of the earliest and most enduring human experiences. From infancy, food is linked to nurturing and connection. We are fed before we understand hunger, and we learn love and safety through bottles, spoons, and shared meals. Even when language fades or cognition deteriorates, the ritual of eating often remains—a spark from the earliest human bond.

Let's take a closer look at the symbolic, clinical, and emotional dimensions of food in serious mental illness. We will examine how hunger, nourishment, and disordered eating manifest across diagnoses; the effects of medication on appetite and metabolism; and the cultural, psychological, and relational meanings food carries. Understanding these layers invites clinicians to respond with more curiosity, compassion, and care—and to recognize food not merely as fuel, but as a profound expression of vitality.

The Neurobiology of Eating and Reward

Eating behavior is governed by a complex network of neurobiological systems that integrate homeostatic needs, emotional states, environmental cues, and reward processing. At the center of this network is the hypothalamus, which regulates hunger and satiety through hormonal signals like leptin, ghrelin, and insulin. These hormones inform the brain about the body's energy status and influence feeding behavior accordingly.

Beyond the hypothalamus, dopaminergic pathways—especially the mesolimbic reward system involving the ventral tegmental area (VTA) and nucleus accumbens—play a key role in the motivation to seek and consume food. Dopamine release in response to palatable food reinforces eating behavior and connects food intake to pleasure and reward. This system is closely linked to the neural circuits implicated in addiction, mood disorders, and psychosis.

Neurobiology of Food Motivation and Reward

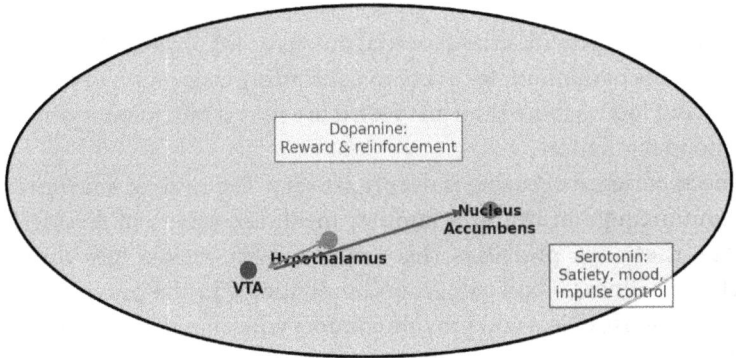

Serotonin, another key neurotransmitter, is involved in satiety, mood regulation, and impulse control. Medications that alter serotonin transmission, like SSRIs or atypical antipsychotics, can significantly impact appetite and weight.

In people living with serious mental illness, these neurobiological systems are often disrupted. For example:

- Antipsychotics, particularly second-generation agents like olanzapine and clozapine, are associated with hyperphagia and weight gain due to their antagonism of histamine (H1), serotonin (5-HT2C), and dopamine (D2) receptors.
- Mood stabilizers like lithium or valproate may also contribute to increased appetite and changes in metabolism.
- Cognitive impairments and negative symptoms can reduce motivation to prepare or consume balanced meals, resulting in malnutrition or erratic eating patterns.
- Stress and trauma—common experiences in people living with schizophrenia and bipolar disorder—can further dysregulate the hypothalamic-pituitary-adrenal (HPA) axis. Elevated cortisol levels are associated with increased cravings for high-calorie, high-fat foods, reinforcing cycles of emotional eating.

Understanding the neurobiology of hunger, reward, and appetite regulation is essential for clinicians. It helps contextualize the eating behaviors of patients with serious mental illness not as laziness or poor choices, but as rooted in complex neurochemical and physiological processes.

A neurobiological lens allows for greater compassion and precision in treatment—one that integrates metabolic monitoring, nutritional counseling, trauma-informed care, and targeted medication adjustments into the broader framework of psychiatric care.

The Psychological Role of Food: More Than Nutrition

Of course, food provides the essential nutrients for physical health, a need that remains paramount for everyone, including those with severe mental illness. But food is more than just fuel, it is a portal into memory, meaning, and mood regulation.

The experience of eating is deeply sensory. The taste of a favorite dish, the comforting warmth of a familiar meal, the aroma of freshly baked goods—these are pleasures that endure, even amidst the turmoil of psychiatric illness. Food can ground individuals in the present moment, rekindle a sense of joy, and provide comfort when language or logic fails.

Food also anchors us socially and culturally. It connects us to our families, our histories, and our identities. Shared meals are a common way to celebrate, mourn, and connect. Yet many people living with severe mental illness eat in isolation—in shelters, group homes, or alone in their rooms. This absence of communal eating magnifies loneliness and disconnect.

Food can serve as a powerful emotional anchor. Comfort foods often soothe distress, providing a symbolic balm for emotional wounds. However, this coping strategy can evolve into unhealthy behaviors, binge eating, obsessive food rituals, or restrictive eating patterns that reflect a struggle for control in a chaotic world. In some cases, eating becomes a secret language of survival, a way to self-soothe or punish, a response to trauma or fear.

Certain meals evoke memories of home, childhood, or lost loved ones. Others may be avoided because they trigger associations with pain or scarcity. For individuals who have experienced neglect, poverty, or institutionalization, food often carries layers of meaning—some tender, some fraught.

Reintroducing the social dimension of food, family-style meals in residential programs, cooking groups in day treatment, shared snacks during therapy—can help reignite the relational spark food naturally holds. These are not just acts of nutrition, but acts of repair. They restore a sense of humanity, dignity, and shared experience.

Food, when understood as more than nutrition, becomes a medium of healing. It touches memory, ritual, pleasure, and pain. To ignore this is to miss one of the most accessible and enduring sparks of life—one that continues to nourish the body and the soul, even in the midst of madness.

Food as Culture, Comfort, and Belonging

Despite the difficulties, food also becomes one of the richest sources of joy and identity for many patients:

- A man in a group home insists on cooking his grandmother's rice and beans recipe every Sunday.
- A woman experiencing auditory hallucinations finds peace while baking—"the voices don't like cinnamon."
- A patient who won't speak in therapy glows while describing his favorite corner deli.

These aren't just anecdotes. They're windows into preserved selfhood.

Food often connects patients to a sense of home—whether it's a literal home they lost, a family they miss, or a cultural identity that grounds them. Through food, many reclaim language, tradition, and pleasure.

These culinary rituals serve as threads of continuity, reminders of who they are and where they come from. In the midst of diagnostic labels and institutional routines, food offers something profoundly human—a space of choice, memory, and connection.

For many people living with serious mental illness, food is one of the few ways they can still express preference and creativity. In environments where autonomy is limited, the ability to choose what to eat, how to prepare it, or whom to share it with becomes a quiet act of resistance and affirmation.

Honoring food traditions and facilitating cultural eating practices within mental health care can strengthen therapeutic alliance and promote dignity. Whether it's offering culturally familiar meals, asking about food preferences, or incorporating food into therapeutic rituals, clinicians can use food as a bridge to trust and identity.

Food is not a distraction from treatment. It is a part of it.

I've watched patients come alive over a shared meal. Food is never just nutrition—it is restoration. There was a woman on the ward who never smiled—except when she helped in the kitchen. Food, I learned, was her form of agency.

On Thanksgiving one year, we served dinner on the inpatient unit. A woman who usually refused meals asked for seconds of sweet potatoes. "Tastes like my grandma's," she said, wiping tears away. That bite of food brought her somewhere memory could still reach. It reminded me how food carries love.

Food as a Symbol of Control

For people living with serious mental illness, food can serve as a means of control over one's environment and body. In disorders like bipolar disorder, schizophrenia, and schizoaffective disorder, food may become a tool to express the illusion of autonomy in an otherwise chaotic or uncontrollable life. Restricting food or binge eating can be ways to exert control over one's body when other aspects of life feel out of control.

For instance, during periods of depression, some individuals may use food restriction as a way to gain a sense of mastery over their internal world. Conversely, binge eating can be an expression of emotional overwhelm or a response to feelings of emptiness, offering temporary relief from difficult emotions or psychotic symptoms.

Food restrictions and rituals are not uncommon in psychosis. Some patients develop beliefs that certain foods are poisoned, or that their thoughts can be read through what they consume. Others become obsessed with purity, only eating organic foods or refusing processed meals. For some, food becomes entangled with religious or moral delusions—fasting for spiritual purification, rejecting certain items as unclean.

In inpatient settings, disordered eating may be subtle or overt. Hoarding is common. So is food refusal. One woman with schizophrenia consistently hid rolls in her pillowcase. Another patient would fast for days, convinced that food was a government tracking device. A third insisted on eating only blue foods—any deviation was intolerable.

Sometimes, the control over food is the only control left. In the chaos of hospitalization, when clothes are chosen for you and lights go out on schedule, the ability to say yes or no to food is an act of autonomy.

Understanding food as a symbol of control helps clinicians move beyond compliance and into compassion. When a patient resists a meal plan or clings to a food ritual, it may not be about calories at all. It may be a way of holding on—of expressing something too deep or dangerous to say aloud. Meeting these behaviors with curiosity, not coercion, creates space for deeper healing.

The Impact of Illness on Eating Habits and Attitudes Towards Food

Serious mental illness can significantly disrupt an individual's relationship with food.

The Relationship Between Mental Health and Appetite Regulation

The intricate interplay between the brain and the gut—often referred to as the gut-brain axis—highlights the profound influence of mental health on appetite and eating behaviors. When this system is disrupted, the impact on daily living can be dramatic.

- Appetite increase or decrease: In depression, appetite may fade to the point of near-starvation, while in mania, overeating or bingeing can emerge alongside heightened energy. Antipsychotic medications may further increase hunger signals, complicating self-regulation.
- Food as comfort or avoidance: Some individuals turn to food as an immediate source of relief from anxiety, loneliness, or intrusive thoughts. Others withdraw from eating altogether, perceiving meals as overwhelming or meaningless.
- Distorted attitudes: Paranoia or delusions can attach themselves to food, leading someone to believe it is poisoned, contaminated, or controlled by outside forces. For others, food may become symbolic—a way of expressing control in an otherwise chaotic life.
- Social disruption: Shared meals often represent belonging and connection. Yet in serious mental illness, social withdrawal, stigma, or institutional routines can fracture this communal experience, leaving eating to become solitary or mechanical.

Taken together, these disruptions illustrate that eating habits are never just about calories or nutrition. They are deeply bound to identity, trust, safety, and meaning. To support recovery, clinicians and caregivers must look beyond weight or appetite charts and ask: *What role does food play in this person's inner life right now?*

Neurotransmitter involvement:
- Serotonin contributes to satiety, and its low levels can trigger cravings for carbohydrates and promote overeating.
- Dopamine influences reward perception, and disruptions may lead to reduced pleasure from food (anhedonia) or increased cravings for calorie-dense foods.
- Gamma-aminobutyric acid (GABA), the brain's main inhibitory neurotransmitter, often implicated in anxiety, can influence appetite by modulating stress responses, contributing to emotional eating in some cases.

Hormonal influences:
- Cortisol, the stress hormone, often elevated in SMI, increases appetite for high-fat, high-sugar foods.
- Ghrelin and leptin, which regulate hunger and satiety, are frequently dysregulated in mental health conditions.

Behavioral patterns:
- Depression may cause a lack of motivation to prepare food, social withdrawal, and reliance on processed options.
- Mania can result in impulsive eating, skipped meals, or poor food choices.
- Psychosis may contribute to disorganized or paranoid beliefs about food, disrupting intake.

Understanding these complex biological and behavioral links underscores the need for integrated approaches that address both mental health symptoms and eating behaviors.

Diagnosis-Specific Considerations

Schizophrenia and schizoaffective disorder:
- Food may become entangled in delusional systems: patients may refuse food due to fears of poisoning or contamination, or believe their thoughts can be read through meals.
- Examples include patients avoiding round foods due to symbolic associations, or eating only red items believed to offer protection.
- Disorganized thinking can lead to erratic or impulsive eating, while negative symptoms reduce the motivation to prepare or consume nutritious meals.
- Cognitive impairments can interfere with meal planning, recipe-following, or even remembering to eat.

Bipolar disorder:
- Manic episodes may bring about impulsive or excessive eating, especially high-sugar, high-fat comfort foods. Conversely, some experience appetite suppression.
- Depressive episodes may lead to either increased food intake as self-soothing or a complete loss of interest in eating.
- In both states, food becomes a domain of control and expression, reflecting internal emotional states.

Depression and Appetite
- Appetite may fluctuate dramatically—either diminished due to anhedonia and low energy or increased as a coping mechanism for emotional distress.

Anxiety and Eating
- Anxiety can cause nervous loss of appetite or, conversely, lead to stress-eating, often resulting in the patient favoring calorie-dense comfort foods.

- In more severe cases, anxiety may contribute to eating disorders.

Sensory Sensitivities
- Individuals on the autism spectrum or with comorbid neurodevelopmental conditions may experience food aversions based on texture, smell, or taste, complicating nutrition management.
- Basic acts of nourishment, like consistently eating meals, can be monumental achievements for patients grappling with severe mental illness.

I once treated a patient whose severe anorexia, intertwined with depression, left him frail. One day, I asked him his favorite childhood meal. His eyes flickered as he described his grandmother's chicken soup. Weeks later, he asked for that soup in the hospital. It wasn't just food—it was a bridge to comfort and memory.

Food and the Body-Mind Interface

Mental illness is experienced in the body as much as the mind. Anxiety churns the stomach. Depression silences hunger. Antipsychotics change metabolism, triggering intense cravings and weight gain.

Many patients describe feeling out of control in their own bodies—betrayed by hunger, dulled by fullness, or punished by every bite. Yet even amid dysregulation, food becomes a form of agency.

Refusing food may express resistance or autonomy in institutional settings. Compulsive eating may attempt to restore grounding or simulate comfort. Clinicians must learn to hear what food is saying.

Hoarding, Scarcity, and the Echo of Poverty

In both inpatient and community settings, food hoarding is common. Crackers under mattresses. Milk cartons in drawers. Rolls stuffed in pillowcases.

Staff may view these actions as irrational—but they often reflect histories of deprivation: childhood hunger, food insecurity, or homelessness.

Even when food is available, the psychological imprint of scarcity remains. Hoarding becomes a survival adaptation, not a pathology. It says: "I've been without before—I won't be again."

Rather than solely enforcing rules, clinicians can engage with empathy:
- Have there been times when you went hungry?
- What helps you feel safe around food?
- What does saving food mean to you?

These questions de-pathologize behavior and build relational safety.

Food as Self-Soothing, Self-Harming, or Self-Expression

Eating can serve many psychological functions:
- Self-soothing: Binging on sweets during a psychotic episode to dull emotional overwhelm.
- Self-harming: Food refusal or purging as punishment or control.
- Self-expression: Adhering to a cultural diet or vegetarian identity as a way to assert individuality and values.

Each food interaction reflects a person's unique body-mind relationship. The core question is never just what someone eats, but why, how, and with whom.

Food as a Source of Routine and Structure: Eating Rituals and Symbolic Order

In the often-chaotic inner world of someone experiencing severe mental illness, the predictability of regular mealtimes can provide a valuable sense of structure and routine. Knowing that there will be breakfast at a certain time, lunch at another, and dinner in the evening can offer a sense of stability and normalcy, which can be particularly grounding for individuals struggling with disorganized thoughts or fluctuating moods.

Many individuals develop rigid or elaborate eating rituals—cutting food into exact shapes, eating only at certain times, separating textures, or demanding sameness day after day. While sometimes dismissed as obsessive or compulsive symptoms, these rituals often provide symbolic structure in otherwise chaotic psychic terrain.

In psychosis, where time dilates and thought fractures, mealtime rituals become anchors. They affirm continuity, identity, and control. Even the act of choosing a meal, in the face of overwhelming internal noise, becomes a reclaiming of self.

Rather than stripping away rituals, clinicians can gently explore them:
- What's the story behind this food pattern?
- What would it feel like to experiment with one small change?
- What does this routine do for you emotionally?

This approach respects food rituals as containers rather than simply symptoms.

Food, often underestimated, can also serve as ritual. One mother described how meals carried her daughter's identity forward. This vignette illustrates how nourishment is not just physical, but emotional and cultural.

Social Isolation and Eating: The Solitary Meal

Reduced Social Interaction
Social withdrawal can lead to eating alone more frequently, which may result in less attention paid to the nutritional value and enjoyment of meals. Eating alone can also diminish the social and emotional benefits associated with shared meals.

Lack of Motivation for Meal Preparation
Cooking for one can feel like a chore, leading to reliance on convenience foods that are often less healthy and more expensive in the long run.

"On the unit, staff often see how food and music intersect as sparks. Nurse educator Danielle Sanzi recalled..." Her account reinforces how shared meals transform treatment into community.

Financial Constraints and Food Access: The Economics of Nourishment

Limited Budgets
Individuals relying on disability benefits often have very limited budgets for food, making it challenging to afford fresh produce, lean proteins, and other nutritious options.

Food Deserts
Some individuals live in areas known as food deserts, where access to affordable and healthy food options—like grocery stores and farmers' markets—is limited. This disproportionately affects low-income individuals and those without reliable transportation.

Reliance on Food Pantries and Assistance Programs
Local food pantries and government assistance programs, like SNAP, play a critical role in food security for people living with mental illness. However, navigating these systems can be complex and stigmatizing.

Medication Side Effects and Food

Antipsychotics and mood stabilizers often disrupt appetite and metabolism. Some patients gain 30, 50, or even 100 pounds within months. Others develop compulsive cravings for sugar, starch, or salt. This weight gain isn't just physical—it's emotional. Patients often feel ashamed, unrecognizable, or betrayed by their bodies. Some stop treatment altogether just to feel like themselves again.

Providers may focus on labs and lipids—but patients focus on pants that no longer fit, faces they don't recognize, and the constant pull of hunger they can't control. These experiences shape how patients relate to food—and to the people who prescribe what they eat, when they eat, and what it does to them.

The impact goes far beyond aesthetics—it erodes self-worth, sexual identity, and motivation. Some patients discontinue medications not because they deny their illness, but because they cannot tolerate what the medications do to their bodies.

Clinicians must address this head-on. Dismissing weight gain as "the price of stability" is not therapeutic—it is invalidating. Instead, patients should be invited into collaborative discussions about nutrition, movement, alternatives, and harm reduction strategies.

Weight should be addressed compassionately, not as a number but as a narrative:
- What has your body been through?
- What does it mean to carry extra weight?
- How can we support your sense of dignity and health?

Clinical Considerations: The Metabolic Burden

A significant number of psychotropic medications commonly prescribed for SMIs have side effects that directly impact weight, appetite, and metabolism. These include:
- Weight gain and appetite increase: Often due to histamine and serotonin receptor blockade, leading to increased appetite and reduced satiety
- Metabolic syndrome: A combination of weight gain, insulin resistance, dyslipidemia, and hypertension that raises the risk for type 2 diabetes and cardiovascular disease
- Taste alterations (dysgeusia): Some medications cause metallic or unpleasant aftertastes, reducing appetite or altering food enjoyment.
- Dry mouth (xerostomia): Can make eating uncomfortable and increase the risk of dental problems
- Self-esteem and adherence: Weight gain can damage self-image and lead to nonadherence to life-saving medications.

Managing Metabolic Side Effects

Given these risks, clinicians must:
- Monitor weight, waist circumference, lipids, blood pressure, and glucose regularly.
- Educate patients about nutrition and the metabolic risks of medications.

- Consider switching to medications with lower metabolic risk profiles when feasible.
- Offer referrals to nutritionists, dietitians, and wellness programs.
- Explore lifestyle interventions collaboratively, emphasizing choice, flexibility, and compassion.

Medication decisions should weigh both psychiatric stability and physical well-being. The goal is not merely compliance but care.

Nutritional choices are often overlooked in psychiatric care, yet poor diet contributes significantly to morbidity. A randomized trial by Teasdale et al. demonstrated that targeted dietary support can lead to significant improvements in mood and cognitive functioning among people with severe mental illness.

Challenges in Accessing Healthy and Affordable Food

Socioeconomic factors can create formidable, significant barriers to accessing nutritious and affordable food for individuals living with severe mental illnesses. Poverty, unemployment, and limited financial resources can make it exceedingly difficult to afford a balanced diet rich in fruits, vegetables, lean protein sources, and whole grains. Lack of reliable transportation can make it difficult to get to grocery stores that offer a wider selection of healthy and affordable foods, especially in areas with limited public transport. Cognitive impairments, like difficulties with planning, organization, and problem-solving, can also make grocery shopping, meal planning, and the preparation of healthy meals a significant challenge. Furthermore, negative symptoms like lack of motivation (avolition) or social withdrawal can further impede an individual's ability to access food resources, like food banks or assistance programs. Limited financial resources often mean that individuals have to prioritize cheaper, less nutritious options.

Food insecurity can lead to inconsistent access to adequate food, resulting in both undernutrition and overconsumption of calorie-dense, nutrient-poor foods when available. Food insecurity, characterized by limited or uncertain access to adequate food, is a significant and often overlooked concern within this population, and it can exacerbate both mental and physical health problems, undermining the fundamental spark of sustenance and well-being. However, the desire for satisfying and enjoyable meals persists. Support in accessing affordable and healthy options, as well as assistance with meal planning and preparation, can help people living with SMIs experience the pleasure and nourishment that food provides.

Addressing these challenges requires a multi-pronged approach, including advocating for increased funding for food assistance programs, improving access to affordable and healthy food options in underserved communities, providing support with grocery shopping and meal preparation (potentially through occupational therapy or community support programs), and addressing transportation barriers.

The Importance of Addressing Food and Nutrition in Treatment

Food sustains more than the body—it sustains meaning. By paying attention to nutrition in treatment, we honor one of the most enduring sparks of life: the need for nourishment, comfort, and strength.

The Role of Nutrition in Managing Symptoms and Overall Health

While nutrition is not a substitute for evidence-based mental health treatment, a well-balanced and nutritious diet plays a crucial supportive role in overall well-being and may have a positive impact on mental health symptoms. Certain nutrients, like omega-3 fatty acids (found in fatty fish, flaxseeds, and walnuts), B vitamins (found in whole grains, leafy greens, and lean proteins), and antioxidants (found in fruits and vegetables), are essential for optimal brain function and may have a positive impact on mood and cognitive function. Adequate hydration is also critical for cognitive function, energy levels, and overall physical health.

Promoting healthy eating habits can contribute to improved energy levels (which can help combat fatigue, a common symptom of many SMIs and a side effect of some medications), greater mood stability, and enhanced physical health, which can indirectly support mental health recovery and an individual's capacity to engage with the enjoyable aspects of life, including the pleasure of good food. Nutritional interventions, often implemented in conjunction with other therapeutic modalities, can be a valuable component of a comprehensive and holistic treatment plan, nurturing the spark of well-being from the inside out. Focusing on enjoyable and nutritious foods can be a positive aspect of self-care. As discussed earlier, good nutrition is essential for preventing and managing the increased risk of physical health conditions in this population.

Emerging research highlights the importance of gut health in mental well-being. A diet rich in fiber and probiotics can support a healthy gut microbiome, which may have positive effects on mood and anxiety—the gut-brain axis phenomenon.

Nutritional education and counseling, provided by registered dietitians with expertise in mental health, can empower individuals to make informed food choices and develop healthy eating habits that support both their physical and mental health.

Culture, Identity, and the Table

Food is also a carrier of culture. Patients from different ethnic, religious, or national backgrounds bring with them food memories that ground their identities.

A Haitian patient may long for spiced griot, rice, and beans. A Puerto Rican woman may mourn the absence of sofrito. A Jewish man may request matzo ball soup. In many cases, psychiatric institutions offer generic menus, devoid of cultural resonance. Patients adapt, but some grieve.

There is also sacred meaning attached to food. Fasting during Ramadan, not eating pork, observing kosher or halal restrictions—all of these must be respected in clinical settings. To ignore them is not just an oversight; it is an erasure of the patient's sense of self.

Clinicians who ask, "What foods remind you of home?" or "Are there any dishes that bring you comfort?" may be shocked at what opens up.

The Psychology of Eating Disorders and Dual Diagnoses

Individuals living with serious mental illnesses may be at increased risk for developing disordered eating patterns. Impulsivity, emotional dysregulation, medication side effects, or trauma can all contribute to maladaptive food behaviors. These vulnerabilities can manifest in specific eating behaviors, such as:

- Binge eating: Consuming large amounts of food in short periods, often accompanied by a loss of control and emotional distress.
- Restrictive eating: Driven by distorted body image or unusual beliefs about food, sometimes linked to weight gain from medication or psychosis-related delusions.
- Pica: The persistent craving and consumption of non-food substances, sometimes seen in people living with psychiatric or developmental disorders.

Many of these behaviors go undiagnosed due to the complexity of psychiatric presentations. Patients with eating disorders may be mischaracterized as manipulative or noncompliant when, in fact, their food rituals reflect trauma histories or neurobiological dysregulation.

Eating disorders often require structured care, while psychosis demands flexibility. The patient may become a battleground between treatment models. The goal is not forced compliance—it is building trust and understanding food as both a site of distress and a site of healing.

Disordered eating is often overlooked in psychotic or mood disorders. Sometimes the eating disorder predates psychotic symptoms; other times it develops as a coping strategy. Trauma, dissociation, and food dysregulation often co-occur.

Examples include:
- A man with schizoaffective disorder who purged in secret. "It's the only time I feel something," he said.
- A woman who starved herself during depressive episodes, describing it as "just how I get when I'm down."

Diagnostic Considerations

In some cases, disordered eating behaviors meet criteria for a formal eating disorder. Recognizing these conditions is essential, as they carry distinct risks and require targeted interventions. Diagnostic considerations include:
- Anorexia Nervosa: Characterized by severe food restriction, intense fear of weight gain, and body image disturbance.
- Bulimia Nervosa: Involves cycles of bingeing and purging, often with emotional triggers and deep shame.
- Binge Eating Disorder: Marked by frequent episodes of uncontrolled overeating without compensatory behaviors.
- Avoidant/Restrictive Food Intake Disorder (ARFID): Involves limited food intake due to sensory sensitivities, lack of interest in eating, or fear of negative consequences (e.g., choking). It is prevalent across the lifespan and is often underdiagnosed.

Integrated Care for Disordered Eating

Screening for disordered eating patterns and providing access to specialized treatment, including therapy and nutritional counseling, is essential to address these potentially life-threatening conditions.

A truly integrated care approach recognizes the central role of food and nutrition in the overall well-being of people living with SMIs. Managing disordered eating behaviors in people living with mental illness requires a comprehensive approach that addresses both the psychological and physical aspects of the disorder. Key interventions include:
- Routine nutritional screening: Mental health professionals should routinely ask about eating habits, weight changes, and any nutritional concerns.
- Psychotherapy: Cognitive-behavioral therapy, mindfulness-based therapies, and dialectical behavior therapy can help individuals identify and challenge distorted thoughts and build emotional regulation skills.

- Pharmacological treatment: Consider medications that support mood stabilization while minimizing metabolic side effects. Monitor weight gain and explore alternative agents when appropriate.
- Nutritional counseling: Collaborate with nutritionists to develop sustainable and balanced eating plans tailored to the individual's needs and preferences.
- Support groups: Peer-led or professional support groups offer validation and reduce isolation.
- Meal planning support: Provide structured meal planning assistance and basic cooking instruction.
- Addressing food insecurity: Help patients navigate resources like food banks and community meal programs.
- Nutritional education: Offer accessible information about healthy eating and hydration.
- Medication management: Discuss potential weight changes, monitor metabolic health, and collaborate on harm-reduction strategies.
- Cooking groups and social meals: Promote social bonding and practical skill-building through communal food activities.
- Accessible cooking skills programs: Develop local initiatives that teach shopping, budgeting, and food preparation skills.
- Community gardens and food pantries: Encourage connection to food through gardening and local food resources.
- Mindful eating practices: Teach skills that enhance awareness of hunger, fullness, and the emotional context of eating.
- Addressing sensory issues: Tailor interventions for people living with heightened sensitivities around food textures and smells.
- A non-judgmental approach: Foster safety and dignity in conversations about food, eating, and body image.

By prioritizing food and nutrition as a fundamental spark of life and integrating nutritional care into the broader mental health treatment plan, we can significantly improve the physical and mental health outcomes and overall quality of life for individuals living with severe mental illnesses.

The Enduring Pleasure of Food: Moments of Joy and Comfort

Food is not only tied to illness and treatment—it also endures as a spark of joy. Even in the midst of suffering, favorite meals, cooking rituals, and sensory experiences can offer comfort and connection. These moments include:

- Favorite foods and comfort meals: Despite adversity, many people living with SMIs retain strong food preferences that anchor them emotionally.
- The act of cooking: For some, preparing food restores a sense of creativity, mastery, and control. Even small acts, brewing tea, assembling a sandwich—can be therapeutic.
- Food as a sensory anchor: The taste, smell, texture, and look of food ground individuals in the present. This sensory stability can calm anxiety, ease dissociation, and spark memory.

In locked wards and institutional settings, food takes on layered meaning. A cup of coffee becomes a ritual. A favorite meal can recall a lost mother, a hometown, a version of the self worth remembering.

For many individuals, food is more than sustenance—it becomes a ritual or creative outlet that helps them navigate the challenges of illness. Consider the following examples:

Juan's Story: Juan, a 35-year-old man with schizophrenia, begins each day with peanut butter toast and black coffee. Any deviation—burnt toast or sweetened coffee—disturbs him. These small rituals offer him control in a world otherwise dictated by voices and fears.

Latasha's Story: Latasha, a woman with bipolar disorder, bakes elaborate cakes during hypomania. Baking is her creative release. Her cakes are sweet symbols of resilience, created during sleepless nights.

Karen's Story: Karen, a young adult navigating medication-induced weight gain, struggles with body image and social anxiety. With support, she begins to develop a balanced eating plan and reclaim a sense of self-worth.

Robert's Story: Robert relies on food pantries and struggles with healthy eating on a tight budget. Community garden access and cooking groups help him regain dignity and obtain nutritional knowledge.

Susan's Story: Despite depressive fatigue, Susan finds meaning in cooking simple meals. The ritual itself becomes self-care.

I've seen people come back to themselves over something as simple as a favorite snack.

There's a quiet dignity in choosing your own meal. I never saw it that way until a patient taught me.

Clinical and Therapeutic Reflections

Food rituals, though sometimes misunderstood, are not mere symptoms to eliminate—they are coping tools, emotional anchors, and clues to deeper needs. Instead of pathologizing them, clinicians can:

- Ask about meaning behind food choices.

- Create space for agency around meals.
- Use food preparation and sharing as therapeutic practices.

Acknowledging the central role of food in psychiatric recovery allows for more empathetic, person-centered care.

Eating with Empathy

Food can be a powerful entry point into the inner world of someone with mental illness. To ask, "What do you eat?" is to ask, "Who are you?" When meals are understood as expressions of identity and survival, supportive approaches may include:
- Respecting food rituals—even unusual ones
- Creating space for joy around meals
- Recognizing that refusal may stem from trauma or fear
- Collaborating, not imposing
- Understanding food as memory, survival, resilience

Sometimes, sharing a snack builds more trust than an hour of talk therapy.

Conclusion

Food lingers in the senses. It encodes the past. It nourishes the body, but also the soul. For patients with severe mental illness, food can be a daily battle—but also a daily act of continuity. A patient who hasn't seen his children in years still makes the pancakes they once loved. A woman who hears accusatory voices still finds peace while peeling potatoes. These are not just coping strategies. They are sparks. They remind us that even amid confusion, the body remembers. And sometimes, healing begins with a warm bowl of something familiar.

Food is far more than just a means of survival for people living with severe mental illness. It is intertwined with pleasure, emotional well-being, social connection, and the establishment of daily rhythms. By recognizing the multifaceted role of food in their lives and addressing their relationship with it in a sensitive and comprehensive manner, we can contribute significantly to their overall health, well-being, and journey toward recovery.

This chapter underscores the critical and multifaceted link between food, nutrition, and the overall health and well-being of individuals living with severe mental illnesses. Addressing their nutritional needs is not only essential for physical health but can also positively influence mental health outcomes and enhance their quality of life, allowing them to more fully experience the enduring spark of sustenance and the simple pleasure of a good meal.

This chapter also emphasizes that despite the challenges, the fundamental need for food and the potential for pleasure and connection through it remain important for people living with severe mental illnesses. Supporting healthy and enjoyable eating experiences is a key aspect of holistic care.

For all the ways that mental illness fractures thought, food remains a primal language of being alive. It can be compulsive or controlled, feared or fantasized, sacred or shameful—but it is never meaningless. Every craving, every bite, every ritual around food tells a story: of who a person was, who they are, and who they might become again. When you see a patient eating cold beans from a can, or refusing every meal tray, or clinging to a single pack of crackers like treasure—pause.

There's always something underneath. Hunger, history, hope. The unyielding spark of life.

Food rituals are not just about the act of eating, but about what food represents. Taste is a sense that offers comfort, memory, and self-expression. In the world of psychiatric illness, where much of what defines a person can feel obscured or lost, food remains a way to reclaim a piece of identity. It is not merely a way to nourish the body; it is a way to remain connected to the past, to memories of family meals or special occasions, or even to simpler moments of solace. For some patients, food is not just fuel—it is the last thread that holds them to the world they once knew.

In the end, food rituals remind us that even in the midst of profound mental illness, the human need for comfort and connection endures. Whether it's the simple pleasure of a meal, the control over taste, or the self-expression in cooking, food provides more than sustenance—it offers a thread of continuity. For those living with severe mental illness, these rituals are not just habits; they are lifelines. They serve as quiet rebellions against a world that often feels alien, reminding us that even when everything else seems lost, the simple act of eating can bring us back to ourselves.

Table 6.1 — Food Across Cultures

Context	Food Meaning	Clinical Relevance
Jewish Sabbath	Shared ritual meal	Community, grounding
Ramadan	Fasting, reflection	Spiritual strength, discipline
U.S. Thanksgiving	Gratitude, family	Identity, belonging

1. Fischler, C. (1988). Food, self and identity. *Social Science Information*, 27(2), 275–292. (Food as ritual, memory, identity.)

2. Morton, G. J., Meek, T. H., & Schwartz, M. W. (2014). Neurobiology of food intake in health and disease. *Nature Reviews Neuroscience*, 15(6), 367–378. (Hypothalamus; leptin/ghrelin/insulin.)
3. Kelley, A. E., & Berridge, K. C. (2002). The neuroscience of natural rewards: Relevance to addictive drugs. *Journal of Neuroscience*, 22(9), 3306–3311. (Dopamine; VTA–nucleus accumbens; food reward.)
4. Halford, J. C. G., Boyland, E., Blundell, J. E., Kirkham, T. C., & Harrold, J. A. (2010). Pharmacological management of appetite expression in obesity. *Nature Reviews Endocrinology*, 6(5), 255–269. (Serotonin & satiety; appetite regulation.)
5. Kroeze, W. K., Hufeisen, S. J., & Roth, B. L. (2003). Molecular biology of serotonin receptors: 5-HT2C and antipsychotic-induced weight gain. *Neuropsychopharmacology*, 28(Suppl 1), S44–S51.
6. De Hert, M., Detraux, J., van Winkel, R., Yu, W., & Correll, C. U. (2012). Metabolic and cardiovascular adverse effects associated with antipsychotic drugs. *Nature Reviews Endocrinology*, 8(2), 114–126. (Olanzapine/clozapine risk; 5-HT2C/H1/D2 links.)
7. American Diabetes Association, American Psychiatric Association, American Association of Clinical Endocrinologists, & North American Association for the Study of Obesity. (2004). Consensus development conference on antipsychotic drugs and obesity/diabetes. *Diabetes Care*, 27(2), 596–601. (Metabolic monitoring guidance.)
8. Adam, T. C., & Epel, E. S. (2007). Stress, eating and the reward system. *Physiology & Behavior*, 91(4), 449–458. (HPA axis; cortisol and palatable-food intake.)
9. Cryan, J. F., & Dinan, T. G. (2012). Mind–altering microorganisms: The impact of the gut microbiota on brain and behaviour. *Nature Reviews Neuroscience*, 13(10), 701–712; Cryan, J. F., et al. (2019). The microbiota–gut–brain axis. *Physiological Reviews*, 99(4), 1877–2013. (Gut–brain axis overview.)
10. Teasdale, S. B., Ward, P. B., et al. (2019). Dietary intervention for people with severe mental illness: A randomized controlled trial. *Schizophrenia Bulletin*, 45(1), 75–83. (Dietary support improves outcomes.)
11. Martin, M. S., Maddocks, E., Chen, Y., Gilman, S. E., & Colman, I. (2016). Food insecurity and mental illness: Disproportionate impacts in the presence of disability. *Social Psychiatry and Psychiatric Epidemiology*, 51(5), 689–699. (Food insecurity ↔ mental health.)
12. Ulfvebrand, S., Birgegård, A., Norring, C., Högdahl, L., & von Hausswolff-Juhlin, Y. (2015). Psychiatric comorbidity in women and men with eating disorders. *BMC Psychiatry*, 15, 36; Hudson, J.

I., Hiripi, E., Pope, H. G., & Kessler, R. C. (2007). The prevalence and correlates of eating disorders. *Biological Psychiatry*, 61(3), 348–358. (Eating-disorder comorbidity/prevalence relevant to SMI.)

13. Serretti, A., & Mandelli, L. (2010). Antidepressants and body weight: A comprehensive review and meta-analysis. *Journal of Clinical Psychiatry*, 71(10), 1259–1272. (SSRI/SNRI effects on weight/appetite.)

Chapter 7:
The Universal Language: Music, Emotion, and Engagement

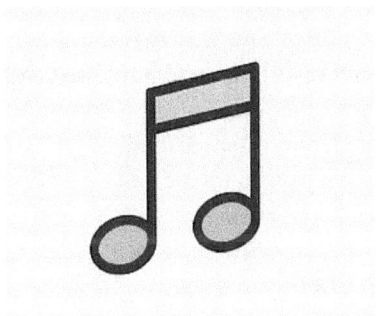

Introduction

Music is the most primal form of time travel. A single chord can transport us to childhood, grief, ecstasy, or safety. Music bypasses language, logic, and often, even the defenses we use to shield ourselves from pain. For people living with serious mental illness, music is not merely entertainment—it becomes internalized, lived, and often sacred.

Music is universal. It transcends language, culture, and even cognition. For people living with severe mental illness, music is not just an auditory experience—it is a lifeline. It can be a source of solace, an outlet for emotion, and a bridge to a world of self-expression that words may fail to reach.

In the face of psychosis, mania, or depression, music provides structure. It offers rhythm to a life that feels chaotic. It offers meaning to a mind that may be struggling to find any. For some, music is the only consistent reality, the only connection to something larger than the self.

Some patients hear music in hallucinations. Others write lyrics as a form of expression. Still others obsess over songs or genres, embedding musical themes into their delusions. But for many, music remains one of the last coherent pleasures in a fragmented world. It is rhythm when life is disorganized. Harmony when thought is chaotic.

Yet for others, music can be a source of confusion or obsession—an overwhelming cacophony of sound that both comforts and disturbs. Music has the power to move us in ways words cannot—it becomes a powerful tool for expression and sometimes, escape.

Music has always been a powerful force, but for people living with mental illness, it often takes on a much more intense role. It can become a way to express emotions that feel too overwhelming to articulate, a way to cope with painful feelings, or a way to escape from the harsh realities of life.

For someone struggling with a mental illness, music can become more than just background noise. It's a way to feel understood, to connect with something that speaks to the heart when everything else seems to fall short. Music provides a sense of comfort; it's familiar, it's soothing, and it offers a way to distract from inner turmoil.

The emotional connection to music can be so deep that it becomes an obsession. For someone who already struggles with emotional regulation, music can sometimes be the only thing that makes sense, that helps them feel grounded, even if just for a moment.

Music is a ubiquitous and deeply human phenomenon, a universal language that transcends cultural boundaries and has a profound impact on the human emotional landscape and well-being. Music resonates deeply within us, offering a powerful spark of self-expression, emotional connection, cognitive engagement, sadness, peace, excitement, sheer joy, and a myriad of other feelings, offering unique avenues for navigating the challenges of the condition and fostering a deeper connection with oneself and the world. Music transcends cultural and linguistic barriers.

For individuals living with severe mental illnesses, music can be a particularly vital resource, providing an accessible and meaningful way to connect with their emotions, express themselves, and engage with the world around them. For individuals who may struggle with verbal communication due to cognitive challenges or social anxiety associated with their mental illness, music can provide an alternative and powerful means of expression and connection. It can offer solace during times of distress, a sense of rhythm and structure in a chaotic inner world, and a bridge to shared human experience.

In a world often filtered through the complex lenses of psychosis and mood dysregulation, music frequently emerges as a universal language, capable of reaching people living with severe mental illness in profound and meaningful ways. It possesses a unique power to bypass cognitive barriers, evoke deep emotions, and foster connections that words alone may fail to achieve. For many, music is not just a passive auditory experience but an active source of comfort, stimulation, and a vital link to their own inner world and the world around them.

Music often appears in the lives of those with severe mental illness not as background noise but as a force—filling silence, shaping identity, bridging realities. Whether through headphones worn constantly on the ward, elaborate playlists for different moods, or references to song lyrics in delusional systems, music functions as both symptom and sanctuary. As a spark, it speaks to the desire for coherence, connection, and transcendence.

This chapter will explore the enduring significance of music in the lives of those with schizophrenia, schizoaffective disorder, and bipolar disorder, highlighting its emotional resonance, its potential for connection, and its role in providing grounding and engagement. Its accessibility and the diverse ways in which it can be experienced make it a valuable resource in supporting the mental health and recovery journey. We will also examine how music can serve as a source of comfort, identity, and emotional expression, and how music therapy can be a valuable tool in psychiatric treatment.

Let's take a closer look at how music becomes a lifeline—an echo of humanity that mental illness cannot silence.

Neurobiological Insights

Neuroscience confirms what experience has long suggested: music stimulates widespread brain regions involved in emotion, memory, reward, and language. In serious mental illness, where neural circuits are disrupted, music may serve as a compensatory organizer—a way to regulate affect, sustain attention, or recall fragmented autobiographical memory.

The science behind why music has such a profound impact on the mind can be traced to its effects on the brain. Music activates multiple areas of the brain simultaneously, including the auditory cortex, the prefrontal cortex, and the limbic system—the emotional center of the brain. These areas are involved in processes like emotion regulation, memory, attention, and reward.

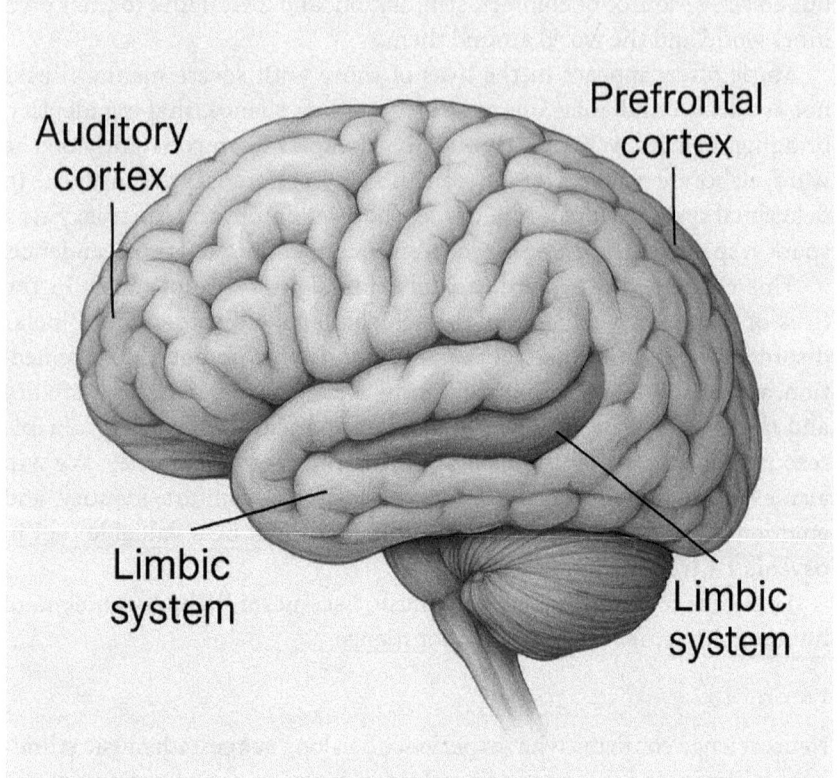

Music's rhythm and structure can provide a sense of predictability and order, which is especially beneficial for individuals whose mental states may feel fragmented or chaotic. The predictable patterns of a song or a melody can help to calm racing thoughts and provide a sense of normalcy in an otherwise unpredictable world. For people living with psychosis, where reality is often experienced as fragmented or uncertain, music offers a rare form of coherence, restoring a sense of unity in the mind. Scientific studies reveal that music:
- Boosts dopamine release, providing pleasurable sensations akin to the experiences of eating or sexual activity.
- Activates memory circuits, helping patients reconnect with positive past experiences.
- Enhances neuroplasticity, potentially supporting recovery and rehabilitation of emotional regulation pathways.

Music becomes more than entertainment; it becomes a neurobiological intervention.

A depressed patient may use melancholic music to match internal despair, creating a paradoxical feeling of comfort through resonance. Someone with mania may chase high-tempo beats to match their inner velocity—or, just as often, use ambient music to calm themselves. A person with schizophrenia might use music to drown out intrusive voices, or as a metaphoric language to express what cannot be verbalized. Recognizing this, clinicians can see musical habits not as distractions or escapes, but as sophisticated self-regulation strategies.

The Impact of Illness on Engagement with Music

For most people, music offers connection, pleasure, and self-expression. But for those living with serious mental illness, the relationship with music can be complicated. Symptoms such as hallucinations, mood swings, or cognitive disorganization may shape how sound is perceived and interpreted. In some cases, music becomes a source of comfort and grounding; in others, it intertwines with psychotic experiences in unsettling ways. One striking example is the phenomenon of musical voices in auditory hallucinations.

Auditory Hallucinations and Musical Voices

"I don't hear voices. I hear radio stations in my head."

Auditory hallucinations are among the most common symptoms of schizophrenia—and while they're often described as voices, a significant minority of patients experience music. Some hear songs from childhood. Others report original music, soundtracks that accompany their daily lives. One patient believed her hallucinated orchestra was assigned by the CIA. Another described a voice that only sang—in German opera, no less.

These experiences can be distressing, especially when they interfere with concentration or sleep. But they can also be oddly comforting. One man described a female voice singing to him in the evenings—he believed she was an angel watching over him. Clinically, this raises complex questions. Are musical hallucinations less pathologic than command hallucinations? Do they offer comfort or confusion? Should we treat them pharmacologically or respect their place in a patient's world?

The answer often depends on whether the music in the mind feels intrusive or intimate.

Schizophrenia and Schizoaffective Disorder

In psychosis, auditory hallucinations may include hearing voices, sounds, or music that isn't there. For some, these sounds can be disorienting or frightening. Yet for others, the experience of music—whether real or perceived—can be emotionally rich. Music may reflect memories, inspire comfort, or become part of a delusional framework.

Some patients describe hearing music that is intensely beautiful, transcendent even. Others may hear repetitive, looping tunes. Still others are convinced they are composers of divine symphonies. Music becomes a form of self-narrative—a communication tool beyond words.

In psychosis, music may become part of the delusional system:
- A patient hears a song on the radio and believes it's a secret message.
- Lyrics are interpreted as divine communication.
- Rhythms become coded instructions.

Clinicians can explore these experiences by asking:
- What does this song mean to you?
- What's the message you're hearing?
- When did music start feeling this way?

Such questions uncover not just symptoms, but deeper longings—for meaning, affirmation, connection.

Music can help quiet intrusive thoughts or hallucinations, but can also be distorted by delusional interpretations. Certain genres, especially intense or dissonant ones, may exacerbate paranoia or agitation. Cognitive impairments may also limit the ability to engage with complex music. Thus, clinicians can work collaboratively to curate music that regulates emotion without overwhelming.

Bipolar Disorder

In mania, creativity often soars—and music becomes a central outlet. Some patients compose, sing, or perform with passion and urgency. A patient may write an entire album in a weekend, believing it will change the world. But the crash can be devastating.

Manic creativity often blends inspiration with delusion. Music may feel like a divine gift or a tool of cosmic importance. Clinicians must walk a line between encouraging expression and managing risk.

During manic or hypomanic states:
- Music may be played loudly, obsessively.
- Patients may become fixated on a song.
- Lyrics or rhythms may take on grandiose significance.

In depressive states, music engagement may wane. Anhedonia may dampen enjoyment. But others may find solace in melancholic music that mirrors their mood.

Depression

In major depression, music can be both a refuge and burden. For some, it becomes a companion to sadness—a safe space to feel. For others, music feels unbearable, emphasizing the chasm between inner emotion and external sound.

Music mirrors depression. It reflects emotional depth, validates grief, and sometimes allows safe confrontation of despair. For others, it may offer distraction or gentle relief.

Obsessive Listening and Its Impact on Behavior

While music can be therapeutic, it can also become an obsessive preoccupation. Some individuals find themselves replaying certain songs or genres over and over, to the exclusion of everything else. This behavior can take several forms:

- Repetitive listening: Individuals may listen to the same song, album, or genre repeatedly, often for hours at a time. This repetitive listening can create a sense of familiarity and comfort but can also lead to isolation from the outside world.
- Psychological dependency: In extreme cases, individuals may develop a psychological dependency on music, feeling as though they cannot function properly without it. They may use music to avoid confronting emotions or trauma and find themselves unable to experience life without the constant presence of sound.

These behaviors may reflect a need for control, ritual, or connection to imagined meanings. Clinicians can work with patients to understand and redirect these fixations. Music isn't eliminated; it's reshaped into something that soothes without consuming.

Clinicians are encouraged to:

- Ask about musical preferences and their meanings.
- Use music in therapy to foster communication.
- Help patients experiment with new genres for emotion regulation.
- Be mindful of music that might trigger trauma or symptoms.
- Promote musical routines as stabilizing rituals.

In many inpatient settings, music becomes a ritual. Patients blast speakers, share headphones, or recite lyrics aloud. It is not mere background—it is declaration, comfort, structure, and sometimes, a symptom.

A woman believed Beyoncé communicated through lyrics. A man claimed he authored every Beatles song. Another believed his raps altered the weather.

These may be delusions—but they also reveal human desires: to be seen, heard, remembered. Music is voice. Music is legacy. Music is spark.

Music as a Tool for Connection and Communication

Shared musical experiences can foster a powerful sense of connection, as they serve as a social bridge for individuals who may otherwise feel isolated due to their psychiatric symptoms. Whether it is listening to a favorite song together, singing along, attending concerts, participating in music therapy groups, discussing favorite artists with peers, or even just being in the same space while music plays, these moments can create a sense of shared humanity, belonging, and help foster social engagement.

Music and Identity: A Way Back to Self

For many patients, music is deeply tied to identity. It carries with it memories of childhood, cultural roots, and past relationships. A song heard in a hospital waiting room may evoke memories of a loved one. A melody may remind someone of a time before they became ill, offering a fleeting sense of normalcy or self.

Patients who are unable to verbalize their feelings may still communicate through their choice of music. A man who cannot speak of his loneliness may put on a love song that conveys his longing. A woman who feels disconnected from her body may dance to music that helps her feel grounded again.

For clinicians, paying attention to a patient's musical preferences can provide important insights into their emotional state and sense of self. Music becomes a map of the patient's inner world, guiding therapeutic interventions and enhancing connection.

Music as a Source of Grounding and Routine

The familiar structure and rhythm of music can provide a sense of grounding and predictability, which can be particularly beneficial for individuals experiencing the internal chaos of psychosis or the fluctuations of mood disorders. Listening to the same playlist or engaging in a regular musical activity can create a sense of routine and stability in an otherwise unpredictable experience. Music can also be a powerful tool for self-soothing and managing anxiety. Certain types of music can have a calming effect, providing a welcome distraction from distressing thoughts or feelings.

Few sparks are as universal as music. Angela Argenzio, a music therapist, described how "rhythm and choice restore connection." Her reflections echo what neuroscience tells us: music reaches where illness cannot.

Music as Identity and Survival

Many individuals build and protect musical identities as core aspects of self:
- A patient may carry notebooks filled with lyrics.
- Another may identify as a rapper, a gospel singer, or a former DJ—even if their performance career only existed in their imagination.
- Favorite genres may reflect cultural roots, family ties, or aspirational selves—hip-hop for power, jazz for sophistication, metal for catharsis.

These identities often endure through illness and hospitalization. They offer continuity. In places where the person's name may be forgotten or distorted, their musical preferences remain firm: "I'm the one who loves Prince"; "I'm the one who sings in Spanish."

Music becomes a tether to identity—before, during, and after the storm.

The Emotional Power of Music: Music as an Emotional Anchor

The profound impact of music on emotions is well-documented. Listening to music can evoke a vast range of feelings, from joy, exhilaration, and excitement to sadness and peace. Individuals with serious mental illnesses can intentionally use music to regulate their mood, choosing upbeat music to lift their spirits or calming music to soothe anxiety and agitation. The predictable structures and patterns in music can provide a sense of order and stability, which can be particularly helpful during times of emotional distress or internal chaos. Furthermore, the release of neurochemicals associated with pleasure when listening to enjoyable music may also contribute to mood enhancement and overall well-being, a readily accessible and potent spark of emotional comfort. Therefore, people living with severe mental illnesses can intentionally use music to regulate their mood, finding solace in calming melodies or energy in upbeat rhythms. This ability to use music for emotional regulation is a significant spark of self-soothing and well-being.

Music provides a safe and creative outlet for emotions. Music can be a potent tool for regulating mood. Upbeat music can be energizing and uplifting, while calming melodies can reduce anxiety and promote relaxation. Individuals may intuitively gravitate towards music that mirrors or contrasts with their current emotional state, providing a sense of validation or a pathway to a different feeling.

Music has an extraordinary ability to tap into the core of human emotion. A familiar melody can instantly evoke feelings of joy, sadness, nostalgia, or peace. For individuals who may struggle to identify, articulate, or process their emotions verbally due to their illness, music can provide a direct and often more accessible pathway to these feelings. A melancholic tune might resonate with underlying sadness, offering a sense of validation or release. An upbeat rhythm can be energizing and uplifting, providing a temporary respite from difficult internal states. Music can act as a container for complex emotions, offering a sense of catharsis without the need for explicit verbalization. Furthermore, music is often intertwined with personal memories and associations, allowing individuals to connect with moments from their past and the emotions tied to those experiences.

Engaging with music, whether through active participation like singing or playing an instrument, or through receptive listening to uplifting or emotionally resonant pieces, can elevate mood, increase feelings of joy, and provide a sense of hope and connection. Music therapy can also offer a safe space for processing difficult emotions associated with depression.

Improved Cognitive Function

Music-based activities, like learning to play an instrument or engaging in rhythmic exercises, can enhance attention, memory, and executive functions, which are often impaired in SMIs.

In the turmoil of psychosis, when reality feels fractured and fleeting, music remains a constant companion. For those living with serious mental illness, music often becomes a lifeline, providing structure, comfort, and a connection to the world that feels increasingly distant. From the soothing sounds of a favorite song to the repetitive rhythms of a calming melody, music has the power to anchor the mind when everything else seems to be slipping away. In this way, music becomes more than just an art form—it becomes a mental anchor that can restore a sense of order, control, and even self-identity in the midst of chaos.

Music has a remarkable ability to bypass cognitive distortions and speak directly to emotional centers in the brain. For individuals living with schizophrenia, schizoaffective disorder, and bipolar disorder, music often serves as an anchor in the storm of their emotional turmoil.

Despite severe disorganization of thought or emotional dysregulation, many retain an intense connection to music, from childhood favorites to melodies that mirror their internal states.

Neurologically, music activates the limbic system, particularly the amygdala and ventral striatum, regions responsible for emotional processing and reward. Even when the world feels fragmented or alien, music provides continuity and familiarity.

For people living with severe mental illness, music can serve as both a soothing balm and a powerful catalyst. It may offer a safe, structured space to process emotions, yet it can also stir intense memories or amplify feelings in ways that are difficult to manage. Music's ability to affect mood, evoke memories, and create emotional resonance can be incredibly powerful. Listening to calming music has been shown to lower heart rate, blood pressure, and levels of stress hormones like cortisol. Music with a slow tempo, predictable rhythms, and calming melodies can promote relaxation, decrease physiological arousal, and alleviate feelings of anxiety and agitation, which are frequently experienced in conditions like schizophrenia, bipolar disorder, and severe depression. The predictable patterns and soothing sounds can create a sense of safety and security.

For some, listening to certain genres or songs provides comfort during anxious or depressive episodes. Classical music, ambient sounds, or even nature sounds can help calm the nervous system and provide a sense of peace.

For others, music can serve as a distraction or form of escapism. It becomes a way to disconnect from the harshness of their reality. Music's rhythmic patterns and lyrics can create a sense of control or order, providing temporary relief from chaotic thoughts.

While music therapy is not a direct treatment for psychotic symptoms like hallucinations or delusions, it can serve as a valuable coping mechanism by providing a positive distraction, promoting relaxation, and fostering a sense of control and self-expression in the face of distressing experiences.

Music therapy isn't just an alternative intervention—it's evidence-based. In a Cochrane review, Gold and colleagues found that music therapy significantly improved negative symptoms, social engagement, and quality of life for people living with schizophrenia.

There are days when music has done what meds could not. I've seen its magic firsthand. I've seen patients in catatonic stupors hum along to Whitney Houston. Music does something medication never could.

There was a man on the unit who never made eye contact, never spoke—until music therapy came around. When the opening chords of a reggae song played, he started tapping his fingers and softly sang along. He didn't stop until the music did. It was the only time we ever heard his voice.

"Peers, too, testify to music as an anchor," one man with schizophrenia explained. His experience shows how music creates continuity of self, even in disorganized states.

Personal Narratives

The lived experiences of people with serious mental illnesses often highlight the deeply personal and significant role that music plays in their lives and recovery journeys. Many describe using music as a constant companion, a source of solace during periods of isolation, a means of coping with difficult emotions, and a powerful way to connect with others. These personal narratives underscore the unique and multifaceted ways in which music can provide comfort, hope, and a profound sense of self, acting as an enduring spark of resilience and connection to their own humanity.

Mark, a teenager with autism spectrum disorder and co-occurring anxiety, finds solace and a means of communication through playing the guitar. His narrative illustrates the power of music as a non-verbal form of expression and connection.

Emily, an older adult with schizophrenia, finds comfort and memory recall through listening to music from her youth. Her story highlights the cognitive and emotional benefits of music.

Jose, who attends a music therapy group, finds a sense of community and emotional release through shared musical experiences.

Marcus, a 35-year-old man with schizoaffective disorder, refused to participate in most group activities. He wore noise-canceling headphones all day, often humming or tapping rhythmically. Staff initially viewed this as isolating behavior. But when a music therapist introduced a weekly lyric-writing group, Marcus volunteered to join. He began writing verses, sharing lines about his childhood, his hallucinations, his loneliness, and his hopes. Eventually, he recorded his lyrics over a beat. For the first time in months, he smiled openly. When he said, "I'm an artist, not just a patient," it became a turning point in his recovery.

Spiritual Songs, Lullabies, and the Echoes of Home

Certain songs hold sacred resonance:
- Hymns and gospel tunes that tether someone to early church experiences
- Lullabies from a grandmother or mother
- Songs played at funerals, birthdays, or pivotal moments in life

Clinicians are encouraged to:
- Ask about musical preferences and their meanings.
- Use music in therapy to foster communication.
- Help patients experiment with new genres for emotion regulation.
- Be mindful of music that might trigger trauma or symptoms.
- Promote musical routines as stabilizing rituals.

In many inpatient settings, music becomes a ritual. Patients blast speakers, share headphones, or recite lyrics aloud. It is not mere background—it is declaration, comfort, structure, and sometimes, a symptom.

These may be delusions—but they also reveal human desires: to be seen, heard, remembered. Music is voice. Music is legacy. Music is spark.

A woman with bipolar disorder may listen to calming classical music during moments of agitation to regain a sense of calm.

A man with schizophrenia may use music to anchor his thoughts, tuning out intrusive voices or chaotic thoughts with rhythmic beats.

A teenager with schizoaffective disorder may listen to the same song over and over, finding solace in its predictability.

James, a 45-year-old man with schizophrenia, found comfort in his guitar. When the voices in his head grew overwhelming, he would retreat into the corner of his room and strum his guitar, playing the same simple chords over and over. To those around him, it seemed like a repetitive exercise, but for James, it was a crucial act of self-soothing. The rhythmic strumming and familiar tunes offered him stability in a world that felt increasingly chaotic. For James, music was a bridge to a calm and orderly space, a mental escape from the overwhelming noise of psychosis.

Clara, a 30-year-old woman with bipolar disorder, would frequently hum songs during manic episodes, often losing herself in the repetition of her favorite tunes. She believed that certain songs held special significance, and she would often speak of them as if they were a direct link to something greater—a sign of hope or a message from a higher power. The songs allowed her to express emotions that she otherwise couldn't articulate, creating a sense of connection to the world around her. During times of intense mania, Clara would sing in an attempt to center herself, finding reassurance and grounding in the music's rhythmic structure.

In these instances, music acts as both a distraction and a stabilizer, providing a predictable pattern that contrasts with the unpredictability of mental illness.

Accessibility and Preferences

Just like anyone else, people living with serious mental illness have diverse musical tastes. Some may find comfort in classical music, others in rock, hip-hop, folk, or electronic genres. Exploring these personal preferences can offer insights into the emotional landscape and provide a basis for connection. One of the remarkable aspects of music is its inherent accessibility and the vast diversity of genres, styles, and ways of engaging with it. Musical preferences are highly individual and deeply personal, ensuring that there is a form of music that can resonate with almost everyone.

What one person finds soothing, another may find irritating. Therefore, music-based interventions should be tailored to the individual's tastes and cultural background.

Accessibility is also key. Accessibility is particularly important for people living with severe mental illnesses, who may face barriers to other forms of engagement. Providing opportunities for individuals to access and engage with music in various settings, whether through formal music therapy sessions, community music groups, or simply having access to personal music listening devices, can make a significant and positive difference in their lives, nurturing this readily available spark of joy and self-expression. The diverse ways in which music can be experienced and the importance of individual preferences make it an accessible and personal spark for everyone. Whether listening to a favorite genre, learning an instrument, or simply humming a tune, music offers a readily available source of pleasure and expression.

Community, Identity, and Soundtracks of Belonging

For many patients, music connects them to something larger—subculture, community, belonging. A punk-rock obsessive sees himself in the rebellious aesthetic of distortion and chaos. A gospel devotee finds transcendence in harmonies that remind her of childhood church. A hip-hop fan studies lyrics for codes, messages, truth. Music can also form the scaffolding of social life. In group homes or inpatient settings, musical taste becomes identity currency. "You like Outkast? Okay, we can hang." In psych units where so much is stripped away—names, possessions, privacy—musical affiliation becomes one of the few remaining badges of self.

And music travels. I've seen unhoused patients carrying USB drives full of curated playlists. I've met people who lost families but never lost their headphones. A man who could not remember his diagnosis knew every word of Bob Dylan's *Blood on the Tracks*.

The Dark Side: Noise, Overstimulation, and Triggers

Not all musical encounters are positive. Some patients become overstimulated by loud or fast music. Others are triggered by certain lyrics or memories tied to songs. A woman who survived trauma would dissociate every time she heard a particular radio jingle. A man spiraled into a manic episode after an all-night rave. For people living with sensory processing vulnerabilities, music can be both medicine and poison. Clinical awareness is key. Not every jam session is therapeutic. Not every headphone moment is safe. But with the right boundaries, music can be tailored to support, not destabilize.

The Enduring Connection: Music as a Lifeline

Music can provide a sense of continuity, identity, and connection that endures even amidst the challenges of mental illness. It can be a constant companion, a source of comfort, and a reminder of shared humanity. For individuals who may experience fluctuations in their thoughts, feelings, and social engagement, music can offer a stable and reliable source of emotional support and connection to themselves and others.

Music Therapy and Its Benefits: The Healing Power of Music in Mental Health

For individuals living with serious mental illness, music is more than just a coping mechanism—it can play a critical role in recovery and treatment. Music therapy, an established therapeutic practice, has been shown to help people living with psychosis reduce symptoms of anxiety and depression, improve social engagement, and even enhance cognitive abilities. In both group and individual therapy settings, music can be used to promote emotional expression and encourage socialization, which are often difficult for those living with severe mental illness.

In psychiatric settings, structured music therapy can provide a non-invasive way to address complex emotional and psychological needs. For instance, patients can be encouraged to participate in group music-making, creating a sense of community and shared experience. Listening to music together in a group setting can offer opportunities for emotional regulation and foster a sense of belonging, helping to combat the social isolation that is often part and parcel of serious mental illnesses.

Music therapy affects both the emotional and cognitive centers of the brain, regulating mood and enhancing emotional well-being. In times of distress, rhythmic patterns can calm, reduce anxiety, alleviate depressive symptoms, and improve cognitive function. For those experiencing psychosis, music can provide structure and connection—a vital way to re-engage with reality.

Music activates the brain's reward system and releases dopamine—offering rare pleasure and relief. For people living with severe mental illness, this can anchor them during internal chaos, offering moments of clarity and joy.

I've seen music pull people out of catatonia and into laughter. It felt like witnessing a resurrection.

Sometimes, I think music speaks the language the rest of psychiatry forgets.

Group Therapy, Rhythm, and the Power of Drumming

Rhythmic synchronization—clapping, tapping, drumming—can regulate neural timing and promote group cohesion. In group therapy settings, even modest music-based activities can reduce agitation, promote expression, and invite emotional resonance.

Drumming circles, in particular, have been shown to:
- Foster nonverbal connection among participants
- Improve mood and decrease dissociation
- Reinforce boundaries and attunement through shared beats

This is not mere recreation. It is repair. Drumming with others says: I exist, I belong, I contribute.

Improving Cognitive Function: Engaging the Mind

Music-based activities, like learning to play a new instrument, engaging in rhythmic exercises, or participating in song-based memory tasks, can enhance various cognitive functions, including attention, concentration, memory, processing speed, and executive functions, which are often areas of difficulty for people living with SMIs.

Listening to familiar songs can evoke vivid memories, while learning to play an instrument can improve focus and coordination. For individuals experiencing cognitive difficulties, music can offer a gentle and engaging form of stimulation.

"Clinicians often observe the preservation of music memory," Dr. Helen Bloomer recalled. Her stories illustrate how music bridges past vitality with present recovery.

Facilitating Communication and Social Interaction: Harmony in Shared Experience

Group music therapy sessions provide structured and often non-threatening opportunities for individuals to interact with others in a supportive environment, fostering social skills, reducing feelings of isolation, and building a sense of community through shared musical experiences, like attending concerts, participating in music groups, or even discussing favorite artists. These shared experiences can reduce feelings of isolation and foster a sense of belonging.

Music possesses a remarkable ability to bridge social divides and foster a sense of connection among individuals, bringing people together. Participating in musical activities with others—singing in a choir, playing in a band, attending concerts, or simply listening to music together—creates shared experiences that build social bonds. The shared enjoyment of music can transcend diagnostic labels and create a sense of community, mutual support, and joy.

Increased Self-Esteem and Self-Expression: Creative Accomplishment

For individuals who may struggle with verbal communication due to illness, cognitive challenges, or negative symptoms like alogia, music can provide a powerful non-verbal outlet for expressing a wide spectrum of emotions, thoughts, and experiences.

Music can be a profound way to express joy, sadness, anger, or peace. This act of self-expression through melody, rhythm, and harmony can be validating and empowering—a vital spark of identity. Creating or listening to resonant music fosters a sense of being understood and seen, even when words fail.

This is especially important for people living with flattened affect. Music remains a channel of emotional life—a thread of continuity and personhood that persists when other forms of communication are impaired.

Music Therapy Techniques and Coping Applications

Music therapists use a diverse range of techniques tailored to the individual's needs and goals, including:
- Active music making (playing instruments, singing, improvising)
- Receptive music listening (listening to selected music for relaxation, emotional processing, or guided imagery)
- Songwriting (creating original songs to express thoughts and feelings)
- Lyric analysis (exploring the themes and emotions within existing songs)
- Music and imagery (listening to music to evoke visual images and explore associated feelings and memories)

Formal music therapy integrates structured musical experiences into psychiatric treatment plans. Techniques include:
- Active music-making: Drumming, singing, improvising music, or playing instruments to express and release emotions.
- Receptive listening: Curating playlists that align with therapeutic goals, like relaxation, emotional processing, imagery, or motivation.
- Songwriting: Helping patients create their own music to process experiences, thoughts, and feelings.
- Lyric Analysis: Discussing the themes and emotions in existing songs.
- Guided imagery with music: Listening to selected pieces to unlock inner imagery and associated feelings.

Studies have found that music therapy can reduce negative symptoms of schizophrenia (like withdrawal or apathy), enhance mood stabilization in bipolar disorder, and foster a sense of agency and self-expression.

Coping Mechanisms

Finding refuge in rhythm and melody: Music can serve as a powerful coping mechanism for managing symptoms. Some may use loud, energetic music to distract from intrusive thoughts, while others might turn to calming instrumental pieces to soothe anxiety or find a sense of peace during difficult times. The predictability and structure of music can provide a sense of control when internal experiences feel chaotic.

Creative Expression

The language beyond words: Engaging in music—singing, playing an instrument, writing lyrics, or creating electronic music—provides a vital outlet for creative expression. This is particularly important for individuals who struggle to articulate feelings verbally. Music becomes the language of the unspoken, the melody of survival.

Music often has the capacity to bypass illness, reaching a core part of the individual that remains connected and receptive to beauty and order.

Maria, a young patient with severe auditory hallucinations, was almost entirely unresponsive. One day, a nurse played classical choral music. Maria's pacing slowed. She began to hum softly. The music didn't cure her, but it created a moment of sanctuary, a brief reconnection to her resilient core.

In therapeutic sessions:
- Patients may write lyrics, improvise rhythms, or compose songs.
- Music becomes more than activity; it becomes identity.

Music helps reconstruct narrative and voice in patients who often feel misunderstood.

Music therapy fosters:
- Emotional expression
- Social connection
- Reduced anxiety and agitation
- Enhanced cognitive function

Whether listening, playing, or singing, music becomes a powerful spark of engagement. It must be used thoughtfully—curated to support healing, not overwhelm. Music therapy isn't just an adjunct—it's a bridge. To emotion. To memory. To self.

Conclusion

In the midst of psychosis, when the mind is overwhelmed and reality seems distorted, music stands as a reliable anchor. Its rhythmic patterns offer structure in a world of disarray, its melodies provide comfort in moments of confusion, and its emotional resonance connects individuals to a deeper sense of self. Whether through the strumming of a guitar, the hum of a familiar song, or the steady beat of a drum, music offers something that words alone often cannot—a sense of hope and connection. For those living with severe mental illness, music is not just a distraction; it is a lifeline, a pathway to mental stability and emotional well-being. In a world where so much can feel uncertain, music remains a constant, helping individuals navigate the stormy seas of psychosis and find moments of peace within the chaos.

Music transcends the boundaries of language and cognition, often reaching people living with severe mental illness in profound and meaningful ways. Its enduring power to evoke emotions, facilitate connection, provide comfort, and offer a sense of grounding underscores its vital role in their human experience. By recognizing and appreciating the significance of music in their lives, and by exploring the potential of music therapy, we can offer more holistic and person-centered care that acknowledges and nurtures this universal language of the human spirit.

We must customize musical interventions to each patient's emotional needs and sensitivities, use music as part of a broader multimodal treatment approach, recognize the potential for music to both heal and harm (assess for overstimulation or triggering content), and incorporate patient preferences to foster agency and engagement.

Music is a unique form of expression that transcends barriers. It offers a language of emotion, a bridge between the mind and the heart. For people living with serious mental illness, music is not just sound—it is a connection to self, to others, and to the world.

Even in the most chaotic minds, the rhythm of music beats on. It carries the potential for healing, for understanding, for expression. And in that, it provides a spark—a glimpse of who the person was, who they are, and who they might yet become.

In conclusion, music offers a powerful, multifaceted, and enduring spark of life for individuals living with severe mental illnesses. By recognizing and harnessing the power of music, we can enhance the lives of those affected by these conditions in meaningful ways. Its therapeutic applications, its capacity for self-expression and social connection, and its profound ability to regulate emotions and bring joy make it an invaluable resource in promoting well-being, fostering recovery, and enriching lives in meaningful and deeply personal ways.

This chapter emphasizes that music is a powerful and enduring spark in the lives of people living with serious mental illnesses, offering therapeutic benefits, a means of self-expression, a pathway to social connection, and a tool for emotional regulation and joy.

Even in the most disorganized minds, rhythm persists. It may not follow a metronome. It may not fit a scale. But it's there.

Music is the heartbeat of identity, the echo of self that illness cannot fully erase.

When patients pace the hallways humming melodies, or stare out windows whispering lyrics, or scribble song ideas in journals—pay attention. They are not lost. They are composing something. Not just noise, but signal. Not just symptom, but soul.

Music is more than entertainment for those with severe mental illness. It is a language of emotion, a rhythm of regulation, and a map of identity. It cuts across delusion and clarity, joy and pain, isolation and community.

When we listen with clinical curiosity and human openness, we hear more than symptoms—we hear story, soul, and spark. And in that shared rhythm, healing becomes possible.

Table 7.1 — Music in Recovery

Use	Example	Effect
Coping	Jazz to calm voices	Reduces hallucination intensity
Memory	Familiar songs in dementia	Enhances recall, identity
Social	Group drumming	Builds connection, reduces isolation

Koelsch, S. (2014). Brain correlates of music-evoked emotions. *Nature Reviews Neuroscience*, 15(3), 170–180. (Distributed network: limbic, paralimbic, prefrontal, hippocampal, auditory.)

Salimpoor, V. N., Benovoy, M., et al. (2011). Anatomically distinct dopamine release during anticipation and experience of peak emotion to music. *Nature Neuroscience*, 14(2), 257–262; Salimpoor, V. N., Benovoy, M., et al. (2013). Interactions between the nucleus accumbens and auditory cortices predict music reward. *PNAS*, 110(28), 10430–10435. (Reward circuitry; dopamine/NAc.)

Large, E. W., & Snyder, J. S. (2009). Pulse and meter as neural resonance. *Annals of the NY Academy of Sciences*, 1169, 46–57; Thaut, M. H., et al. (2015).

Rhythmic entrainment in rehabilitation. *Frontiers in Human Neuroscience*, 9, 444. (Temporal predictability; entrainment aiding regulation.)
Geretsegger, M., Mössler, K., et al. (2017). Music therapy for people with schizophrenia and schizophrenia-like disorders. *Cochrane Database of Systematic Reviews*, CD004025. (Improvements in negative symptoms, functioning, QoL; dose/quality effects.)
Thoma, M. V., et al. (2013). The effect of music on the human stress response. *Psychoneuroendocrinology*, 38(11), 2674–2681; Bernardi, L., Porta, C., & Sleight, P. (2006). Cardiovascular, cerebrovascular, and respiratory changes induced by different music styles. *Heart*, 92(4), 445–452. (Reductions in cortisol/HR/BP with calming music.)
Särkämö, T., et al. (2008). Music listening enhances cognitive recovery after stroke. *Brain*, 131(3), 866–876; Särkämö, T., et al. (2013). Emotional responses to music in dementia. *Journal of the American Geriatrics Society*, 61(12), 2156–2158. (Memory/affect retrieval via familiar music.)
Schlaug, G. (2015). Music, musicians, and brain plasticity. *The Neuroscientist*, 21(5), 495–500; Herholz, S. C., & Zatorre, R. J. (2012). Musical training as a framework for brain plasticity. *Neuron*, 76(3), 486–502. (Experience-dependent plasticity with music.)
Fancourt, D., & Perkins, R. (2018). Effect of group drumming on mental health. *Public Health*, 167, 140–146; Bittman, B., et al. (2001). Recreational music-making modulates immune parameters. *Alternative Therapies*, 7(1), 54–63. (Group rhythm: mood, cohesion, regulation.)
Evers, S., & Ellger, T. (2004). The clinical spectrum of musical hallucinations. *Journal of the Neurological Sciences*, 227(1), 55–65; Vitorovic, D., & Biller, J. (2013). Musical hallucinations: A systematic review. *Journal of the Neurological Sciences*, 338(1–2), 5–17. (Phenomenology, causes, management.)
Magee, W. L., Davidson, J. W., et al. (2017). Music therapy assessment and outcome measures in mental health. *The Arts in Psychotherapy*, 54, 62–70; Chanda, M. L., & Levitin, D. J. (2013). The neurochemistry of music. *Trends in Cognitive Sciences*, 17(4), 179–193. (Clinical use, playlisting, coping mechanisms.)

Chapter 8:
Spirituality: The Enduring Search for Meaning

Even amid chaos, the soul continues to pray.

Among the most persistent, and often misunderstood, sparks in severe mental illness is spirituality. The language of God, the presence of spirits, visions, prayers, divine missions, and moral reckonings appear frequently in the narratives of people living with psychosis, mood disorders, and trauma-related conditions. Some clinicians instinctively pathologize these experiences; others avoid them entirely. But when approached with care and curiosity, spiritual themes reveal powerful truths about suffering, identity, hope, and meaning.

In the heart of psychosis or depression, when cognition is scattered and functioning impaired, something often endures, a pull toward the sacred, a longing for connection with something greater. This is not merely religious observance. It's the enduring human impulse to find meaning, to seek order in chaos, and to feel held by something beyond the self. For many people living with severe mental illness, spirituality is not a byproduct of delusion; it is an anchor through it.

Spirituality refers to a person's internalized connection to something greater, whether defined as God, nature, the universe, love, or existential truth. It may be structured through organized religion or exist as a deeply personal set of rituals, beliefs, or practices. Spirituality, whether expressed through organized religion, personal rituals, or existential questioning, often remains one of the last inner structures to erode in severe mental illness, often persisting long after other structures have crumbled. Even individuals whose cognitive organization is fragmented may still pray, take part in rituals, call upon a higher power, or ponder their place in the universe.

Spirituality is a persistent connection to faith, rituals, or existential meaning. Spirituality is not a delusion. It is a system of sense-making that may become entangled with illness, but also serves as a vital lifeline for many who are otherwise drowning.

For many individuals, a connection to something larger than themselves can be a profound source of comfort, strength, and meaning. This spark of spirituality can manifest in various ways:

- Faith: A deep belief in a particular religion or spiritual tradition, finding solace and guidance in its teachings, community, and practices. Engaging in religious services, prayer, or studying sacred texts can be deeply meaningful.
- Rituals: Finding comfort and stability in repetitive practices, whether they are formal religious ceremonies or personal routines that provide a sense of order and connection to something familiar.
- Existential Meaning: A persistent quest to understand the bigger questions of life, one's place in the universe, or a personal philosophy that provides a framework for understanding experiences and finding purpose. This might involve contemplation, reading philosophical texts, or engaging in discussions about life's meaning.
- Connection to Nature: For some, spirituality is deeply intertwined with the natural world, serving as a way of experiencing awe, peace, and a sense of the sacred in landscapes, animals, or natural phenomena.
- Inner Peace: A persistent seeking of inner tranquility through practices like meditation, mindfulness, or contemplative prayer.

Mental illness often forces individuals to confront profound existential questions, but I've seen how spiritual faith can act as an anchor amid internal chaos.

This dynamic can be seen in the story of Elijah, who, during a manic episode, experienced intense religious delusions. His family worried he had lost his faith. As he stabilized, his delusions faded but his spiritual core remained. "Even when my mind was racing, I held onto the idea that there was a plan," he said. Spirituality, for him, was not a symptom, but a source of resilience.

Nurturing this spark may involve practical support, such as encouraging attendance at religious services, providing access to spiritual materials, or creating quiet spaces for reflection. Sometimes it is as simple as acknowledging and respecting an individual's beliefs and practices. For caregivers and clinicians, understanding a person's spiritual background

and current connection is not an add-on to treatment—it is a vital part of person-centered care. In the lives of those with schizophrenia, bipolar disorder, or major mood disorders, spirituality may take many forms:
- Reciting prayers, even when speech is disorganized
- Engaging in rituals for protection or forgiveness
- Grappling with existential questions about suffering, death, and hope

Neurobiological Mechanisms

Research suggests that spiritual practices, including prayer and meditation, can alter brain chemistry and reduce symptoms of depression and anxiety. Studies on mindfulness-based interventions show that regular meditation can lead to changes in areas of the brain related to emotion regulation, stress response, and cognitive flexibility These neurobiological changes are important for people living with severe mental illness, who often face difficulties in managing emotions and thoughts.

Spirituality and Mental Health: A Pathway to Resilience

Spirituality has long been a cornerstone of healing for many, and research in psychiatry and psychology supports its role in improving mental health outcomes.

Spirituality and Coping

A key role of spirituality in mental health is its function as a coping mechanism. Numerous studies have shown that spirituality helps people living with severe mental illness, like schizophrenia and bipolar disorder, cope with distressing symptoms. In a study published in the *Journal of Clinical Psychology*, it was found that people living with schizophrenia who reported a strong spiritual or religious connection experienced lower levels of distress and better overall functioning. Spirituality provides a sense of meaning and a framework for making sense of suffering, often leading to enhanced coping strategies.

Spirituality as a Protective Factor

Studies have shown that spirituality can act as a buffer against suicide. A review by emphasized that individuals who integrate spirituality into their lives often have better psychological well-being and lower rates of suicide. This finding is particularly important for people with severe mental illnesses, who are at an elevated risk for suicidal thoughts and behaviors.

Spirituality and Mental Well-Being

A growing body of research indicates a positive association between spirituality and improved mental health outcomes. For example, a meta-analysis found that higher levels of religiousness and spirituality were significantly associated with lower rates of depression, anxiety, and substance abuse. Furthermore, longitudinal studies have shown that regular participation in religious activities can predict greater resilience and better coping skills in the face of life stressors (George, et al., 2002).

Spirituality in the Context of Serious Mental Illness

Research suggests that spirituality can be a significant coping mechanism for people living with severe mental illness. A study by Mohr (2010) highlighted that many people living with schizophrenia and other psychotic disorders report using their spiritual beliefs to understand their experiences and find comfort. However, it's also important to acknowledge that spiritual struggles, like feeling abandoned by God or questioning one's faith, can occur and are associated with poorer mental health outcomes.

Chaplain Melissa Hayes-Kolakowski emphasized faith as anchor: "For many, spirituality becomes the most enduring spark." Her perspective highlights how faith sustains identity even amid delusion.

Faith Under Fire: The Intersection of Illness and Belief

Serious mental illness often upends an individual's worldview. Faith systems are tested. Some patients believe they are being punished by God; others feel chosen or possessed. Still others use prayer, ritual, and religious frameworks as ways to ground themselves or make sense of their symptoms.

Common presentations include:
- Religious delusions (believing one is a prophet, messiah, or demon)
- Apocalyptic fears and guilt-ridden moral themes
- Hyper-religiosity during manic or psychotic episodes
- Use of prayer or scripture for comfort, order, and protection

Rather than reflexively labeling these as religiously themed psychosis, clinicians should ask:
- What role does spirituality play in your life?
- Has faith been a comfort to you, or has it caused distress?
- Do you feel closer to or further from the divine during times of illness?

These questions respect spiritual identity while providing a lens for therapeutic engagement.

When a patient told me angels were guarding his bed, I didn't argue. I asked what the angels were protecting him from.

A patient once told me she didn't trust psychiatrists—only God. At first, I tried to reason with her. Later, I just listened. Her prayers weren't obstacles to treatment; they were her treatment. They gave her a language for her fear and a structure for her hope.

Spirituality is not peripheral in mental illness—it is often central. Huguelet and Mohr demonstrated that spiritual beliefs frequently remain intact and meaningful for people living with schizophrenia, shaping identity and guiding recovery narratives.

Other chaplains describe similar experiences. One recalled how "even small rituals restored hope." These voices remind us that spirituality is not a luxury but a core pathway to healing.

Spirituality vs. Psychosis: The Diagnostic Tension

Spirituality and psychosis often occupy adjacent space. A belief in unseen forces, voices from beyond, or divine intervention may be signs of profound faith or signs of florid psychosis. Distinguishing between pathological content and meaningful spiritual experience requires nuance.

Rather than rushing to interpret all spiritual statements as symptoms, it's essential to ask:
- Is the belief distressing or comforting?
- Does it impair functioning or give purpose?
- Is it shared by a faith community or is it idiosyncratic?

Distinguishing Spiritual Experience from Psychosis

One of the most nuanced clinical challenges is differentiating between a culturally or personally normative spiritual experience and a psychotic symptom.

Key points of differentiation often include:
- Shared framework: Is the belief held within a broader community of faith, or is it idiosyncratic?
- Functionality: Does the experience support well-being and connection, or does it lead to isolation, fear, or harm?
- Flexibility: Is the belief open to discussion and reflection, or is it rigid and all-consuming?

For example, a patient who feels "called" to serve the poor may be drawing from deep spiritual purpose. A patient who believes they are the only true savior, and must act on divine command to harm others, is likely experiencing a dangerous distortion. Clinicians can validate spiritual yearning while gently assessing for risk and delusion.

Clinical Insight

Even clearly delusional content can be symbolically spiritual. A man who believes angels speak to him may also find peace and direction in prayer. We must not rob him of that source of comfort.

Clinical Observations

- Patients with schizophrenia who struggle with disorganized speech may nonetheless articulate coherent prayers.
- Individuals with bipolar disorder often report a heightened sense of spiritual connection during manic or depressive episodes.
- Persons with schizoaffective disorder may maintain private rituals of forgiveness, protection, or thanksgiving, even when delusions are active.
- Patients experiencing psychosis may offer prayers with remarkable coherence even as their speech elsewhere deteriorates.
- Some individuals cling to rituals (crossing themselves, repeating sacred phrases, lighting candles) as a way to create order amid chaos.
- Existential themes—"Why me?" "What is my purpose?" "Is there redemption for my mistakes?"—often emerge even when logic is compromised.

Maria's Story

Maria, a woman with chronic schizophrenia, was hospitalized repeatedly for paranoid delusions. Staff often noted her habit of whispering at sunset, facing east, and holding an imaginary candle. When gently asked about this, she explained: "This is how I keep watch for the children I left behind. God knows where they are. I light a prayer for them."

Maria had lost custody of her children years earlier during a manic episode. The candle was not a symptom—it was a sacred practice of remembrance, of hope. When clinicians respected this ritual rather than dismissing it, her agitation decreased.

I used to dismiss spiritual language in psychosis. Now I listen for the need beneath the words. Many of my patients pray—not as a symptom, but as a form of survival. I've learned that spirituality can't be dismissed, even when it appears tangled with delusions.

Clinicians also note "how spiritual practices like prayer and journaling provide structure." Such sparks offer resilience, grounding patients even during relapse.

Spiritual Coping and Moral Injury

Many people living with chronic illness experience what has been called "moral injury—the sense that they have failed themselves, others, or God. They may feel cursed, unworthy, or unforgivable. Others struggle with forgiveness, rage at the divine, or disillusionment with once-beloved religious institutions.

Spiritual coping includes:
- Seeking forgiveness or redemption
- Attending religious services or reading sacred texts
- Engaging in ritual for healing and order
- Turning toward spiritual mentors or communities

Clinicians should be prepared to address spiritual trauma: abuse by clergy, rejection by faith communities, or internalized shame related to sexuality, substance use, or illness itself. In these cases, the spark of spirituality may still burn—but it burns through grief.

Identifying and Nurturing the Spark of Spirit

While directly measuring the impact of nurturing spirituality can be complex, research on related practices offers insights. For instance, studies on mindfulness and meditation, often integral to spiritual practices, have demonstrated their effectiveness in reducing anxiety and improving emotional regulation Supporting an individual's spiritual engagement may indirectly leverage these benefits.

The Crucial Role of Caregivers and Clinicians

Evidence-based guidelines increasingly recommend that mental health professionals conduct a spiritual history as part of a comprehensive assessment. Understanding a patient's spiritual background and beliefs can inform treatment planning and enhance the therapeutic relationship. Respecting and supporting these beliefs, where appropriate, aligns with person-centered care principles.

Therapeutic Engagement and Clinical Applications

Even outside formal religion, many patients turn to spiritual practices for grounding. Repetitive prayer, mindfulness, guided imagery, and nature-based rituals all serve as stabilizing forces. These practices may regulate breathing, create internal space, and provide a sense of containment in the midst of fragmentation.

Clinicians can support this dimension of care through the following approaches:

- Validate expressions of faith and spirituality without pathologizing them, even if unconventional.
- Listen carefully and non-judgmentally to spiritual expressions, even when they seem unusual.
- Invite patients or families to share meaningful spiritual practices if appropriate.
- Recognize that delusions with religious content (e.g., believing oneself to be a prophet or demon) can complicate assessments. When psychotic content intertwines with religious ideas, discern gently between pathological distortion and healthy, authentic spiritual yearning.
- Collaborate with chaplains, pastoral counselors, or spiritual care providers when appropriate.
- Explore spirituality as a resource for resilience without dismissing it as delusion or magical thinking.

Possible therapeutic modalities include:
- Trauma-informed mindfulness groups
- Music or art therapy with spiritual themes
- Nature immersion for eco-spirituality

These practices should be offered with openness, not prescription. The goal is not to convert but to connect. Spirituality, when honored thoughtfully, becomes a potent ally in recovery work. Faith—whether in God, in humanity, or in the possibility of recovery—is often the very thing that allows survival.

Conclusion

Spirituality offers a framework for hope, a reason for endurance, and a sense of connection beyond isolation. It can function both as an anchor (grounding a fragmented mind) and as a bridge (connecting self to others and to a greater meaning).

Spirituality provides a framework for survival, a compass for dignity, and often, a language for endurance. It taps into a part of the self that seeks coherence, purpose, and hope—needs that often intensify, not diminish, when the mind is under siege. It can reduce shame, foster community, and help people make sense of their experiences. In the absence of a stable ego or intact cognition, a spiritual identity can remain, offering continuity through chaos.

When clinicians and families support this spark, they validate not only the person's belief system but their humanity.

Spirituality in severe mental illness is not a sideshow. It is central. It is where the most profound questions live: Why me? What is my purpose? Is there anything beyond this pain? When we walk into these questions with our patients—not to provide answers, but to accompany them—we embody the very spark we seek to support: presence, reverence, and radical human connection.

Table 8.1 — Spirituality vs. Spiritual Delusion

Expression	Spirituality	Spiritual Delusion
Content	Faith, meaning, belonging	Persecution, control, voices
Impact	Hope, recovery anchor	Fear, distress
Care	Chaplaincy, peer groups	Clinical support, meds + therapy

Huguelet, P., & Mohr, S. (2004). Spirituality and meaning in persons with schizophrenia. *Journal of Nervous and Mental Disease*, 192(11), 660–667.

Zeidan, F., et al. (2010). Mindfulness meditation improves cognition and reduces stress. *Consciousness and Cognition*, 19(2), 597–605; Newberg, A., & Iversen, J. (2003). The neural basis of religious experience. *Trends in Cognitive Sciences*, 7(1), 31–33.

Goyal, M., et al. (2014). Meditation programs for psychological stress and well-being: A systematic review and meta-analysis. *JAMA Internal Medicine*, 174(3), 357–368.

Koenig, H. G., King, D., & Carson, V. (2012). *Handbook of Religion and Health* (2nd ed.). Oxford University Press; Smith, T. B., et al. (2003). Religiousness and depression: A meta-analysis. *Psychological Bulletin*, 129(4), 614–636.

George, L. K., et al. (2002). Spirituality and health: What we know, what we need to know. *Public Health*, 116, 92–101; VanderWeele, T. J., et al. (2016). Religious service attendance and health outcomes. *JAMA Internal Medicine*, 176(6), 777–785.

Mohr, S., et al. (2010). The role of religion and spirituality in coping with schizophrenia: A qualitative study. *Social Psychiatry and Psychiatric Epidemiology*, 45(11), 1235–1242; Huguelet, P., et al. (2011). Spirituality and religious practices among outpatients with schizophrenia. *International Journal of Social Psychiatry*, 57(4), 327–337.

Exline, J. J., Pargament, K. I., Grubbs, J. B., & Yali, A. M. (2014). The religious and spiritual struggles scale: Development and initial validation. *Psychology of Religion and Spirituality*, 6(3), 208–222.

Pargament, K. I., et al. (2013). *APA Handbook of Psychology, Religion, and Spirituality*, Vol. 2. APA; Wu, A., et al. (2015). Religion and completed suicide: A meta-analysis. *PLOS ONE*, 10(6): e0131715.

Hodge, D. R. (2007). A systematic review of spiritual assessment tools. *Social Work*, 52(2), 139–149.

Fox, K. C. R., et al. (2016). Functional neuroanatomy of meditation and religious practice. *Neuroscience & Biobehavioral Reviews*, 65, 208–228.

Hölzel, B. K., et al. (2011). Mindfulness practice leads to increases in regional gray matter density. *Psychiatry Research: Neuroimaging*, 191(1), 36–43.

Puchalski, C. M., et al. (2009). Improving the quality of spiritual care as a dimension of palliative care: The FICA tool. *Journal of Palliative Medicine*, 12(10), 885–904.

Chapter 9:
Creativity: The Urge to Express and Transform

When words fail, the imagination steps in.

When ordinary language collapses, creativity offers a bridge.

Creativity, in its many forms, often emerges as both refuge and revelation in the lives of people living with serious mental illness. Whether through painting, poetry, costume design, story-making, collage, or even elaborate interior decorating in institutional rooms, creative expression is not ancillary—it is vital. In a world often ruled by diagnostic criteria and deficits, creativity provides a rare and resilient form of agency.

In the face of overwhelming mental illness, when words fail and the mind fractures, creativity becomes an unspoken language. It is a way of expressing what words cannot, a channel for emotions that might otherwise remain hidden. Art, music, writing, and other creative outlets provide people with a lifeline—not just a distraction, but a vital connection to self and the world around them.

Creativity encompasses any act of imaginative expression—drawing, painting, sculpting, writing, music-making, fantasy storytelling—that translates internal experiences into tangible form. Creative expression—whether through art, music, writing, or storytelling—is another resilient spark. For many individuals, creating offers a way to externalize inner experiences that defy ordinary language. Creativity offers a pathway for

emotional expression and identity preservation. Creativity is not merely a symptom of disorganized thought. It is a form of organized hope. Even amid cognitive fragmentation, many individuals create:
- Drawings, paintings, collages that externalize internal states
- Stories or poems that give structure to chaos
- Imaginary worlds that offer safety or empowerment

The urge to create and express oneself is a fundamental human drive. For individuals who may struggle with verbal communication or processing complex emotions, creative outlets can become powerful sparks of life. These outlets may take many forms, including:
- Drawing and visual arts: Using colors, shapes, and lines to communicate feelings, ideas, or simply to engage with the sensory experience of creating. This can range from detailed artwork to simple doodles.
- Writing: Allows individuals to express thoughts, feelings, and experiences through words—whether in the form of poetry, journaling, short stories, or even simple lists—and can provide a private, powerful way to process emotions and make sense of inner experiences.
- Storytelling: Sharing narratives, whether real or imagined, can be a way to connect with others, explore different perspectives, and find meaning in experiences. This can be verbal storytelling, creating narratives through art, or even acting out scenarios.
- Music Creation: Composing melodies, writing lyrics, or experimenting with sounds can be a deeply personal and expressive outlet.
- Crafting: Engaging in hands-on activities like knitting, sculpting, or building can provide a sense of accomplishment and a tangible form of self-expression.

Supporting this spark might involve providing access to art supplies, writing materials, quiet spaces for creative work, or opportunities for patients to share their creations, if they wish. Encouraging experimentation without judgment is key. For caregivers and clinicians, observing the themes and emotions expressed through creative work can offer valuable insights into the individual's inner world.

Neurobiological Mechanisms of Creativity

Creativity is not merely a psychological or emotional process—it is also deeply biological. Neuroimaging studies have shown that engaging in creative activities activates multiple brain regions associated with emotion regulation, executive function, and reward processing.

Research has identified the default mode network (DMN)—a network of interacting brain regions including the medial prefrontal cortex, posterior cingulate cortex, and temporoparietal junction—as crucial in the process of creative thinking. This network is associated with self-referential thought, imagination, and the generation of new ideas.

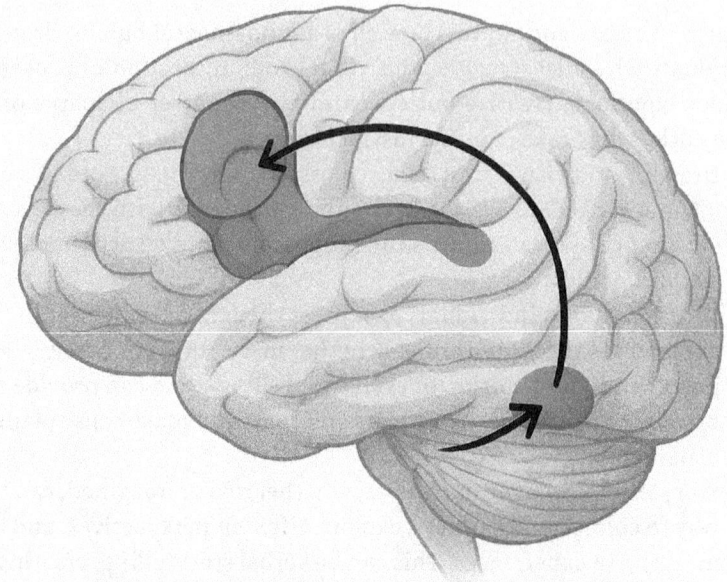

Default Mode Network
- Medial prefrontal cortex
- Posterior cingulate cortex
- Temporoparietal junction

Creative flow states, often reported by individuals when fully immersed in artistic activities, are linked to increased dopamine release in the brain's reward pathways. Dopamine, a key neurotransmitter associated with pleasure, motivation, and cognitive flexibility, is also implicated in mood disorders, schizophrenia, and other severe mental illnesses.

Psychologist Dr. Daniel Latendresse explained how psychodrama reignites agency: "Creativity often flourishes in flow states." His emphasis on flow echoes broader research on recovery through immersive expression.

Functional MRI studies have found that when individuals take part in creative tasks, there is increased connectivity between the DMN and the executive control network, which includes the dorsolateral prefrontal cortex. This suggests that creativity involves a balance of spontaneous and deliberate thinking—an interplay between free-flowing imagination and structured planning.

In patients with serious mental illness, especially bipolar disorder and schizophrenia, some researchers have observed heightened activity in associative networks of the brain. While this may lead to disorganized thinking in extreme cases, it also allows for unique and novel connections that underlie creative breakthroughs.

In short, the brain's architecture for creativity is intimately tied to the same systems affected by mental illness. When channeled constructively, creative expression can tap into these circuits in ways that foster healing, insight, and resilience.

Creativity in the Context of Serious Mental Illness

Studies on the effectiveness of creative arts therapies for people living with severe mental illness have shown promising results. For example, music therapy has been found to reduce negative symptoms and improve social interaction in people living with schizophrenia. Art therapy has also been shown to enhance self-esteem and provide a non-verbal outlet for emotional distress in this population.

Clinical Observations:

- Nonverbal patients sometimes communicate vividly through drawing or painting.
- Journals kept during manic episodes often reveal layered emotional landscapes, even when outward behavior appears chaotic.
- A manic individual writes hundreds of pages of poetry overnight, touching on themes of love, loss, and immortality.
- Storytelling—whether verbal, written, or through fantasy—can serve as an emotional processing tool.
- A mute patient suddenly sketches vivid scenes of emotional turmoil.
- Someone in the throes of paranoia builds intricate models or collages that symbolically represent fears and hopes.

Jamal, a 26-year-old with schizoaffective disorder, often isolated himself in the corner of the dayroom. During one hospitalization, a nurse offered him a simple art project: cutting images from magazines to create a collage. At first, Jamal was resistant, but over time, he became absorbed in the process.

His collage began as a jumble of random images, but slowly, it began to form a narrative: broken clocks, bridges, open doors, and faces looking up to the sky. When asked to describe it, Jamal said, "The clocks are all stopped. Time is broken. The bridge leads to where I'm supposed to go, but I don't know how to cross."

The act of creating something tangible from his inner chaos helped Jamal understand his feelings of fragmentation and yearning for connection. His art became a symbolic language through which he could process and articulate his distress. His story illustrates a larger truth: art can bypass clinical language and access something more intimate. I've seen a single poem reveal more about a person than months of chart notes. Providing Jamal with art supplies led to fewer aggressive episodes and greater engagement with therapy.

Clinical Takeaway: Art can create symbolic order when verbal thought is fragmented, and engaging this creativity can reduce behavioral disturbances.

Psychiatric vulnerability may enhance creative expression. Research suggests a link between bipolar spectrum traits and divergent thinking, artistic creativity, and risk-taking. Kay Redfield Jamison's seminal work explores this overlap, both statistically and narratively.

Imagination as Survival Strategy

The human imagination allows individuals to transcend circumstance. For many patients living with severe mental illness, imaginative activity offers sanctuary from trauma, stigma, boredom, and institutionalization. It is a space in which they are no longer patients but creators—authors of their own mythologies, stories, and internal universes.

Sometimes these creative worlds are fluid and expansive:

- A man who believes he is inventing a machine to purify water for the homeless
- A woman who creates an entire cast of fictional characters she speaks to for guidance and comfort
- A youth who draws futuristic cities where everyone has a safe place to live

Rather than dismissing these as mere delusion or fantasy, we can ask: What purpose does this imagination serve? What is it trying to restore, preserve, or protect?

Creativity as a Therapeutic Outlet: A Bridge to Self-Expression

Creativity has long been used as a therapeutic tool in mental health care. Scientific evidence supports the role of artistic expression, whether through drawing, writing, or music, in reducing the impact of mental illness.

Art and Self-Expression

The therapeutic use of art is well-documented in the field of psychology. Art therapy allows individuals to express emotions that may be difficult to verbalize. A study by Kramer (1971) demonstrated that art therapy could help people living with schizophrenia process complex emotions, thereby reducing symptoms of anxiety and depression. In particular, creative expression provides a non-verbal outlet for experiences of fear, isolation, and confusion, common among those with severe mental illness.

Improved Cognitive and Emotional Outcomes

Engaging in creative activities can also enhance cognitive flexibility. In a study published in the *Journal of Affective Disorders*, individuals who engaged in structured art therapy showed significant improvements in mood and cognitive functioning, including better problem-solving skills and emotional regulation. For people with conditions like bipolar disorder or schizoaffective disorder, creativity provides an important tool to manage symptoms and find balance during emotional extremes.

Music as Emotional Regulation

Music therapy has been shown to be particularly effective for people living with severe mental illness. A meta-analysis concluded that music therapy significantly reduces symptoms of anxiety, depression, and agitation in psychiatric patients. Music can facilitate emotional processing, improve self-expression, and provide a sense of connection to others. This is particularly beneficial in helping people living with severe mental illness reconnect with their emotions and the external world.

The Profound Connection Between Creativity and Emotional Well-Being

Scientific studies have increasingly demonstrated the therapeutic benefits of engaging in creative activities. For instance, a meta-analysis of art therapy interventions found significant reductions in anxiety and depression across various populations. Furthermore, neuroimaging studies suggest that creative engagement activates brain regions involved in emotional regulation and reward processing, contributing to feelings of well-being and flow.

Creativity as a Form of Communication and Connection

Research in communication studies and art therapy highlights how creative expression can serve as a powerful communication tool, particularly for people living with communication challenges. Shared creative endeavors, like community art projects or music groups, have been shown to foster social connection and a sense of belonging.

I've read poetry written on napkins in psych wards that humbled me more than anything published in journals.

One patient spent weeks in near silence, refusing groups and barely engaging—until we started an art group. She asked for charcoal pencils and began sketching faces: haunted, vivid, alive. When I asked who they were, she said, "These are all the people I've lost." Her art spoke grief she couldn't put into words.

The innate drive to create often remains a stubborn, defiant spark, even when identity is under siege.

Leonard, a patient with chronic depression, rarely engaged verbally. One day, I noticed a paper bird on his bedside table. He had been folding origami since childhood. As he shared more of his creations, it became clear that this was not just art—it was a therapeutic outlet and a sign of a preserved self.

A woman with bipolar disorder shared how journaling gave her a voice: "Writing, too, becomes a spark." Her account illustrates how creativity externalizes chaos and restores coherence.

The Many Faces of Creativity in Serious Mental Illness

Creativity takes many forms in the lives of people with serious mental illness, offering both relief and revelation. One of the most visible and accessible of these is art.

Art as Expression of Inner Worlds

Art therapy—whether formal or informal—can become a crucial tool in restoring self-narrative. It allows for expression beyond what linear language can often convey. Some patients who cannot articulate their trauma or symptoms in words will create visual representations that hold complexity, ambiguity, and truth. For many individuals, drawing, painting, or sculpting can allow them to express emotions or experiences they cannot put into words. Whether it's a vivid image of fear, a comforting symbol, or abstract colors that reflect inner turmoil, the art becomes a narrative that transcends the limitations of the verbal mind.

Clinicians can observe:
- Color choices and patterns
- Recurring themes or symbols
- Changes in style, intensity, and affect over time

Art becomes a diagnostic and therapeutic window. But more importantly, it becomes a space where the patient's truth is honored without interruption.

Writing as Catharsis

For others, writing serves as a form of release. This might include poetry, journaling, or storytelling. Writing allows individuals to craft their own narrative, reclaiming ownership of a mind that may feel fractured by psychosis or depression.

Clinical Insight: Even if the writing doesn't make perfect sense, it still allows the individual to experience a sense of control and coherence. The very act of organizing thoughts can be therapeutic.

Music as Emotional Regulation

(Discussed in more detail in Chapter 7) Music, whether listening or playing, has a profound effect on emotional regulation. Individuals with serious mental illness often turn to music to soothe themselves or to release pent-up emotions. Music's repetitive, rhythmic nature can also help ground individuals in the present moment, breaking cycles of rumination or distress.

Offer Unstructured Creative Time

Provide many creative materials (art supplies, writing journals, musical instruments, etc.) without imposing any requirements. Creativity should be free of judgment, expectations, or assessment. Let the individual create for the sake of creating, without pressure to produce a finished product.

Introduce Creative Prompts

For individuals who are unsure how to begin, offer simple prompts:
- "If today were a color, what color would it be?"
- "Write a letter to your future self."
- "Can you draw how you feel right now?"

Let these prompts serve as gentle guides but avoid steering their creativity in a particular direction.

Celebrate the Process, Not the Product

Engage with the art without evaluating its "quality." Focus on the process, the act of creation itself. Ask about what inspired the work, what emotions or thoughts came up, and how the process felt.

The Line Between Creative Genius and Madness

The history of psychiatry is filled with tension around the so-called "mad genius." From Van Gogh to Sylvia Plath, society has long romanticized the suffering artist while often institutionalizing or marginalizing them in life. Many people living with serious mental illness do show heightened aesthetic sensitivity, original vision, or synesthetic perception. Mania can produce surges of inspiration and flow; psychosis can give rise to metaphoric brilliance. But we must be careful not to glamorize suffering or reduce creativity to symptomatology.

The goal is not to mine illness for art. It is to recognize that the creative impulse may be part of what helps individuals survive illness—and sometimes transform it.

Therapeutic Engagement: The Therapeutic Power of Creation

Creativity has long been used as a therapeutic tool. Its importance is reflected in practices like art therapy and music therapy, which are designed to help patients access emotional truths that might be hard to express verbally.

Clinical Insight:

Creativity is not simply a diversion. It taps into deep cognitive processes, from motor skills to emotional regulation. In doing so, it can help individuals reclaim parts of themselves that illness often obscures.

Clinicians and caregivers can encourage the therapeutic power of creation in the following ways:
- Offer materials for artistic expression (art, writing, or music): journals, colored pencils, clay.
- Encourage storytelling without immediate judgment or clinical interpretation.
- Recognize that metaphor, fantasy, and abstraction often carry profound emotional truths.
- Honor symbolic content without rushing to clinical interpretation.
- Celebrate the act of creation itself as a therapeutic success.

Clinicians may be tempted to overanalyze creative works, seeking hidden diagnostic clues. Yet a more supportive approach involves guiding principles such as:
- Creative productions may sometimes contain disturbing themes (violence, sexuality, despair) that require careful, empathetic handling.
- Offer opportunities for non-verbal expression: art supplies, journals, musical instruments.

- Celebrate the act of creating rather than critiquing the content.
- Recognize that symbolic creations often provide insight into emotional needs without needing immediate interpretation.

To create is to affirm, "I exist. I feel. I matter." Even when mental illness obscures identity, creative expression reclaims it. Creative sparks are often flickering signs of autonomy and resilience, worthy of careful protection.

Ethical Considerations

- Respect the art's integrity: Creativity is deeply personal. Do not force individuals to explain or interpret their work, especially if they seem hesitant or uncomfortable.
- Avoid art therapy overload: While creativity is a powerful tool, it should not be used as a replacement for clinical treatment. Ensure that creative activities are supplemental to, not a substitution for, psychiatric care.
- Cultural sensitivity: Different cultures have distinct ways of expressing creativity. Be mindful of cultural context when interpreting or engaging with creative works.

Case Example: Ruben

Ruben, a 42-year-old man with schizophrenia, spent most of his time alone in his room at a long-term care facility. Staff described him as withdrawn and "flat." But one therapist noticed Ruben constantly doodled on napkins. After encouragement, Ruben began participating in a weekly art group. Over time, he produced a large series of paintings—abstract, vivid, and filled with repeating symbols. In therapy, he revealed these images represented different "states of mind" he had experienced: storms, silences, awakenings. He said, "When I can't talk about it, I paint it out of me." Eventually, his work was featured in a local gallery show on outsider art. The pride he felt reshaped how others saw him, and how he saw himself.

Making Space for Creativity in Clinical Settings

Institutional environments are rarely designed for creativity. Schedules, medications, risk assessments, and behavior charts dominate the agenda. But when space is made for expression, even briefly, profound shifts can occur.

Ways to encourage creativity in mental health care:
- Journaling prompts in group therapy
- Access to art supplies or musical instruments
- Poetry readings, open mics, or gallery displays
- Collaborative murals or collective storytelling projects

These do not need to be framed as therapy to be therapeutic. They are ways to affirm the spark of originality, expression, and voice.

"In community programs, art often unlocks expression," one volunteer recalled. Such testimonies confirm that creativity transcends symptom and diagnosis.

Conclusion

Creativity enables the preservation of agency and identity assertion. It allows patients to transform overwhelming experiences into something visible, something shaped, and ultimately, something shareable. It allows an individual to externalize suffering, reshape confusion, and assert presence in a world that might otherwise feel flattening or dehumanizing.

Creativity fosters agency, self-expression, and symbolic healing. When control is lost in other areas of life, creative expression restores a sense of mastery. It can transform the internal chaos of mental illness into something meaningful and tangible. Creativity provides a voice when words fail and a sense of stability in an often-uncontrollable world.

For clinicians and families, fostering creativity is not just an activity; it is a way to honor resilience and potential that endure even in the depths of illness. By respecting and nurturing creative expression, we allow individuals to reclaim their humanity and agency in a world that often seeks to define them by their diagnosis.

Creativity offers more than distraction; it offers transformation. It is where meaning is born, identity is explored, and agency is reclaimed. In severe mental illness, where so much is taken—time, autonomy, relationships—creativity gives something back. It gives story. It gives shape. It gives self.

When clinicians honor the creative spark—not as excess, but as essence—they open the door to healing that is not just clinical, but deeply human.

Table 9.1 — Creativity and Recovery

Outlet	Example	Benefit
Writing	Journals, poetry	Identity, coherence
Art	Painting, crafts	Expression, calm
Performance	Theater, music	Confidence, connection

Glăveanu, V. P. (2014). *Thinking Through Creativity & Culture: Toward an Integrated Model*. Routledge. (Creativity as agency within constraints.)

Beaty, R. E., Benedek, M., Silvia, P. J., & Schacter, D. L. (2016). Creative cognition and brain networks. *Trends in Cognitive Sciences*, 20(2), 87–95; Beaty, R. E., et al. (2015). Creativity and the default–executive coupling. *PNAS*, 112(47), 14738–14743.

Dietrich, A. (2004). The cognitive neuroscience of creativity. *Psychonomic Bulletin & Review*, 11(6), 1011–1026; Ulrich, M., & Ziemssen, T. (2016). Flow experience and autonomic activity. *Biological Psychology*, 115, 54–60.

Kinney, D. K., Richards, R., Lowing, P. A., LeBlanc, D., Zimbalist, M. E., & Harlan, P. (2001). Creativity and psychosis: A shared vulnerability model. *American Journal of Psychiatry*, 158(11), 1733–1741; Jamison, K. R. (1993). *Touched with Fire: Manic-Depressive Illness and the Artistic Temperament*. Free Press.

Geretsegger, M., Mössler, K. A., et al. (2014). Music therapy for people with schizophrenia and schizophrenia-like disorders. *Cochrane Database of Systematic Reviews*, CD004025.

Stuckey, H. L., & Nobel, J. (2010). The connection between art, healing, and public health. *American Journal of Public Health*, 100(2), 254–263; De Witte, M., Spruit, A., et al. (2021). Effects of arts therapies on mental health: A systematic review. *Frontiers in Psychology*, 12, 664–726.

Pennebaker, J. W., & Smyth, J. M. (2016). *Opening Up by Writing It Down* (3rd ed.). Guilford; Forgeard, M. J. C., & Eichner, K. V. (2014). Creativity and mental health: A profile of evidence. *Psychology of Aesthetics, Creativity, and the Arts*, 8(3), 241–253.

Fancourt, D., Perkins, R., Ascenso, S., et al. (2016). Group drumming modulates anxiety, depression, and social resilience. *PLOS ONE*, 11(3), e0151136.

Crawford, M. J., Killaspy, H., et al. (2012). Group art therapy as adjunctive treatment for schizophrenia: MATISSE trial. *BMJ*, 344, e846 (see discussion and secondary outcomes/qualitative insights despite neutral primary outcome); Sandmire, D. A., et al. (2012). Psychological effects of art making. *Art Therapy*, 29(2), 68–73.

MacGregor, J. M. (1999). *The Discovery of the Art of the Insane*. Princeton University Press;

Rhodes, C. (2000). *Outsider Art: Spontaneous Alternatives*. Thames & Hudson.

Chapter 10:
Movement: The Body's Enduring Language

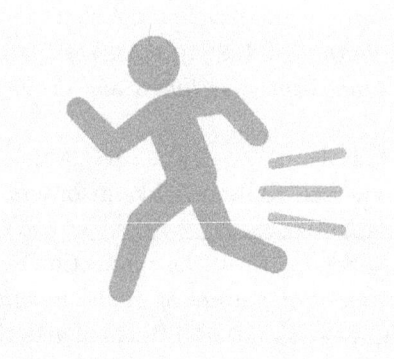

The body carries wisdom the mind cannot always speak.

The body knows, even when the mind forgets.

The body in motion is often overlooked in the treatment of serious mental illness, even though it speaks volumes—through pacing, rocking, dancing, flinching, or stillness. Long before words are formed, the body expresses suffering, longing, regulation, and release. Movement, like music and creativity, emerges as both symptom and spark—a deeply encoded language through which individuals navigate distress and reclaim vitality.

To move is to be alive. And in serious mental illness, movement is often a lifeline to coherence and control. In the landscape of serious mental illness, movement often becomes a language of its own. When words fail, the body moves—pacing, rocking, swaying, tapping, or gesturing. These movements are not merely physical actions; they are expressions of inner states, ways of coping with emotional turmoil, and attempts to communicate what the mind cannot say. For people living with severe mental illness, the body itself can become a sanctuary, an instrument of release, and even a form of resilience.

Movement includes everything from conscious dancing to unconscious swaying or repetitive motions. It is the body's way of regulating, expressing, and processing emotion. Movement—both conscious and unconscious—often persists when verbal communication falters. We see this in:

- Rocking, pacing, or rhythmic swaying
- Spontaneous dance, gestures, or hand movements
- Somatic rituals: bodily practices such as rhythmic breathing, rocking, stretching, or repetitive movement that help regulate emotional storms.

I once watched a man dance barefoot in the hallway. It was disarming, raw, and beautiful.

Movement is not just physical; it's a fundamental aspect of being, a primal spark that can persist and offer a pathway back to connection.

Sophie was in a profound catatonic state. A physical therapist began moving her limbs in rhythmic patterns. Sophie's fingers twitched in response. It was fleeting, but meaningful. Even when her mind seemed locked, the body's drive to respond endured.

The body is not just a vessel but also a powerful means of communication and emotional expression. For individuals who may have difficulty articulating their feelings verbally, movement can become a vital spark of life:

- Dance: Expressing emotions and connecting with rhythm and music through structured or free-form movement. Dance can be a powerful release and a source of joy.
- Pacing: While sometimes associated with anxiety, rhythmic pacing can also be a way of processing thoughts and emotions, providing a sense of grounding or release.
- Gestures: Expressive hand movements or body language that accompany or even replace verbal communication. Observing and understanding these gestures can provide insights into the individual's emotional state.
- Repetitive body motions: Rocking, hand flapping, or other repetitive movements can serve various functions, including self-soothing, sensory regulation, or a way of expressing internal feelings that are difficult to articulate verbally.
- Exercise: Engaging in physical activity, even simple movements like stretching or walking, can be a way to release tension, improve mood, and connect with one's body.
- Movement rituals: These include repeated sequences of motion like clapping, humming while walking, or rhythmic body tensing. Such behaviors may have protective, spiritual, or grounding meaning to the individual.

The Neurobiology of Movement and Emotion

Movement is deeply rooted in the brain's architecture. The motor cortex, basal ganglia, cerebellum, and brain stem coordinate to initiate and regulate voluntary and involuntary movements. These structures are also closely connected to emotional and cognitive processing regions like the amygdala, prefrontal cortex, and limbic system.

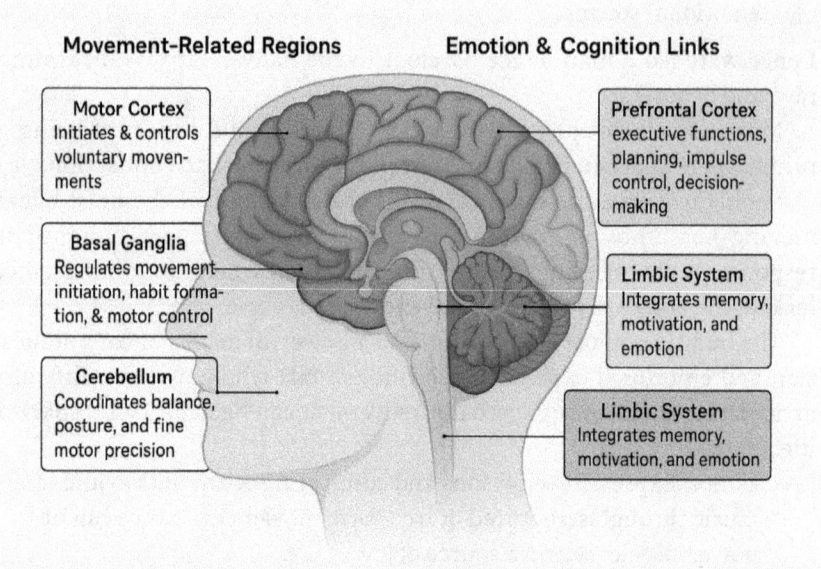

Basal Ganglia: Often implicated in psychiatric disorders, this cluster of nuclei plays a critical role in initiating movement and also intersects with circuits involved in motivation and reward. In schizophrenia and bipolar disorder, dysfunction in dopaminergic signaling in the basal ganglia can result in both motor symptoms (like catatonia or agitation) and emotional dysregulation.

Cerebellum: Traditionally known for its role in balance and coordination, recent research also links the cerebellum to emotional regulation and cognitive processing. Its dysfunction may contribute to affective and psychomotor disturbances seen in severe mental illness.

Mirror Neuron System: Found primarily in the premotor cortex and inferior parietal lobule, mirror neurons are activated both when a person performs an action and when they observe someone else performing that action. This system may underlie the capacity for empathy and social learning—and may explain why movement therapies in groups can foster connection and reduce isolation.

Vagus Nerve and Polyvagal Theory: The vagus nerve mediates the body's parasympathetic responses. Polyvagal theory suggests that rhythmic, soothing movements can stimulate the vagus nerve, promoting calm and social engagement states—key goals in trauma-informed care.

Endorphins and Neuroplasticity: Physical activity increases endorphin release and supports neurogenesis. Movement-based therapies can promote emotional resilience by enhancing synaptic plasticity and modulating stress pathways.

These systems together illustrate that movement is not just a mechanical process but a deeply integrated neurobiological phenomenon with implications for mood regulation, sensory integration, and relational attunement.

Recent brain imaging studies show that mindful movement activates the default mode network (DMN), a set of interconnected brain regions involved in self-reflection, memory, and the integration of past experiences with present awareness. It is often overactive in depression and rumination. Rhythmic movement has also been linked to decreased amygdala activation during stress, suggesting a calming effect on fear-based circuits. The insula—responsible for interoception and bodily awareness—is strengthened through consistent movement practices, enhancing emotional insight and bodily integration.

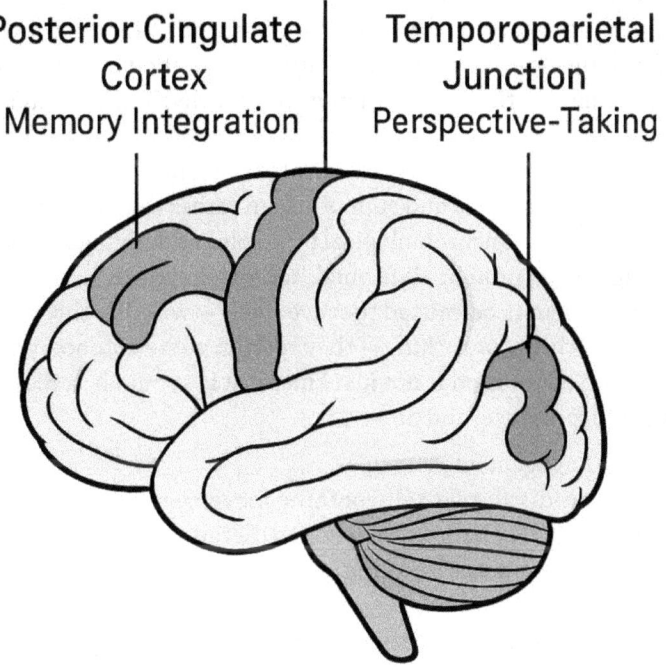

Expanded Implications for Clinical Care

Movement should be assessed and encouraged not only as a symptom to monitor but as a clinical tool to empower. Clinicians can:

- Incorporate movement logs to track emotional and behavioral correlations.
- Introduce gentle movement as part of psychoeducation and skill-building.
- Create individualized movement routines as part of recovery planning.
- Pair movement with verbal therapies to enhance trauma processing.
- Collaborate with occupational therapists to design sensory-informed movement spaces.
- Use movement as a check-in: "Where do you feel tension? Can you move that part of your body?"

I once watched a man pace for hours—not agitated, but grounded. That rhythm gave him peace.

For some, movement takes the form of ritual. One peer explained how daily walks provided control. This account reminds us that even modest routines can spark autonomy.

Movement is a form of language I've come to respect. I used to think movement was about exercise. Now I know it's about reclaiming the body.

I once had a patient who refused all therapy but would pace the halls every morning at dawn. One day, I walked with him. Step by step, he started talking—first about the weather, then about the voices. Those walks became our therapy. Motion gave him rhythm, and rhythm gave him voice.

Family members and care staff can also be trained to recognize beneficial movement behaviors and support them rather than discourage them. An understanding of neurobiological principles underlying movement can reduce stigma and promote informed, compassionate care.

When a patient is permitted to move freely—whether through pacing, dancing, stretching, or rocking—they reclaim some autonomy over their inner world. That motion is not just kinetic; it is symbolic: a reclaiming of rhythm, will, presence, and power.

Therapeutic Engagement Strategies

- Allow non-disruptive, self-soothing movements.
- Incorporate rhythmic activities into therapeutic work.
- View movement as a meaningful communication, not merely as a symptom.
- Reframe movement not simply as pathology but as communication.

- Encourage safe rhythmic activities: drumming, walking, mindful breathing, dance therapy.
- Allow non-harmful repetitive behaviors unless they interfere with safety or health.
- Use movement breaks during sessions to regulate affect.
- Provide fidget tools or stress balls as proxies for larger movement needs.

Engagement Strategies

- Create space for movement: Offer opportunities for movement in a safe and structured environment. If a person tends to pace, designate walking space. If they enjoy dancing, provide a quiet area where music and movement are welcome.
- Encourage rhythmic activities: Introduce activities like swaying to music, tapping feet, or guided stretching with breathing. Rhythmic sensory input can soothe and stabilize.
- Use movement to promote emotional awareness: Prompt individuals to reflect on their movement:
    o How does it feel when you move like that?
    o What is your body asking for right now?
- Incorporate mindfulness with movement: Integrate practices like Tai Chi or yoga to help individuals engage both body and awareness, fostering emotional regulation and interoception.

Through movement, individuals reconnect with sensation, autonomy, and life force.

As Director Louis Pachlin described, "Recreation therapy often begins with the body." His reflections show that movement anchors identity as much as expression does.

Ethical Considerations

- Respect boundaries: never compel someone into movement-based activities.
- Be culturally sensitive: recognize that movement practices may hold cultural or spiritual meaning.
- Be nonjudgmental: what may seem purposeless may serve critical emotional or regulatory functions.
- Avoid pathologizing coping movements unless they cause harm.
- Promote autonomy by asking permission before inviting movement.

Exercise improves not only cardiovascular health but also psychiatric outcomes. Vancampfort's meta-analysis shows strong evidence that physical activity improves mood, cognition, and functioning in schizophrenia, while also reducing the metabolic side effects of antipsychotics.

Conclusion

Movement is not merely a physical act; it is a form of expression, regulation, and communication. For many people living with severe mental illness, movement allows them to bridge the gap between their inner experiences and the outside world. By providing a space where movement is allowed and even encouraged, clinicians and families can support the emotional well-being of individuals in ways that words cannot.

Movement is a spark that cannot be extinguished. It is a way to engage with the world—and with oneself—when other pathways of expression are blocked. By recognizing the importance of movement, we affirm the person's autonomy, provide a channel for emotional expression, and support their ongoing resilience.

In the landscape of severe mental illness, movement tells the story of survival. It is how the body remembers, how it defends, and how it seeks freedom. Sometimes chaotic, sometimes graceful, movement is the original language of trauma, and one of its most accessible paths to healing.

To honor movement is to honor the body as a site of wisdom, not just pathology. It is to say: Your gestures matter. Your pacing tells us something. Your dance is not a distraction—it's a declaration.

Table 10.1 — Movement and Mental Health

Activity	Effect	Clinical Use
Walking	Calms, regulates	Grounding, accessible
Yoga	Reduces anxiety	Trauma recovery
Dance	Builds joy, social bonds	Group therapy

Sheets-Johnstone, M. (2011). *The Primacy of Movement* (2nd ed.). John Benjamins. (Movement as foundational human "language"/sense-making.)

Hutt, C., Hutt, S. J. (1968). *Stereotypies in Human Subjects*. Pergamon; Kappeler, L., et al. (2013). Repetitive behaviors as self-regulation in stress. *Developmental Psychobiology*, 55(6), 569–583.

Haber, S. N., & Knutson, B. (2010). The reward circuit: linking primate anatomy and human imaging. *Neuropsychopharmacology*, 35, 4–26; Howes, O. D., & Kapur, S. (2009). Dopamine in schizophrenia—revisited. *Schizophrenia Bulletin*, 35(3), 549–562.

Schmahmann, J. D. (2019). The cerebellum and cognition. *Neuroscience Letters*, 688, 62–75; Stoodley, C. J., & Schmahmann, J. D. (2009). Functional topography of the cerebellum for motor, cognitive, and affective processing. *NeuroImage*, 44(2), 489–501.

Rizzolatti, G., & Craighero, L. (2004). The mirror-neuron system. *Annual Review of Neuroscience*, 27, 169–192; Iacoboni, M. (2009). *Mirroring People*. Picador.

Porges, S. W. (2011). *The Polyvagal Theory*. Norton; Dana, D. (2018). *The Polyvagal Theory in Therapy*. Norton. (Use with nuance—clinical utility despite ongoing debate.)

Boecker, H., et al. (2008). The runner's high: opioidergic mechanisms in humans. *Cerebral Cortex*, 18(11), 2523–2531; van Praag, H., et al. (1999). Running enhances neurogenesis, learning, and LTP. *PNAS*, 96(23), 13427–13431.

Brewer, J. A., et al. (2011). Meditation experience is associated with deactivation of the DMN. *PNAS*, 108(50), 20254–20259; Fox, K. C. R., et al. (2016). Meta-analysis of meditation's brain effects. *Neuroscience & Biobehavioral Reviews*, 65, 208–228; Thoma, M. V., et al. (2013). Music and stress reduction: autonomic/endocrine responses. *PLoS ONE*, 8(8), e70156.

Vancampfort, D., et al. (2012). Physical activity & sedentary behavior in major mental illness: systematic review. *Acta Psychiatrica Scandinavica*, 125(5), 352–362; Firth, J., et al. (2015). Aerobic exercise improves cognition and functioning in schizophrenia: meta-analysis. *Schizophrenia Bulletin*, 41(3), 486–496; Stubbs, B., et al. (2018). EPA guidance: physical activity in severe mental illness. *European Psychiatry*, 54, 124–144.

Koch, S. C., et al. (2019). Effects of dance movement therapy: meta-analysis across populations (depression/anxiety). *Frontiers in Psychology*, 10, 936; Ren, J., & Xia, J. (2013/2014). DMT for schizophrenia—pilot evidence for negative symptom/social function gains. *The Arts in Psychotherapy*, 40(3), 269–274.

Dauwan, M., et al. (2016). Physical exercise for schizophrenia: systematic review and meta-analysis of walking/aerobic programs. *Journal of Nervous and Mental Disease*, 204(9), 620–631; Soundy, A., et al. (2015). The experiences of walking in people with severe mental illness. *International Journal of Therapy and Rehabilitation*, 22(3), 131–141.

Chapter 11:
Rituals as Spark: A Clinical Reframe

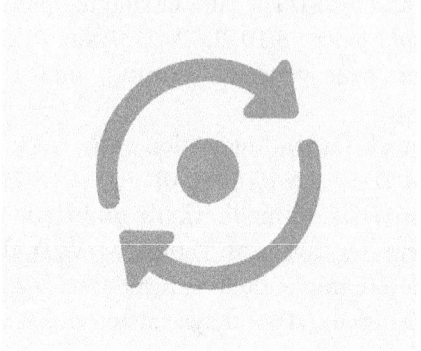

Having explored the sparks of spirit, creation, and movement, we now turn our attention to another fundamental aspect of human experience that can serve as a significant source of comfort and engagement: rituals. Often ingrained in our daily lives, both consciously and unconsciously, rituals provide a sense of predictability and stability. For individuals navigating the complexities of severe mental illness, these familiar routines and repetitive actions can be particularly anchoring, acting as subtle yet powerful sparks that foster a sense of normalcy and well-being.

Rituals are the architecture of safety. They are repeated behaviors, sometimes simple, sometimes complex—that bring order to an otherwise disordered world. In serious mental illness, rituals can take on outsized significance. They are not always pathological; often, they are lifelines—structures that hold meaning, preserve identity, and offer continuity through chaos.

Rituals helped me understand how people survive chaos. They aren't just habits; they're anchors. Rituals, I've learned, are not superstitions; they're scaffolding. They help people hold their days together. I've seen patients find meaning in the smallest routines: folding clothes, blessing a meal, lighting a candle.

In clinical settings, we often encounter rituals that manifest as routines: patients who pace in rhythmic patterns, who pray at exact times, who arrange their possessions in precise order. These actions are often interpreted as compulsions or symptoms, but they may also reflect the person's attempt to find grounding, structure, and meaning.

Rituals are cultural, spiritual, and personal. They appear in the way people dress, eat, greet, and grieve. Even in the throes of psychosis, patients may adhere to sacred practices passed down through generations. A Haitian man may recite a morning prayer, a Jewish woman may light a Friday candle, a secular artist may draw the same shape each day. These patterns matter—they are the soul's choreography.

When everything else felt out of control, rituals helped my patients feel like something still belonged to them. A woman in the unit would light an imaginary candle every night before sleep. She said it was for her mother. Staff used to redirect her, until we realized this ritual calmed her more than any sedative. Eventually, we placed a small electric candle by her bedside. It flickered quietly, and so did her peace.

While some rituals interfere with function or safety, many do not. The task of the clinician is not to eliminate ritual, but to discern which rituals heal and which harm. Those that bring calm, identity, or hope can be integrated into treatment plans as stabilizing forces.

Ritual is one of humanity's oldest arts of survival, a technology for managing uncertainty, trauma, and transition. Whether religious or secular, private or communal, rituals serve to anchor the psyche in time, structure the day, and affirm identity. In the lives of people living with severe mental illness, rituals often emerge not only as cultural artifacts, but as deeply personal survival strategies.

Rather than dismissing ritualistic behavior as pathology (e.g., in OCD or catatonia), clinicians can inquire about meaning, support adaptive rituals, and co-create healing ones. A morning walk, a prayer chant, a nightly journaling session—all can serve as sparks of continuity and selfhood. Rituals absolutely qualify as a distinct and powerful spark in the lives of people living with severe mental illness. They often serve as anchors of structure, identity, and meaning—especially when internal reality feels fragmented or chaotic.

Rituals, religious or secular, offer stability in the chaotic inner world of psychosis. Tanya Luhrmann's anthropological research reveals how structured rituals provide coherence, identity, and comfort in the face of illness. Director Michelle Goscinsky described how, "At the Recovery Center, ritual became structure." Her account illustrates how predictable routines foster community and stability.

Neurobiology of Rituals

Rituals are not just cultural practices; they are embodied behaviors with measurable effects on the brain. Neuroscience shows that they influence three major systems:

1. Activate the Reward System
   The repetitive and structured nature of rituals stimulates the brain's reward circuitry, releasing dopamine, a neurotransmitter linked to pleasure and reinforcement. This creates a positive feedback loop, encouraging continued engagement.
   ▶ *Why this matters:* Rituals often feel comforting because they provide small, predictable bursts of satisfaction, much like the relief of completing a familiar habit.

2. Engage the Prefrontal Cortex
   Rituals demand focus and organization, activating the prefrontal cortex, the brain's hub for planning and self-regulation. This activation can downregulate the limbic system, reducing emotional reactivity and fostering calm.
   ▶ *Why this matters:* By occupying the brain's "planning center," rituals can quiet emotional storms, creating a felt sense of order and stability.

3. Reduce Neural Response to Failure
   Electroencephalogram (EEG) studies show that rituals decrease error-related negativity (ERN), a neural signal tied to performance anxiety and self-monitoring. This buffering effect may help protect people with serious mental illness from excessive self-criticism.
   ▶ *Why this matters:* Rituals can soften the impact of mistakes, helping individuals feel steadier and more resilient in the face of setbacks.

Together, these processes explain why rituals endure across cultures and history—and why, in the lives of people with serious mental illness, they remain a powerful spark for survival, meaning, and stability.

Even clinicians observe the resilience of rituals. One psychiatrist noted prayer and journaling as...

These sparks provide continuity, even in relapse.

Anxiety Reduction: Rituals offer predictability, activating the parasympathetic nervous system and quieting the limbic brain, leading to reduced physiological arousal and emotional distress.

Cognitive Efficiency: Ritualized behavior lowers cognitive load by minimizing decision fatigue and freeing up mental bandwidth—a benefit for those struggling with attention or executive function.

Social and Emotional Benefits: Engaging in rituals can foster belonging and social cohesion, key protective factors for individuals at risk of isolation.

Default Mode Network and Interoception: Rituals may engage the DMN, which supports narrative identity, and the insula, enhancing bodily awareness through structured behavior. These effects improve integration of self and emotion.

Pachlin emphasized ritual as an anchor of stability in patient lives. His words highlight how rituals transform unease into rhythm.

Psychiatric Anthropology and the Deep Logic of Repetition

Psychiatric anthropology has long observed how rituals serve as adaptive tools for individuals experiencing psychosis. Tanya Luhrmann's ethnographic research illustrates how people living with schizophrenia use ritual to shape voices, tame hallucinations, and preserve identity amidst chaos.

Repetitive acts—while sometimes labeled pathological—can reflect an effort to impose structure, regulate affect, or preserve memory.

Rituals may also serve as metaphoric anchors, helping individuals enact themes of cleansing, transition, or safety. The repetition is not mindless; it is often purposeful, carrying emotional logic even when unspoken.

Ritual vs. Compulsion: A Clinical Distinction

Understanding the difference between adaptive ritual and distressing compulsion is crucial. The distinction often lies in:
- Intentionality: Is the behavior meaningful or symbolic?
- Distress: Does interruption cause excessive anxiety?
- Flexibility: Is the behavior rigid or adaptable?
- Functionality: Does it support or impede daily life?

While some rituals are symptoms, others offer grounding and comfort in the midst of illness.

Mr. Chang, with severe OCD, had many compulsions. Yet each night, he gently arranged photos of his late wife and listened to the same symphony. These were not compulsions—they were sacred acts of remembrance and peace. Ritual, at its core, was a tether to meaning.

Clinicians should approach all ritualized behaviors with curiosity, not dismissal. Even maladaptive rituals can be reframed into more supportive routines with therapeutic guidance.

Rituals in Institutional Settings

In hospitals, where control is often externally imposed, patients may create personal rituals to regain agency such as:
- Folding clothes in specific ways
- Saying a repeated phrase before meals
- Walking specific routes before therapy

These rituals, when not harmful, can be adaptive coping mechanisms. Instead of suppressing them, clinicians can explore their significance and, when appropriate, integrate them into treatment routines.

Cultural and Spiritual Rituals: Honoring Identity

Rituals rooted in culture or faith carry deep personal meaning. Psychiatric systems that ignore or disrupt these rituals risk compounding distress or causing spiritual injury.
Clinicians should:
- Understand the patient's cultural and spiritual framework
- Explore how rituals may have been disrupted by illness or trauma
- Seek to preserve or co-create rituals as stabilizing anchors

Case Example: Marcos, a man with schizoaffective disorder, became distressed when his mealtime ritual—prayer and tray arrangement—was disrupted. A culturally sensitive staff member asked about its meaning. Marcos explained the ritual reminded him of his grandmother and gave him comfort during hunger. Allowing the ritual to continue decreased his agitation and improved engagement. The ritual became a therapeutic bridge, not a barrier.

Creating New Rituals in Recovery

Rituals are not only inherited—they can be created. In recovery, individuals can develop new rituals that affirm identity, mark transitions, and celebrate growth:
- Lighting candles for sobriety milestones
- Starting each day with a gratitude journal
- Weekly music sessions
- Anniversary rituals for progress

Clinicians can help design rituals that are:
- Personal and meaningful
- Simple and sustainable
- Flexible and growth-oriented
- Celebratory rather than symptom-focused

Rituals need not be elaborate to be effective. What matters is choice, meaning, and consistency. Like other sparks, rituals illuminate what endures in the human spirit—even in the face of profound illness.

Coffee, Cigarettes, and Other Ritual Sparks

In the landscape of serious mental illness, rituals take many forms—some soothing, some repetitive, some socially discouraged but nonetheless deeply human. Among the most common and persistent are the consumption of coffee, tea, and cigarettes. While often viewed clinically as habits or dependencies, these practices can also be understood as sparks—small, rhythmic acts that provide comfort, structure, and identity.

Consider the patient who begins each day with three cups of coffee before engaging in any group therapy, or the individual who times their cigarette breaks with remarkable precision, using each smoke as a marker of time, emotion, or interpersonal space. These behaviors are not always random. They carry significance—symbolic, sensory, neurochemical—and serve as familiar anchors in an unpredictable world.

Neurobiologically, both caffeine and nicotine engage key neurotransmitter systems implicated in schizophrenia, bipolar disorder, and depression. Nicotine, in particular, stimulates acetylcholine receptors and modulates dopamine pathways—both of which are involved in attention, reward, and mood regulation. It is no coincidence that smoking rates are disproportionately high among people living with schizophrenia and schizoaffective disorder.

In clinical care, these rituals can be frustrating, especially when they compete with medication regimens or health interventions. But dismissing them as merely unhealthy misses the deeper meaning. For some patients, the morning cup of coffee or the evening cigarette is not just a craving—it is a ritual of continuity. It is a way to assert control, maintain rhythm, and feel a thread of normalcy.

These practices may also be social. Coffee shared in a group home, tea served during a therapy session, or a cigarette offered on the ward patio may create micro-moments of connection and community. For individuals whose illness isolates them from typical social cues, these rituals offer a shared language—a pause in which to exist alongside others without pressure or judgment.

That is not to say we should ignore the health consequences or dependency risks. But in a recovery-oriented model, we recognize that healing must coexist with autonomy. If these small rituals provide comfort or clarity, they can be gently supported, even as alternative coping tools are introduced.

Coffee and cigarettes, like prayer beads, music playlists, or daily walks, are sometimes the most stable aspects of a person's routine. They remind us that sparks do not have to be dramatic or idealized—they can also be found in the ordinary. In the smell of fresh coffee, the warmth of a tea mug, the shared silence of a smoke break. These, too, are human. These, too, endure.

Conclusion: The Sacred in the Everyday

Rituals endure not because they are rigid, but because they adapt. They move with the person, flex around suffering, and hold the soul when words fail. In the lives of people with severe mental illness, rituals are often the bridge between fractured mind and continuous self. They are not quirks to be erased, but sparks to be honored—each one a small, flickering act of reclaiming life.

Where words falter and logic breaks down, ritual continues. It is the body's language of meaning. In severe mental illness, rituals may appear as fragments—but when seen through the right lens, they are often threads of coherence in a world gone loose. Supporting and understanding these rituals is not just good care—it's an act of respect for the person's core humanity.

Assessing for sparks in people living with severe mental illness—those enduring preoccupations or passions, such as sex, money, food, music, spirituality, creativity, movement, rituals, nature, humor, touch, storytelling, hope, and freedom—requires curiosity, sensitivity, and structure. These sparks often remain alive even when much else is impaired, and uncovering them can be clinically and relationally transformative.

In serious mental illness, so much feels fragmented: time, memory, identity, relationships. Ritual provides a counterweight. It restores rhythm where there is disarray, continuity where there is rupture, and sacredness where there was once only survival.

When we honor ritual, we do more than reduce symptoms. We help rebuild the architecture of self. We affirm that behind every repeated gesture is a story and often, a yearning to belong.

Table 11.1 — Rituals vs. Compulsions

Feature	Ritual	Compulsion
Intent	Meaning, identity	Anxiety relief only
Flexibility	Adaptive	Rigid
Emotional Effect	Comfort, belonging	Distress if interrupted

1. Kirmayer, L. J. (2007). Psychotherapy and the cultural concept of the person. *Transcultural Psychiatry*, 44(2), 232–257. (Rituals as meaning-holding structures in distress.)
2. Luhrmann, T. M. (2012). *When God Talks Back: Understanding the American Evangelical Relationship with God*. Knopf. (Ritual/practice providing coherence and identity in anomalous experience.)
3. Graybiel, A. M. (2008). Habits, rituals, and the evaluative brain. *Annual Review of Neuroscience*, 31, 359–387. (Basal-ganglia loops; dopaminergic reinforcement in ritualized habits.)
4. Tang, Y.-Y., Hölzel, B. K., & Posner, M. I. (2015). The neuroscience of mindfulness meditation. *Nature Reviews Neuroscience*, 16(4), 213–225. (Top-down control/limbic modulation via prefrontal systems in structured practices.)
5. Hobson, N. M., et al. (2018). The psychology of rituals: An integrative review and process-based framework. *Personality and Social Psychology Review*, 22(3), 260–284. (Summarizes evidence including ERN reductions following ritualized acts.)
6. Norton, M. I., & Gino, F. (2014). Rituals alleviate grieving. *Journal of Experimental Psychology: General*, 143(1), 266–272; Brooks, A. W., et al. (2016). Don't stop believing: Rituals reduce anxiety by decreasing uncertainty. *Organizational Behavior and Human Decision Processes*, 137, 71–85.
7. Lally, P., et al. (2010). How are habits formed in the real world? *European Journal of Social Psychology*, 40(6), 998–1009; Baumeister, R. F. (2012). *Willpower*. (Decision fatigue & the value of routinization.)
8. Wiltermuth, S. S., & Heath, C. (2009). Synchrony and cooperation. *Psychological Science*, 20(1), 1–5; Xygalatas, D., et al. (2013). Extreme rituals promote prosociality. *Psychological Science*, 24(8), 1602–1605.
9. Brewer, J. A., et al. (2011). Meditation deactivates the default mode network. *PNAS*, 108(50), 20254–20259; Farb, N. A. S., et al. (2013). Interoception, insula, and self-regulation in contemplative practice. *Social Cognitive and Affective Neuroscience*, 8(1), 15–26. (Analogous mechanisms likely shared by structured ritual practices.)
10. American Psychiatric Association. (2022). *DSM-5-TR*. (Criteria and clinical differentiation of OCD compulsions vs. nonpathological routines); Veale, D. (2007). Cognitive–behavioural conceptualisation of compulsive behaviours. *Advances in Psychiatric Treatment*, 13(6), 438–446.

11. Deegan, P. E. (2005). The importance of personal medicine. *Scandinavian Journal of Public Health*, 33(66 Suppl), 29–35. (Self-devised routines/rituals as adaptive "personal medicine".)
12. Koenig, H. G. (2012). *Religion, Spirituality, and Health: The Research and Clinical Implications. ISRN Psychiatry*, 2012, 278730. (Clinical guidance on honoring religious/cultural practice.)
13. Wood, W., & Rünger, D. (2016). Psychology of habit. *Annual Review of Psychology*, 67, 289–314. (Designing sustainable, flexible rituals/habits in recovery.)
14. de Leon, J., & Diaz, F. J. (2005). A meta-analysis of smoking in schizophrenia. *Schizophrenia Research*, 76(2–3), 135–157; Hartz, S. M., et al. (2018). Comorbidity of smoking in serious mental illness. *JAMA Psychiatry*, 75(2), 164–172; Dalack, G. W., et al. (1998). Nicotine and schizophrenia: neurobiological hypotheses. *Biological Psychiatry*, 43(3), 187–193; Lara, D. R. (2010). Caffeine, mental health, and psychiatric disorders. *Journal of Alzheimer's Disease*, 20(s1), S239–S248.
15. Vancampfort, D., et al. (2012). Physical activity in major mental illness: systematic review. *Acta Psychiatrica Scandinavica*, 125(5), 352–362. (Exercise routines as stabilizing rituals with psychiatric and metabolic benefits.)

Chapter 12:
Nature: The Spark of Vitality and Connection to the Living World

There is something deeply primal and healing about being in the presence of trees, water, sky, and soil. For individuals living with serious mental illness, nature can serve as both witness and balm—a silent companion that offers sensory regulation, symbolic meaning, and spiritual grounding. In settings often stripped of natural elements, reconnection to the earth may be one of the most overlooked forms of care.

To be in nature is to remember one's own vitality. To feel wind on the face, sun on the back, dirt under fingernails—this is to reclaim a body often alienated by illness, stigma, or medication. The natural world offers a wordless welcome that many people living with psychiatric conditions seldom encounter in clinical environments. There are no intake forms in a forest, no evaluations by a river. Nature simply allows.

Neurobiology of Nature

Nature is not only emotionally grounding—it has measurable effects on the brain and body:

Amygdala Deactivation: Studies using fMRI have shown that spending time in nature can decrease activity in the amygdala, a brain region involved in processing stress and negative emotions. This reduction is associated with lower levels of anxiety and a decreased likelihood of rumination, particularly important in psychotic and mood disorders. (Bratman et al., 2015).

Attention Restoration: Natural environments promote soft fascination, which gently engages the mind and allows the directed attention system to rest. This contrasts sharply with the demands of modern environments, which often overload people living with cognitive impairments. (Kaplan & Kaplan, 1989).

Increased Brain Connectivity: Time spent in nature enhances connectivity between regions involved in executive function, emotional regulation, and sensory integration—networks often disrupted in schizophrenia and bipolar disorder (Bratman et al., 2015; Bratman, Anderson, Berman, Cochran, de Vries, et al., 2019).

Autonomic Nervous System Balance: Nature exposure triggers the parasympathetic nervous system, decreasing heart rate, lowering blood pressure, and stabilizing cortisol levels. These changes promote a restorative physiological state (Park et al., 2010; Antonelli, et al., 2019).

Improved Sleep and Circadian Rhythms: Exposure to natural light regulates melatonin production and helps synchronize sleep cycles—often severely disrupted in people living with psychiatric illness (Fischer et al., 2017; Grigsby-Toussaint, et al., 2015).

Brain and Body Effects of Nature

Amygdala Deactivation: Studies using fMRI have shown that spending time in nature can decrease activity in the amygdala, a brain region involved in processing stress and negative emotions. This reduction is associated with lower levels of anxiety and a decreased likehood of rumination, particularly important in psychotic and mood disorders.

Attention Restoration: Natural environments promote "soft fascination," which gently engages the mind and allows the directed attention system to rest. This contrasts sharply with be- demands of modern environments, which ofiten overload people living with cognitive impairments.

Increased Brain Connectivity: Time spent in nature enhances connetivity between regions involved in executive function, emotional regulation, and sensory integration - networks often disrupted in psychiophrenia and bipolar disorder

Autonomic Nervous System Balance: Nature exposure triggers the parasympathetic nervous system, decreasing heart rate, lowering bloud pressure, and stabilizing cortisol levels.

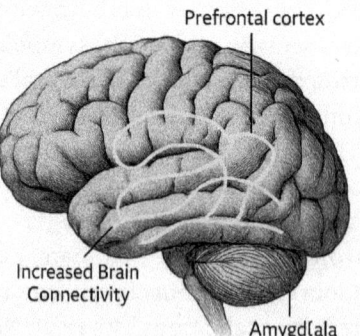

Nature as Grounding and Reconnection

The sensory language of nature bypasses the verbal mind. For individuals whose thinking may be disorganized or whose speech is muted by medication or trauma, nature becomes a place of direct, embodied experience.

Touching bark can become a ritual of grounding. Watching a leaf float may represent letting go. Feeling the rhythm of rain might mirror the rising and falling of emotion. Nature communicates through sensory metaphor. Its patterns—cycles, rhythms, emergence—reflect the psyche's own attempts at healing.

Symbolism and Metaphor: Nature as Inner Mirror

Nature is a mirror of internal states. When patients speak of drowning, being lost in the woods, or needing to "grow roots," they are often describing emotional landscapes through ecological metaphor. These metaphors can become powerful therapeutic tools.
Clinicians can:
- Use seasonal metaphors to talk about change and recovery.
- Explore landscape imagery in dreams, writing, or hallucinations.
- Use nature-based guided imagery or art therapy to externalize emotional states.

This symbolic use of nature enables people to narrate complex internal experiences that may be difficult to express otherwise.

Solitude Without Isolation

Nature offers a space for solitude without the social stigma of withdrawal. Unlike the silence of a hospital room, which may feel empty or confining, the quiet of a forest or a garden is rich and alive. It affirms presence rather than absence.

For people living with severe mental illness, this distinction is crucial. Many crave time alone but are labeled as isolative. Nature allows for restoration without alienation.

Therapeutic Applications: Ecotherapy and Beyond

Wilderness Therapy: Structured programs involving hiking, camping, or outdoor challenges have shown improvements in self-esteem, mood regulation, and group cohesion.

Horticultural Therapy: Gardening programs improve sensory integration, motor skills, and emotional regulation. The act of tending to life becomes an act of reclaiming one's own.

Green Exercise: Physical activity in natural settings produces greater reductions in depression and anxiety than indoor activity alone. This dual effect—movement and nature—compounds therapeutic benefits.

Forest Bathing (Shinrin-Yoku): Originating in Japan, this practice involves intentional, mindful immersion in nature. Clinical trials show decreased cortisol, reduced pulse rate, and improved mood (Park et al., 2010; Song, Ikei, & Miyazaki, 2016).

Cultural Context: In Japan, Shinrin-Yoku has been formally recognized as part of national health promotion. The Japanese Ministry of Agriculture, Forestry, and Fisheries promoted it as a public health initiative, and designated "forest therapy bases" were established across the country where physicians could recommend visits as adjunctive treatment for stress-related conditions. Unlike in Western countries, where nature exposure is often viewed as lifestyle advice, in Japan, Shinrin-Yoku is embedded in preventive medicine and integrated into clinical care as a culturally endorsed, evidence-based practice.

Comparative Perspectives: Nature as Medicine

Japan (Shinrin-Yoku)
- Origin: Formalized in the 1980s as a public health practice
- Integration: Endorsed by the Ministry of Agriculture, Forestry, and Fisheries
- Infrastructure: Over 60 official forest therapy bases with guided programs
- Clinical Use: Physicians recommend Shinrin-Yoku for stress reduction, hypertension, depression, and burnout.
- Cultural Framing: Nature immersion is seen as both a spiritual and medical practice, blending Shinto traditions with modern science.

United States/Europe
- Origin: Increasingly promoted in the 2000s under "ecotherapy," "green exercise," and "nature prescriptions"
- Integration: Driven largely by grassroots advocacy and research; not formally embedded in public health systems
- Infrastructure: Local parks, nonprofit programs, and nature prescription initiatives (e.g., ParkRx America)
- Clinical Use: Often adjunctive, used in wellness and psychotherapy rather than mainstream medicine
- Cultural Framing: Seen primarily as lifestyle modification or preventive care, rather than a medical intervention

Nature as Medicine

Japan (Shinrin-Yoku)	United States/ Europe
Origin Formalized in the 1980s as a public health practice	Increasingly promoted in the 2000s under "ecotherapy," "green exercise," and "nature prescriptions."
Integration Endorsed by the Ministry of Agriculture, Forestry, and Fisheries	**Integration** 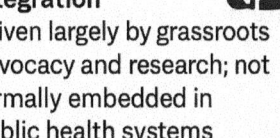 Driven largely by grassroots advocacy and research; not formally embedded in public health systems
Infrastructure Over 60 official "forest therapy bases" with guided programs	**Infrastructure** 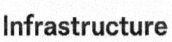 Local parks, nonprofit programs, and nature prescription initiatives (e.g., „ParkRx America")
Clinical Use Physicians recommend Shinrin-Yoku for stress reduction, hypertension, depression, and burnout	**Clinical Use** Often adjunctive, used in wellness and psychotherapy rather than mainstream medicine
Cultural Framing Nature immersion is seen as both a spiritual and medical practice, blending	

Nature in the Institutional Frame

Many psychiatric environments are nature-deprived. Windows are sealed. Courtyards are concrete. The absence of natural light and living systems mirrors the psychological lifelessness many patients feel.

Yet even small interventions can restore vitality, such as:
- Indoor plants
- Water features
- Nature murals
- Soundscapes of birds or rain
- Fresh air breaks in green spaces

These changes are not aesthetic—they are therapeutic. They signal to patients that life continues, even in confinement.

The natural world has a measurable impact on mood and cognition. Bratman, et al., found that time in nature reduces rumination and dampens neural activity in the subgenual prefrontal cortex, a region linked to depression.

Tina, a 26-year-old with bipolar disorder, stabilized not through medication alone but through daily time in the courtyard garden. There, she spoke freely for the first time in weeks—about flowers, then her mother, then her fear. Nature served as relational glue.

A patient once asked to sit outside for five minutes. She didn't need words afterward. Just that moment.

Nature does something no ward can. I've witnessed that again and again.

David, a veteran with schizoaffective disorder, began tending a small herb garden at his group home. His paranoia lessened as his focus shifted to the fragile plants. He began describing his symptoms as "weeds I'm pulling out."

These are not isolated stories. They echo a larger truth: that nature invites connection, not just to the earth, but to self and others.

I've watched concrete walls close in on people and seen trees open something back up.

We once took a group of long-term inpatients to a nearby garden. One man, usually mute, knelt beside a sunflower and whispered, "This is the first beautiful thing I've seen in years." That day, dirt under nails and sun on faces meant more than a hundred therapy sessions.

"For some, nature itself became sanctuary," a neighbor described, "a spark nurtured on porches, in gardens, and in a small community of care." This account underscores how green spaces and gardens provide belonging and calm.

Barriers and Equity

Not everyone has access to safe, green spaces. Racial and economic disparities often determine proximity to parks, gardens, and wilderness.

Urban areas, where many with serious mental illness reside, are especially deprived.

Mental health systems can:
- Advocate for access to nature as a health right.
- Design facilities with integrated green spaces.
- Partner with local gardens, farms, or nature centers.
- Create mobile nature therapy units or bring plants and natural materials into inpatient settings.

Nature as a Spark of Identity

For many, nature is not just therapeutic—it is cultural, ancestral, and spiritual. From Indigenous traditions to agrarian memories, the land holds personal and collective history.

Engaging with nature allows individuals to:
- Reclaim traditions and land-based rituals.
- Connect to lineage and resilience.
- Establish a sense of place and belonging.

Nature's quiet power to ground and inspire can endure even the most isolating of illnesses.

Elena, with severe agoraphobia, hadn't left her home in years. We began talking about the oak tree outside her window. Over weeks, she became curious about it. One day, she called me: "I opened the window. The tree… It's so green." That single tree had become a bridge to life beyond her fear.

Conclusion: Returning to the Living World

In a world of diagnosis and disorder, nature is a reminder that healing is organic. It does not rush, but it persists. It is patient and whole.

To walk among trees is to remember what it means to be alive. To sit by a stream is to hear the mind slow down. To plant something, water it, and watch it grow is to participate in one's own restoration.

Nature is not supplemental—it is fundamental. For those living with severe mental illness, nature is not only a setting, but a partner in healing. It is not a luxury. It is a right. A spark. A mirror. A medicine.

Let us bring nature back into the heart of care—not as a backdrop, but as a central figure in the journey toward wholeness.

Table 12.1 — Nature's Benefits

Setting	Effect	Clinical Application
Forest walk	Reduces cortisol	Nature-based therapy
Gardening	Routine, patience	Recovery programs
Water views	Calms, restores	Hospital design

Williams, F. (2017). *The Nature Fix: Why Nature Makes Us Happier, Healthier, and More Creative*. (Accessible synthesis on why "nature simply allows," grounding clinical intuition.)

Sudimac, S., Sale, V., & Kühn, S. (2022). How nature nurtures: Amygdala activity decreases after a walk in nature. *Molecular Psychiatry*, 27, 4765–4770.

Bratman, G. N., Hamilton, J. P., Hahn, K. S., Daily, G. C., & Gross, J. J. (2015). Nature experience reduces rumination and subgenual prefrontal cortex activation. *PNAS*, 112(28), 8567–8572; Bratman, G. N., Anderson, C. B., Berman, M. G., Cochran, B., de Vries, S., et al. (2019). Nature and mental health: An ecosystem service perspective. *Science Advances*, 5(7), eaax0903.

Kaplan, R., & Kaplan, S. (1989). *The Experience of Nature: A Psychological Perspective*. (Attention Restoration Theory—"soft fascination".)

Park, B.-J., Tsunetsugu, Y., Kasetani, T., et al. (2010). The physiological effects of Shinrin-Yoku. *Environmental Health and Preventive Medicine*, 15(1), 18–26; Antonelli, M., Barbieri, G., & Donelli, D. (2019). Effects of forest bathing on stress: A systematic review. *International Journal of Biometeorology*, 63, 1117–1132; Song, C., Ikei, H., & Miyazaki, Y. (2016). Physiological effects of nature therapy. *Frontiers in Public Health*, 4, 80.

Fischer, D., et al. (2017). Light exposure & sleep timing: links with circadian phase. *Current Sleep Medicine Reports*, 3, 201–210; Grigsby-Toussaint, D. S., et al. (2015). Sleep insufficiency and the natural environment: a population study. *Preventive Medicine*, 78, 78–84.

Barton, J., & Pretty, J. (2010). What is the best dose of nature and green exercise for mental health? *Environmental Science & Technology*, 44(10), 3947–3955.

Ministry of Agriculture, Forestry and Fisheries (Japan). Shinrin-Yoku/Forest Therapy initiatives; see also Tsunetsugu, Y., Park, B.-J., & Miyazaki, Y. (2010). Trends in research related to "forest bathing." *International Journal of Environmental Research and Public Health*, 7(7), 2912–2933.

Soga, M., Gaston, K. J., & Yamaura, Y. (2017). Gardening is beneficial for health: A meta-analysis. *Preventive Medicine Reports*, 5, 92–99.

Bowen, D. J., & Neill, J. T. (2013). A meta-analysis of outdoor education/wilderness therapy outcomes. *Journal of Outdoor and Environmental Education*, 17(1), 15–29.

Gillis, K., & Gatersleben, B. (2015). A review of biophilic design in the built environment. *Frontiers in Psychology*, 6, 921.

Jennings, V., & Gaither, C. J. (2015). Approaching environmental health disparities and green spaces: An ecosystem services perspective. *International Journal of Environmental Research and Public Health*, 12(2), 1952–1968

Chapter 13:
Humor: Laughter, Absurdity, and the Spark of Play

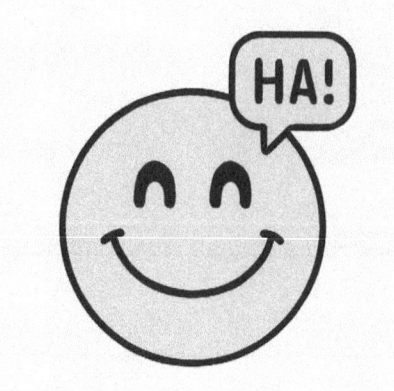

I've been struck by the power of unexpected humor to pierce through the darkest moments, offering a brief, vital release for patients.

Thomas, in the depths of a depressive episode, rarely spoke. One day, I asked about his sleep. He replied: "Doctor, I'm getting so much rest, I think I'm starting to remember my past lives." I stifled a laugh. He didn't smile, but a flicker of pride crossed his face. Even in the dark, humor can survive—a sign of enduring humanity.

Amid the weight of psychosis, depression, and trauma, it may seem surprising to find laughter. Yet humor is one of the most resilient and underappreciated human faculties in the landscape of severe mental illness. It offers both psychological oxygen and existential commentary. In moments of absurdity, parody, or playful connection, individuals can reclaim power, perspective, and presence. Humor, even in the darkest hours, says: I still see the irony. I still see the humanity. I am not erased.

Humor thrives not in the absence of suffering, but often because of it. For many individuals navigating severe mental illness, humor becomes a lifeline—an anchor of identity, a form of expression, and a safe way to engage with the world.

Neurobiology of Humor

Humor engages a complex network of brain regions that support emotional regulation, reward, language processing, and social cognition:
- Reward Pathway Activation: Humor and laughter stimulate the brain's mesolimbic dopamine pathway—the same reward system activated by pleasurable experiences like eating and social connection. This can generate joy, motivation, and bonding.
- Endorphin Release: Laughter triggers the release of endogenous opioids (endorphins), creating natural pain relief and an overall sense of well-being.
- Cortisol Reduction: Humor helps reduce cortisol, the stress hormone, thereby promoting relaxation and reducing the physiological wear and tear often associated with chronic stress and psychiatric illness.
- Prefrontal Cortex Engagement: Understanding and appreciating humor involves cognitive functions like irony detection, theory of mind, and language nuance—functions rooted in the prefrontal cortex. Stimulating this area can strengthen cognitive flexibility.
- Temporal Lobe and Limbic System: The ability to process and respond to humor involves the temporal lobes (for language and emotional memory) and limbic structures like the amygdala, which are crucial for emotional interpretation.

Humor's activation of these integrated systems contributes to emotional modulation, interpersonal connection, and even insight generation.

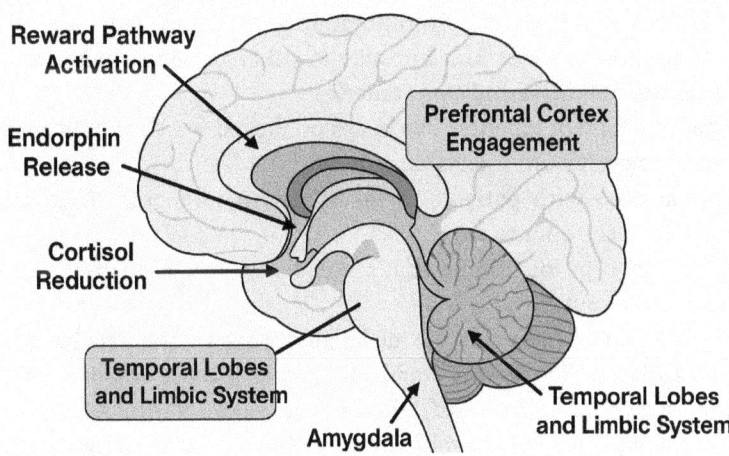

Humor as a Psychological Spark

Humor functions as a powerful and multidimensional tool of survival and recovery in the following ways:

- Cognitive reframing: Humor allows individuals to reinterpret threatening or painful experiences, creating emotional distance while maintaining engagement. This is especially helpful in trauma, where humor can defuse overwhelming affect.
- Resistance and defiance: Humor can be a subtle—or overt—form of protest. Jokes about symptoms, hospitalization, or psychiatry allow individuals to critique the systems that have labeled or confined them.
- Agency and control: In environments where autonomy is limited, being funny is a way to control narrative and social perception. To make others laugh is to reassert power.
- Narrative continuity: Humor helps preserve a sense of narrative self—a person who is more than a patient, more than a set of symptoms. It bridges past identities and current roles.
- Spontaneity and creativity: In contrast to the rigidity often imposed by mental illness, humor fosters spontaneity. Wordplay, impersonations, and surreal commentary reconnect the individual to creative freedom.

Clinical Vignettes and Examples

Devon, a 45-year-old man with chronic schizophrenia, was described as "flat" and unengaged. But during a group discussion on hospital meals, he quipped, "I've had delusions that taste better than this." The room erupted in laughter. From then on, Devon's humor became his identity—he was the comic sage of the ward. Staff noted increased engagement and social connection, not only in him but also in other patients, who responded with greater openness and camaraderie.

There's a kind of laughter I've heard on locked wards that is both pain and resistance. It's unforgettable.

I've laughed with patients at the strangest moments. That laughter often opened the door to trust.

There's a type of humor that's not escape—it's survival. And I've learned to honor it.

The first time a patient made me laugh during a crisis, I realized humor wasn't a distraction; it was survival. During a tense moment in group therapy, a patient deadpanned, "If they ever make a Netflix show about us, I want to be played by Denzel." Everyone burst out laughing—including staff. That moment cracked something open. It reminded us all that levity can be sacred, too.

Maya, a 28-year-old woman with bipolar disorder, experienced intense mood swings and interpersonal conflicts. But in manic episodes, she often took on comedic personas: a dramatic news anchor, a rebellious therapist, a "psychiatric DJ." Her therapists began using these personas in sessions, helping her explore identity safely and humorously.

Jorge, a young man with schizoaffective disorder, used dark humor to narrate his hallucinations: "The voices are like roommates who never pay rent." Humor helped him externalize the experience, reducing fear and shame. In therapy, this metaphor became a doorway to empowerment.

Humor Styles: Helpful vs. Harmful

Not all humor is created equally. Clinicians must understand the function and tone of humor to assess its therapeutic value:

- Affiliative Humor: Strengthens social bonds through jokes and storytelling
- Self-Enhancing Humor: Supports resilience and reframing
- Aggressive Humor: Targets others and may reflect underlying anger or trauma
- Self-Deprecating Humor: Can be empowering or a mask for low self-worth

Therapists can use the Humor Styles Questionnaire to explore patterns and intentions behind humor.

Humor as Communal Medicine

Laughter binds groups together. In psychiatric units, where tension runs high, shared humor reduces fear, dissolves hierarchy, and builds solidarity.

- Group Therapy: Laughter builds cohesion. Clients who laugh together are more likely to trust and support one another.
- Peer Support: Humor is often used in peer-run groups to challenge stigma and connect over shared struggle.
- Staff Culture: Clinicians who model appropriate levity can de-escalate crises and humanize the clinical environment.

Humor can be therapeutic. A review by Gelkopf, et al., found that humor interventions decrease anxiety, improve pain tolerance, and support social bonding in patients with serious mental illness.

Humor in Psychosis and Delirium

In psychosis, humor may emerge in strange or uncanny ways. Individuals might pun on delusional themes, use ironic metaphors, or laugh inappropriately.

Rather than dismiss this, clinicians can ask:
- What's the joke about?
- What might this humor be protecting against?
- How does this form of expression relate to meaning-making?

Sometimes, humorous expression during psychosis serves as an organizing mechanism, helping the person maintain coherence in a chaotic perceptual world.

Therapeutic Use of Humor

Therapists can integrate humor into care in the following ways:
- Naming absurdity: "We really expect you to function in here without decent coffee?"
- Exaggeration: "I think your anxiety is at an Olympic level today."
- Improv and drama therapy: Role-play and humor-based exercises can explore trauma, identity, and emotional range.
- Comedic journaling: Patients can document absurdities of their week or write fictional headlines about their lives.

Humor as a Bridge to Insight

Laughter and insight often arise together. The moment one sees the contradiction in a situation, a new perspective opens. In therapy, these "comic insights" can be transformative:
- "So you're saying my plan to cure depression with Oreos might need tweaking?"
- "If my paranoia had a business card, what would it say?"

These reframings open doors for further exploration.

"Humor often cuts through silence." A sibling recalled how jokes about sports... This illustrates how humor restores bonds when words fail.

"Clinicians, too, witness humor as healing," one psychiatrist recalled. These stories reveal how laughter is a spark of resilience.

Case Reflection: Healing Through Comedy

Tony, a 36-year-old former stand-up comic, was hospitalized for severe depression with psychotic features. He avoided groups and rarely spoke. A therapist invited him to co-lead a "Comedy Hour" for other patients. Initially hesitant, Tony eventually delivered a five-minute monologue.

Laughter rippled through the room. That night, he wrote in his journal: "Today, I remembered who I am." That moment didn't cure his illness—but it reawakened his will to live.

Humor and Cultural Context

Cultural norms deeply shape what is considered funny. Clinicians must be attuned to humor that may:
- Reflect community storytelling traditions
- Serve as resistance to historical trauma
- Include sarcasm, parody, or slapstick unique to cultural identity

Understanding humor through a cultural lens affirms identity and reduces misinterpretation.

Conclusion: Humor as Sacred Play

To laugh while suffering is not denial—it is transformation. Humor holds the absurdity of life gently, without solving it. It makes pain bearable and beauty visible.

In the fog of psychosis, a single joke can be a beacon. In the heaviness of depression, a shared chuckle can lift the veil. In the isolation of stigma, humor says: "I'm still here. And I'm still me."

Humor is not frivolous—it is sacred play. It is rebellion, resilience, and renewal. For people living with severe mental illness, humor is often the last light to go out—and the first to return.

Let us honor it as one of the most vital sparks of all.

Table 13.1 — Humor Functions

Type	Example	Clinical Value
Coping	Laughing at absurdity	Stress relief
Bonding	Inside jokes	Peer connection
Self-reflection	Irony, satire	Identity, insight

1. Mobbs, D., Greicius, M. D., Abdel-Azim, E., Menon, V., & Reiss, A. L. (2003). Humor modulates the mesolimbic reward centers. *Neuron*, 40(5), 1041–1048.
2. Dunbar, R. I. M., Baron, R., Frangou, A., Pearce, E., van Leeuwen, E. J. C., Stow, J., ... van Vugt, M. (2012). Social laughter is correlated with elevated pain thresholds. *Proceedings of the Royal Society B: Biological Sciences*, 279(1731), 1161–1167.
3. Martin, R. A., Puhlik-Doris, P., Larsen, G., Gray, J., & Weir, K. (2003). Individual differences in uses of humor and their relation

to psychological well-being: Development of the Humor Styles Questionnaire. *Journal of Research in Personality*, 37(1), 48–75.
4. Gelkopf, M., Gonen, B., Kurs, R., Melamed, Y., & Bleich, A. (2006). The effect of humor on psychiatric patients: A review and meta-analysis. *Evidence-Based Complementary and Alternative Medicine*, 3(2), 159–164.

Part III – The Hidden Sparks

Chapter 14:
Sparks in the Shadow: Hidden Drives That Survive Mental Illness

The light we seek is not always loud. What we call symptoms may be smokescreens for something more sacred—what endures in the dark, burning low, smoldering in the corners of the mind, waiting to be seen and to be named.

Introduction: Not Lost, Just Hidden Beneath Symptoms

Not every spark announces itself. Some are easy to spot—appetites for food, music, money, or sex. They surface in behaviors, obsessions, and fixations. But others dwell in shadow. These are the sparks that don't always look like desire. They may look like silence, withdrawal, ritual misunderstood, or gesture overlooked. Yet underneath them lies something persistent: quieter truths. The human need for freedom, hope, touch, and story.

These truths rarely appear on checklists. They whisper rather than shout. They are not always requested, but they are always needed. For individuals living with schizophrenia, bipolar disorder, or other serious mental illnesses, overt expressions of vitality are often obscured. What remains are faint signals: a hand reaching toward the sun through a locked ward window, a worn Bible tucked into a pillowcase, a muttered joke no one else hears.

These signals are not mere noise. They are remnants of vitality. They persist not because illness spares them, but because they are woven into the human condition. I call them *sparks in the shadow*. They flicker beneath the surface, and if we pay attention, they can illuminate the most obscured aspects of survival and humanity.

Why Sparks Hide

The first ten sparks—sex, money, food, music, spirituality, creativity, movement, rituals, nature, and humor—tend to show themselves in visible ways. They are easier to chart, easier to code, easier to manage. The hidden sparks often evade notice. Why?

1. Clinical Blindness
   Psychiatry is trained to measure symptoms. When a patient refuses meals, refuses medication, or speaks in fractured narratives, we often see pathology, not yearning. Resistance is labeled oppositional, not protective. Silence is charted as flat affect, not wounded communication.

2. Institutional Suppression
   Hospitals and group homes are designed for safety, not self-expression. Touch is discouraged, choice is limited, personal items are controlled. Narrative is often treated as irrelevant if it cannot be easily aligned with diagnostic categories.

3. Symptom Masking
   Psychosis, depression, or negative symptoms cloak underlying human needs. A paranoid refusal of medication may be framed as delusion, but often it is an assertion of autonomy. A delusional story may appear incoherent, but it is often a disguised truth.

4. Stigma and Fear
   Patients quickly learn which parts of themselves are "acceptable" and which will be dismissed, punished, or pathologized. Hidden sparks stay hidden because the world has taught people to protect them.

Clinical Vignette: Resistance or Spark?

A man in long-term care refused showers for weeks. Staff saw it as defiance. When I sat with him, he finally said: "They tell me when to sleep, eat, even poop. This is the one thing I still control." That wasn't defiance. It was a spark—an insistence on agency.

Shadows in Practice

The hidden sparks emerge not in loud declarations but in fragments, often misinterpreted.
- A muttered joke in the dayroom, charted as "inappropriate behavior"
- A Bible hidden under a pillow, called "contraband"
- A patient's claim to be the "last survivor of a galactic war," dismissed as delusion
- A blanket clutched tightly in seclusion, labeled as regression

To the untrained eye, these look like symptoms. But through a different lens, they are survival signals: humor, spirituality, storytelling, the need for touch.

Extended Vignette

One woman, mute for weeks, began tearing napkins into thin strips and braiding them together. Staff noted "bizarre behavior." But when asked what she was making, she whispered, "A story." Each braid represented a memory of her childhood. What was charted as pathology was, in fact, narrative persistence.

The Neurobiology of Hidden Sparks

Science confirms what patients quietly demonstrate: the brain retains its architecture for hidden sparks, even when illness disrupts cognition.

- Touch. Gentle tactile input activates C-tactile afferents, oxytocin release, and amygdala downregulation.[1] The skin itself is a social organ.[2] Even in psychosis, tactile craving endures.
- Storytelling. Narrative identity engages the medial prefrontal cortex and posterior cingulate—areas linked to self-referential thought.[3] Patients construct stories even when language coherence falters.
- Hope. The mesolimbic dopamine pathway underlies reward prediction and future orientation.[4] Even fragile or "irrational" hopes represent intact circuitry for persistence.
- Freedom. Neuroimaging shows that opportunities for choice activate the ventral striatum and prefrontal cortex.[5] Agency itself is rewarding, even in low-stakes decisions.

These circuits are not erased by illness. They persist, waiting for recognition.

The Cost of Neglect

When hidden sparks are ignored, the results are devastating: despair, disengagement, and resistance. Patients who feel unseen often retreat further, compounding institutional cycles of isolation.

When sparks are honored, outcomes shift. Research confirms:

- Autonomy supports treatment adherence and recovery.[6]
- Hope predicts functional improvement, even in schizophrenia.[7]
- Narrative therapies increase insight and self-esteem.[8]
- Safe tactile interventions reduce anxiety, agitation, and stress.[9]

The difference lies in whether we treat behavior as noise—or as signal.

Reframing Clinical Practice

Engaging hidden sparks requires listening beyond symptoms.
- Attend to choice. Ask, "Would you prefer water or juice with your meds?" Small choices restore autonomy.
- Value metaphor. Listen to delusional narratives for the truths they contain.
- Name hope. Even improbable hopes can anchor treatment plans.
- Respect touch. Offer safe sensory grounding when physical touch isn't possible.

The task is not to eliminate sparks, but to kindle them.

Clinical Vignettes

- A patient was convinced he would win the lottery. Staff dismissed it as grandiose delusion. But in treatment, we reframed it: *What does winning represent?* For him, it was security and family connection. That spark fueled a vocational plan.
- A woman who stayed mute for weeks whispered "thank you" when a nurse placed a warm towel in her hands. That towel was not a medical tool. It was human connection.
- A man who refused therapy began attending when given a choice of session times. What he needed wasn't less therapy—it was more freedom.
- A woman with chronic depression kept hiding candy bars in her room. Staff called it hoarding. But she explained: "It's for when I need to feel a little normal." A spark of self-soothing was disguised as defiance.

Reflection Prompts for Clinicians

1. When have I dismissed a patient's behavior as a "symptom" without asking what need it might express?
2. How might silence, resistance, or ritual be signals of a hidden spark?
3. What structures in my setting suppress touch, storytelling, hope, or freedom—and how might I soften them?
4. Which spark do I most easily miss in my patients, and why?
5. How can I create micro-choices, micro-moments of hope, or micro-opportunities for connection in my practice?

Transition: Preparing for the Hidden Sparks

This chapter has traced why some sparks remain in shadow. They are easy to miss, yet impossible to extinguish. The next four chapters explore them in full:

- Chapter 15: Touch: The Forgotten Language
- Chapter 16: Storytelling: Making Meaning Amid Madness
- Chapter 17: Hope: The Improbable Light
- Chapter 18: Freedom: Autonomy in Constraint

These sparks are not secondary. They are central. And they may be the most important ones to honor, precisely because they so often go unseen.

Closing Reflection

Not all sparks shine. Some smolder. Some whisper. Some wait in the corners of the mind, disguised as symptoms. But when we learn to see them, we discover that even in shadow, the human spirit burns on.

To engage with hidden sparks is to do more than treat illness. It is to restore dignity, honor survival, and remind patients—and ourselves—that humanity endures in places we once thought void.

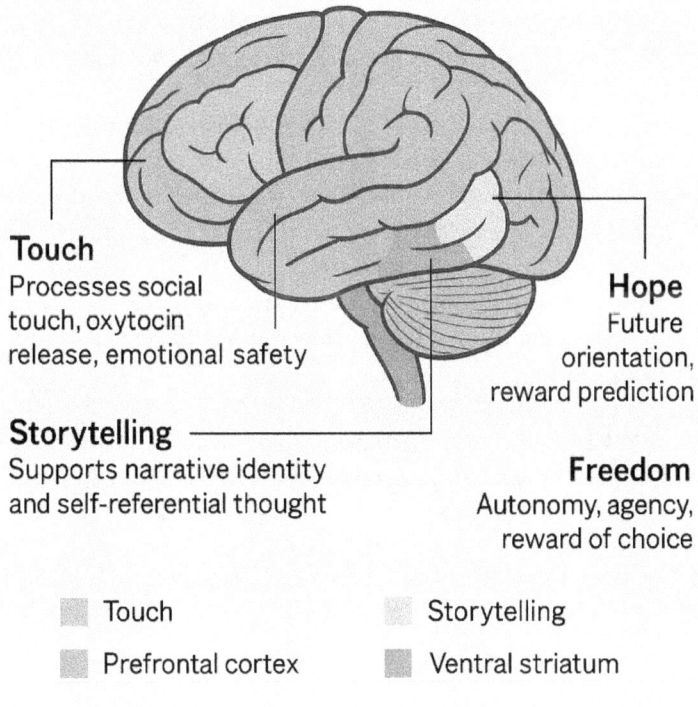

Even in serious mental illness, the brain circuits underlying hidden sparks—touch, storytelling, hope, and freedom—remain active. Recognizing them helps us see symptoms not as voids, but as signals of enduring human drives.

Table 14.1 — Shadow Sparks Examples

Spark	Healthy Expression	Shadow Expression
Sex	Intimacy, love	Hypersexuality, coercion
Money	Budgeting, autonomy	Delusional wealth, gambling
Rituals	Grounding, identity	OCD-like rigidity
Hope	Future orientation	Unrealistic denial

1. Field, T. (2010). *Touch for socioemotional and physical well-being: A review.* Developmental Review, 30(4), 367–383.
2. McGlone, F., Wessberg, J., & Olausson, H. (2014). *Discriminative and affective touch: Sensing and feeling.* Neuron, 82(4), 737–755.
3. Lysaker, P. H., Buck, K. D., Carcione, A., Procacci, M., & Dimaggio, G. (2007). *Narrative enhancement in schizophrenia: Contributions to self-esteem, insight, and quality of life.* Psychiatry, 70(3), 191–201.
4. Snyder, C. R. (2002). *Hope theory: Rainbows in the mind.* Psychological Inquiry, 13(4), 249–275.
5. Leotti, L. A., & Delgado, M. R. (2011). *The inherent reward of choice.* Psychological Science, 22(10), 1310–1318.
6. Ryan, R. M., & Deci, E. L. (2000). *Self-determination theory and the facilitation of intrinsic motivation, social development, and well-being.* American Psychologist, 55(1), 68–78.
7. Schrank, B., Stanghellini, G., & Slade, M. (2008). *Hope in psychiatry: A review of the literature.* Acta Psychiatrica Scandinavica, 118(6), 421–433.
8. Lysaker et al., 2007 (see note 3).
9. Chen, Y. W., et al. (2013). *Therapeutic touch in psychiatric care: Effects on agitation and anxiety.* Journal of Psychiatric and Mental Health Nursing, 20(7), 646–653.

Chapter 15:
Touch: The Forgotten Language

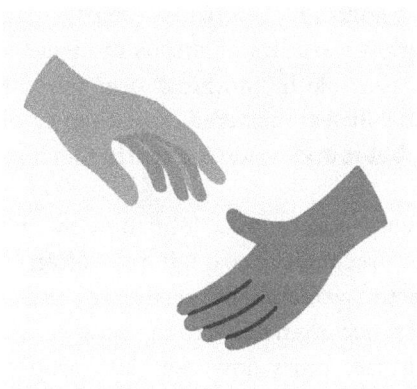

I used to think healing was only cognitive—until I saw what a warm hand could do. In psychosis, what people crave most isn't understanding. It's presence. It's touch.

The Primal Spark

Touch may be the most primitive spark of all. It is among our first languages. It predates speech, and for many, it outlasts language itself. From the moment of birth, human development depends on it. So does emotional regulation.

In serious mental illness, touch is complicated—often absent, sometimes feared, occasionally pathologized. But its absence leaves a mark. In psychiatric settings—especially those shaped by trauma, risk management, and institutional coldness—touch is often avoided. And so patients hunger quietly.

Mental illness can often lead to isolation, either self-imposed or resulting from stigma and misunderstanding. Yet the fundamental human need for touch, for physical comfort and reassurance, often endures.

A gentle hug from a loved one can cut through the isolation of severe depression. A comforting hand on the arm can offer a moment of grounding amidst the chaos of anxiety. For individuals in institutional settings, the simple, non-judgmental touch of a caregiver can be a profound reminder of their humanity. This enduring need speaks to our primal desire for connection—for feeling seen and held, both literally and figuratively. It is a spark that reminds us we are not alone, even when illness tries to convince us otherwise.

Historical and Developmental Roots of Touch

The story of touch begins long before modern psychiatry. In the mid-20th century, Harry Harlow's studies of rhesus monkeys showed that infant monkeys preferred soft cloth "mothers" over wire ones that dispensed food.[1] Warmth and softness mattered more than calories. Harlow's work was controversial, but it underscored a truth: touch is a biological necessity, not a luxury.

Attachment theory echoes this. John Bowlby and Mary Ainsworth showed that safe, responsive caregiving—often mediated through touch—shaped secure attachment, resilience, and emotional health.[2] Infants deprived of touch often failed to thrive, even when fed adequately.[3] Neonatal intensive care units now use "kangaroo care"—skin-to-skin holding—to improve survival, stabilize breathing, and strengthen parent-infant bonds.[4]

Cross-cultural studies show wide variation in touch practices. Mediterranean and Latin American cultures emphasize physical closeness and frequent touch, while Anglo and Northern European cultures often prefer more distance.[5] Yet across cultures, the absence of touch is consistently linked to loneliness, depression, and impaired development.

For patients with serious mental illness, these early lessons matter. Many grew up in environments where touch was inconsistent—sometimes nurturing, sometimes neglectful, sometimes abusive. In adulthood, psychiatric hospitalization often compounds deprivation. The very spark that builds safety in infancy is systematically restricted in institutions.

The Neurobiology of Touch

Touch is not merely a physical sensation—it is a neurobiological event. When activated, touch triggers the release of oxytocin, the so-called "bonding hormone," which promotes trust and connection.[6] Touch also reduces levels of cortisol, the stress hormone, and modulates amygdala activity, reducing fear and hypervigilance.

The skin itself is a social organ. Specialized C-tactile afferents, discovered in the last few decades, are tuned to gentle, caress-like contact.[7] These nerve fibers project to the insula, a brain region involved in emotion and interoception. This makes touch uniquely capable of generating comfort, soothing distress, and reinforcing social bonds.

Polyvagal theory, developed by Stephen Porges, highlights touch's role in regulating the social engagement system.[8] Safe touch increases vagal tone, activates parasympathetic pathways, and helps individuals shift from defensive states (fight, flight, freeze) into states of connection and calm. For patients with trauma histories, this can be life-changing—though it must be offered with care.

For people with serious mental illness, the absence of safe touch can be profoundly destabilizing. In trauma survivors or those living long-term in institutional settings, deprivation of touch often contributes to dissociation, dysregulation, and loneliness.[3] Without tactile reassurance, stress responses heighten, which can exacerbate psychiatric symptoms such as paranoia, agitation, or despair.

Even when direct interpersonal touch is not possible or appropriate, substitutes often emerge. Patients rock themselves, fold linens, clutch blankets, or hold objects close. These behaviors are not meaningless—they are signals of the neurobiological drive for tactile regulation.

Research Insights

A growing body of evidence supports therapeutic touch:
- A study in *Neuroscience & Biobehavioral Reviews* found that affective touch interventions reduced stress and enhanced well-being across populations.[9]
- In psychiatry, therapeutic touch has been shown to reduce agitation and anxiety in schizophrenia and mood disorders.[10]
- Frequency matters more than duration. Even brief, repeated gestures of safe touch—placing a warm towel in a patient's hand, offering a weighted blanket—can lower arousal.
- Sensory integration therapies (weighted blankets, deep pressure stimulation) reduce hyperarousal, lower heart rate, and calm the autonomic nervous system, particularly in trauma-affected populations.[11,12]

Clinical Vignettes

- **The warm towel.** A man on our unit had been mute for weeks. He didn't speak, gesture, or make eye contact. One nurse placed a warm cloth in his hands during daily care. The next day, he whispered, "Thank you." He hadn't spoken in months. That towel wasn't a medical device—it was human contact.

- The "inappropriate" hug. A woman with schizoaffective disorder would attempt to hug staff. She was repeatedly reprimanded. When I asked why she reached out, she said, "Because no one here touches me unless they have gloves on." Her behavior wasn't inappropriate—it was a plea for recognition. We reframed staff training to validate her need while setting safe boundaries.
- The substitute blanket. Another patient refused to attend groups without a blanket wrapped around her shoulders. Staff called it regression. She explained: "It's the only way I feel held." The blanket became a therapeutic tool, not a symptom.

Touch, Trauma, and Boundaries

Touch is never neutral. For trauma survivors, it can be both healing and threatening. Many patients carry ambivalence—yearning for touch while fearing it. A hand on the shoulder can soothe one person and retraumatize another.

This duality demands careful navigation. Professional guidelines in psychiatry strongly discourage routine physical touch because of risks of misinterpretation, retraumatization, or boundary violation.[13] Yet an overly rigid avoidance of touch can strip care of its humanity.

The middle path lies in attuned, trauma-informed practices:
- Always seek explicit consent before offering touch.
- When uncertain, use verbal validation ("I know this is hard—I'm here") instead of physical gestures.
- Offer safe substitutes (weighted blankets, fidget objects, rocking chairs, sensory rooms).
- Normalize self-directed tactile regulation (wrapping in blankets, holding objects).

The paradox is clear: touch may be restricted in psychiatric care, yet patients invent their own ways to meet this need. Clinicians must respect this and respond creatively.

Clinical Applications

- Offer safe sensory grounding. Warm towels, textured objects, weighted items.
- Validate tactile needs verbally. Acknowledge the yearning for comfort even if physical touch isn't possible.
- Train staff in trauma-informed physical care. Teach gentle approaches, consent practices, and predictability.
- Respect ambivalence. Explore the *meaning* of both reaching for and avoiding touch.

- Use substitutes wisely: weighted blankets, deep pressure therapies, and tactile rituals that approximate holding.
- Engage families. Teach caregivers how to reintroduce safe, meaningful touch at home.

Reflection Prompts

1. How do I personally feel about touch in clinical practice—comfortable, cautious, or conflicted?
2. When have I seen a patient respond powerfully to something tactile, even in a small way?
3. What structures in my setting encourage or discourage safe touch?
4. How can I meet patients' tactile needs without violating boundaries or ethical safeguards?
5. What role did touch play in my own development—and how might that shape my comfort with it in others?
6. How can I expand the range of safe, creative substitutes for touch in my practice?

Closing Reflection

Touch is often underestimated in psychiatry. It can be minimized as "non-essential" or pathologized as risky. Yet patients continue to seek it—in blankets, in small gestures, in moments of presence.

To honor the spark of touch is to remember that healing is not only cognitive or chemical. It is relational, embodied, and profoundly human. When we attend to this spark—carefully, ethically, but without fear—we restore something elemental.

Touch is a forgotten language, but not a lost one. Patients are speaking it still, in ways subtle and profound. Our task is not only to listen, but also to respond.

Neurobiology of Touch

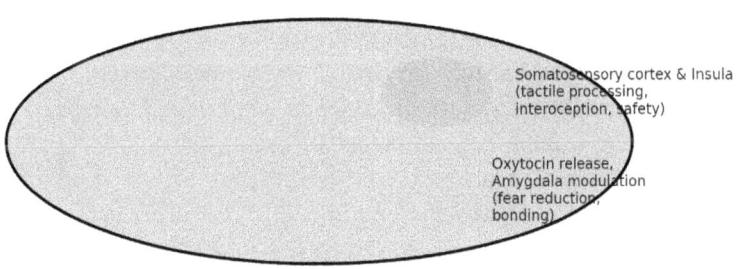

Touch engages the somatosensory cortex and insula, releasing oxytocin and modulating the amygdala to reduce fear and foster bonding. Even in serious mental illness, these pathways remain active, making touch a profound source of safety and connection.

"Touch often speaks louder than words." One daughter explained how holding her mother's hand... Her account demonstrates how physical presence conveys love when cognition falters.

Table 15.1 — Touch in Clinical Settings

Safe Expression	Risk Area	Clinical Note
Handshakes	Boundaries blurred	Clarify consent
Weighted blanket	Comfort	Trauma-informed use
Hugs (consensual)	Abuse history	Always optional

1. Harlow, H. F. (1958). *The nature of love.* American Psychologist, 13(12), 673–685.
2. Bowlby, J. (1969). *Attachment and Loss: Vol. 1. Attachment.* Basic Books.
3. Cascio, C. J., et al. (2019). *Tactile processing in autism and psychiatric conditions: A review.* Neuroscience & Biobehavioral Reviews, 99, 49–57.
4. Feldman, R., et al. (2002). *Kangaroo care and mother–infant bonding.* Pediatrics, 110(1), 16–26.
5. Jourard, S. M. (1966). *An exploratory study of body-accessibility.* British Journal of Social and Clinical Psychology, 5(3), 221–231.
6. Field, T. (2010). *Touch for socioemotional and physical well-being: A review.* Developmental Review, 30(4), 367–383.
7. McGlone, F., Wessberg, J., & Olausson, H. (2014). *Discriminative and affective touch: Sensing and feeling.* Neuron, 82(4), 737–755.
8. Porges, S. W. (2011). *The polyvagal theory: Neurophysiological foundations of emotions, attachment, communication, and self-regulation.* Norton.
9. Morrison, I. (2016). *Keep calm and cuddle on: Social touch as a stress buffer.* Adaptive Human Behavior and Physiology, 2(4), 344–362.
10. Chen, Y. W., et al. (2013). *Therapeutic touch in psychiatric care: Effects on agitation and anxiety.* Journal of Psychiatric and Mental Health Nursing, 20(7), 646–653.
11. Champagne, T., & Stromberg, N. (2004). *Sensory approaches in inpatient psychiatric settings.* Journal of Psychosocial Nursing, 42(9), 34–44.
12. Eckstein, M., et al. (2020). *Weighted blankets and sleep quality in psychiatric inpatients: A randomized controlled trial.* Occupational Therapy in Mental Health, 36(1), 1–16.
13. American Psychiatric Association. (2013). *Practice guidelines for the psychiatric evaluation of adults.* APA.

Chapter 16:
Storytelling: Making Meaning Amid Madness

Sometimes the delusion is the story—and sometimes it hides and protects the story underneath.

The Spark of Story

Humans are storytelling beings. We do not merely experience life; we narrate it. We explain, embellish, and imagine our way into coherence. We are authors—sometimes unreliable, sometimes poetic, but always reaching for meaning.

Every patient has a narrative, even if it is fractured, chaotic, or embedded in hallucinations. The need to tell one's story is as old as language, and it persists even in the most disorganized minds. For individuals living with serious mental illness, the act of storytelling becomes both a survival strategy and a route toward healing.

Storytelling takes many forms: a conversation in therapy, diary entries scrawled in notebooks, artwork, music, or the metaphorical layers of delusions. Patients are not just symptomatic—they are narrators. Listening for story means listening beyond symptoms, which allows us to become allies in recovery rather than recorders of deficits.

"Writing is also a form of storytelling," one peer described. Her reflection shows how stories reclaim coherence and dignity.

The Neurobiology of Narrative

Narrative engages a distributed set of brain regions known collectively as the default mode network (DMN)—including the medial prefrontal cortex (mPFC), posterior cingulate cortex (PCC), and hippocampus.[1] These areas coordinate autobiographical memory, self-referential processing, and the ability to imagine possible futures.[2]

- Medial Prefrontal Cortex (mPFC): Involved in evaluating personal relevance, sense of self, and autobiographical detail
- Posterior Cingulate Cortex (PCC): Helps integrate memory with identity and contributes to self-continuity
- Hippocampus: Critical for memory consolidation—binding fragments into a coherent timeline
- Default Mode Network (DMN): Active when the brain is at rest, daydreaming, or telling stories. It allows us to weave past experiences into future possibilities.[3]

Disruptions in the DMN are linked to schizophrenia, depression, and PTSD.[4] Patients may struggle with temporal coherence, fractured memory, or narrative disorganization. Yet even within psychosis, the drive to narrate persists—often through metaphor or fantasy. Delusions can thus be reframed as narrative attempts: protective myths the mind creates to restore meaning in the face of chaos.

Research Insights

- Narrative enhancement therapy: Patients with schizophrenia who participated in narrative enhancement and cognitive therapy showed improved self-esteem, insight, and quality of life. Stories foster coherence, even when lives feel incoherent.
- Narrative identity theory: McAdams emphasizes that identity itself is a story—an internalized, evolving life narrative that gives a sense of unity and purpose. Serious mental illness may fracture continuity, but the underlying narrative drive remains.
- Recovery narratives: Research shows that patients who construct personal recovery stories (even if non-linear) experience greater empowerment, adherence to treatment, and resilience.[7]
- Clinical outcomes: Narrative work has been shown to reduce internalized stigma, strengthen therapeutic alliance, and improve long-term functioning.[8]

Clinical Vignettes

- **The Galactic Survivor:** A patient once told me he was the last survivor of a galactic war. Most staff dismissed it as psychotic. I asked, "What did you fight for?" He replied, "So the children could sleep safely." Later, we learned he had endured childhood abuse. His "war" was metaphor. His delusion was survival encoded in myth.
- **The Manic Author:** A woman with bipolar disorder, in a manic episode, declared she was writing a book that would save humanity. She filled notebooks with fragments of poetry and prophecy. At first, it seemed grandiose. But in her story, she located herself as powerful, purposeful, and needed—counterweights to the helplessness she felt when depressed.
- **The Trauma Re-Teller:** A veteran with PTSD told his story as if it had happened to "someone else." This distancing allowed him to narrate horrors without being overwhelmed. Over time, he shifted to "I," reclaiming authorship of his pain.
- **The Diary Pages:** Another patient brought journals filled with fragments: "I am broken glass," "the music stopped," "I am still here." Staff dismissed them as nonsense. But when we read together, he explained each fragment symbolized a chapter of trauma. His diary became a bridge between chaos and coherence.
- **The Silent Artist:** A woman with chronic psychosis drew cages and open doors. Asked about the meaning, she said: "These are the times I was locked in, and the times I was free." Her art was narrative—visual, but coherent.

"Nonverbal storytelling also emerges in art," a community volunteer recalled. This moment illustrates how hands can narrate when voices cannot.

Cultural and Collective Storytelling

Storytelling is not only personal; it is cultural and collective.

- **Indigenous and religious traditions:** Many cultures use myth, ritual, and oral storytelling as healing practices. Narratives of ancestors and deities frame suffering as survivable and meaningful.[9]
- **Immigrant narratives:** For displaced individuals, telling stories of homeland and migration preserves identity and fosters resilience.
- **Peer and recovery groups:** Programs like Alcoholics Anonymous rely on personal storytelling—"sharing"—to transform isolation into solidarity. Psychiatric peer groups similarly use narrative to reframe stigma into strength.

- Illness vs. recovery narratives: Sociologists distinguish between "illness narratives," which describe suffering, and "recovery narratives," which reframe illness as survivable.[10] Both are essential; both keep sparks alive.

Psychiatric Implications

Clinicians are trained to gather history but not always to honor it. Narrative identity theory suggests that meaning-making is central to recovery. Illness may distort timelines or coherence, but the core desire—to be heard, to be known—remains intact.

Documenting only "flight of ideas" or "loose associations" risks missing the deeper truths. Delusions, metaphors, or disorganized speech may carry kernels of purpose. Patients are more than symptoms; they are narrators.

Clinical Applications

- Invite storytelling. Ask: "Can you tell me how it all began?"
- Value metaphor. Don't rush to flatten symbolic speech into literal reality.
- Build narrative capacity. Encourage journaling, art, roleplay, digital storytelling.
- Reframe delusion as story. Ask: "What wish or fear might this belief be holding?"
- Integrate families. Help caregivers honor patient narratives rather than correcting them.
- Narrative Medicine. Incorporate patient stories into clinical charts and team discussions, not just symptoms.

Reflection Prompts

1. How often do I treat patient speech as noise, rather than as story?
2. What metaphors from patients have I overlooked or dismissed?
3. How do my biases shape which stories I accept?
4. What role does my own narrative identity play in the way I hear patients?
5. How can I expand opportunities for patients to tell their stories in my setting?
6. In what ways can I invite *collective* stories—family, peer groups—into recovery?

Closing Reflection

Storytelling is not just what patients do; it is who they are. To invite story is to invite humanity. When we listen for stories rather than symptoms, we become witnesses to survival, not just custodians of illness.

These hidden sparks—freedom, hope, touch, and story—are often missed in diagnosis, dismissed in treatment, or muted in institutional care. Yet they endure, whispering in journals, metaphors, drawings, and delusions.

To honor story is to affirm that even in madness, there is meaning. What patients need is not only medication or management, but the chance to author themselves again.

Neurobiology of Storytelling

- Default Mode Network (Imagination, storytelling, internal narrative)
- Medial Prefrontal Cortex (Self-reference, identity)
- Posterior Cingulate Cortex (Autobiographical memory, continuity of self)
- Hippocampus (Memory consolidation, timeline coherence)

Storytelling engages the brain's default mode network, including the medial prefrontal cortex, posterior cingulate, and hippocampus. Even in serious mental illness, these circuits remain active, underscoring the human drive to make meaning through story.

Table 16.1 — Storytelling in Recovery

Narrative Type	Role in Recovery	Example
Illness narrative	Coherence, meaning	Journaling symptoms
Cultural story	Identity, belonging	Folklore, family tales
Recovery story	Peer support	NAMI peer group sharing

1. Northoff, G., & Heinzel, A. (2006). *First-person neuroscience: Imaging the self and its disorders.* Consciousness and Cognition, 15(4), 708–739.
2. Spreng, R. N., et al. (2009). *The common neural basis of autobiographical memory, prospection, navigation, theory of mind, and the*

default mode: A quantitative meta-analysis. Journal of Cognitive Neuroscience, 21(3), 489–510.
3. Andrews-Hanna, J. R. (2012). *The brain's default network and its adaptive role in internal mentation.* The Neuroscientist, 18(3), 251–270.
4. Whitfield-Gabrieli, S., & Ford, J. M. (2012). *Default mode network activity and connectivity in psychopathology.* Annual Review of Clinical Psychology, 8, 49–76.
5. Lysaker, P. H., et al. (2007). *Narrative enhancement in schizophrenia: Contributions to self-esteem, insight, and quality of life.* Psychiatry, 70(3), 191–201.
6. McAdams, D. P. (2001). *The psychology of life stories.* Review of General Psychology, 5(2), 100–122.
7. Roe, D., & Davidson, L. (2005). *Self and narrative in schizophrenia: Time to author a new story.* Medical Humanities, 31(2), 89–94.
8. Hamm, J. A., et al. (2019). *Narrative identity in schizophrenia: Implications for recovery.* Psychiatry Research, 272, 703–708.
9. Gone, J. P. (2013). *Redressing First Nations historical trauma: Theorizing mechanisms for Indigenous culture as mental health treatment.* Transcultural Psychiatry, 50(5), 683–706.
10. Frank, A. W. (1995). *The wounded storyteller: Body, illness, and ethics.* University of Chicago Press.

Chapter 17:
Hope: The Improbable Light

I've sat with people whose thoughts made no sense—but their hope, somehow, still did. And I've seen hope survive in places where reason could not.

The Spark of Hope

When darkness descends, hope can feel like a distant, almost unattainable star. Yet even in the deepest valleys of despair, a tiny ember of hope often remains. For someone battling chronic depression, hope might be the quiet thought that the medication might eventually work, or the belief that a connection with a therapist could offer some solace. For an individual navigating the complexities of bipolar disorder, it could be the yearning for stability, a respite from the extreme swings of mood.

This persistent flicker of hope, however faint, is a testament to the human spirit's resilience. It is the whisper that says, "This too shall pass," even when the storm rages.

Hope is not always rational. It is not merely a cognitive exercise; it is an emotional necessity. Clinicians often caution against "false hope," but in psychiatry, any hope is often preferable to none. Hope does not need to be factually accurate to be therapeutic. It just needs to exist.

A man experiencing homelessness believes he will win the lottery. A woman with chronic delusions insists her family will return. These may appear symptomatic, but they are also signals of endurance. Hope often survives where cognition collapses—and that matters.

The Neurobiology of Hope

Hope is deeply rooted in neurobiology. It is not only a philosophy but a system of circuits and chemicals that orient us toward the future.

- Mesolimbic dopamine system: Hope is closely tied to the mesolimbic pathway, which runs from the ventral tegmental area (VTA) to the nucleus accumbens. This pathway governs reward prediction, motivation, and reinforcement.[1] Dopamine neurons fire not only in response to immediate rewards but also in anticipation of future ones—a key mechanism for hope.[2]
- Prefrontal cortex: The prefrontal cortex integrates agency (belief in one's capacity to act) with pathways (the ability to envision steps toward a goal).[3] This aligns with Snyder's psychological model of hope, where hope is both a belief and a plan.
- Hippocampus and episodic future thinking: The hippocampus supports memory consolidation and simulation of possible futures.[4] In other words, hope relies on the ability to imagine a different tomorrow based on yesterday's experiences.
- Serotonin and persistence: While dopamine drives reward anticipation, serotonin regulates patience and mood stability.[5] Serotonergic pathways contribute to the persistence of hope even when rewards are delayed.
- Reward prediction error: Hope depends on learning from mismatches between expected and actual outcomes.[6] Even in psychosis, when predictions may be distorted, the underlying mechanism of adjusting anticipation remains active.

Together, these circuits explain why hope endures even in serious mental illness. Though symptoms may alter perception, the biology of expectancy—rooted in dopamine, memory, and future simulation—remains intact.

Research Highlights

- Snyder's Theory of Hope: Psychologist C. R. Snyder described hope as two interwoven components:
1. Agency: belief that one can initiate and sustain action
2. Pathways: ability to imagine routes to desired outcomes[3]
- Hope in schizophrenia: Studies show that people with schizophrenia who report higher levels of hope demonstrate better treatment adherence, greater motivation, and improved quality of life.[7]

- Hope and recovery outcomes: Higher hope scores predict reduced hospitalizations, enhanced resilience to relapse, and stronger functional outcomes across psychiatric diagnoses.[8]
- Protective effects: Hope buffers against suicide risk, strengthens therapeutic alliance, and promotes trust in care. Even fragile hope can tilt outcomes toward survival.[9]

Clinically, nurturing hope is as essential as prescribing medication. It strengthens motivation, sustains engagement, and helps patients envision futures worth striving toward.

Clinical Vignettes

- The Chef's Dream: A patient once told me, "I know I'm not well. But someday, I'll be a chef again." His delusions were active, but this vision anchored him. We structured his discharge plan around a culinary skills group. He flourished. Hope was not a lie; it was a compass.
- The Lottery Belief: A man experiencing homelessness insisted he would win the lottery. Staff dismissed it as delusional. Yet the hope within this conviction kept him alive. Instead of extinguishing it, we reframed the question: "What else might feel like a winning ticket to you right now?"
- The Fragile Flame: A woman with chronic depression taped a note to her mirror: "It might still get better." She did not believe it fully, but reading it daily kept her going. Sometimes, hope does not roar. It flickers. And that flicker sustains life.
- Mania and Grand Hope: A patient in a manic episode declared she was destined to lead a global movement. At first this sounded like delusion, but her narrative revealed an unmet longing for significance. With support, her grandiose vision was reframed into activism in her local community—her hope became grounded without being extinguished.
- Institutional Hope: A man institutionalized for decades clung to one hope: "One day, I'll walk outside these gates." Even when discharge seemed improbable, this hope gave him purpose. Staff began offering supervised walks on the hospital grounds, honoring the essence of his hope in a smaller form.
- Family-Anchored Hope: A mother with schizophrenia endured repeated relapses. What kept her alive was the hope of reconnecting with her children. Treatment was reframed not only around symptom reduction, but around steps to restore contact. Hope became the therapeutic engine.

"Sometimes hope comes through staff presence," Paulette Heslop explained. Her words echo the evidence that micro-moments of agency sustain recovery.

Cultural and Spiritual Dimensions of Hope

Hope is not only individual but also cultural, spiritual, and collective.
- Faith traditions: Many religions frame hope as sacred. In Christianity, hope is one of the three theological virtues. In Islam, hope (*raja*) balances fear in the relationship with God. In Buddhism, hope is tethered to the impermanence of suffering. These frameworks shape how patients understand their endurance.
- Collective hope: Marginalized groups often sustain hope through shared narratives. African American spirituals, Indigenous rituals, and immigrant storytelling traditions transmit resilience across generations. Hope here is not only personal—it is communal survival.
- Cultural psychiatry: Clinicians must ask, "What does hope mean in this culture?" For some, it is tied to family honor; for others, to spiritual destiny. Respecting these frameworks prevents reducing hope to a purely Western, individualistic construct.

Psychiatric Implications

Hope is not the same as delusion. Delusion may distort reality, but hope orients the psyche toward possibility. In practice:
- A delusion about winning the lottery may symbolize yearning for security.
- A belief about family returning may reflect a hunger for belonging.
- A dream of becoming a chef may decode a need for dignity and agency.

To treat without nurturing hope risks leaving patients biologically stable but existentially adrift.

Clinical Applications

- Ask future-facing questions, e.g., "What's something you still want to do one day?"
- Anchor treatment in personal dreams. Even symbolic aspirations can guide recovery.
- Reframe delusions with dignity. Look for the wish embedded in the belief.
- Foster micro-hopes. Support small, achievable goals—a call, a meal, a walk.

- Build hope maps. Collaboratively chart goals, pathways, obstacles, and supports.[10]
- Leverage peer support. Patients often borrow hope from those further along in recovery.
- Model authentic optimism. Clinicians' belief in possibility strengthens alliance.

"Forgiveness, too, becomes a spark of hope," Kelly-Ann Fairweather noted. Her story shows how hope often grows out of compassion and community.

Reflection Prompts

1. Do I treat patient hope as naïve, or as a vital sign worth protecting?
2. How have I witnessed hope sustain a patient even when symptoms were overwhelming?
3. How do I distinguish between distorted delusion and enduring hope?
4. What role do my own hopes play in shaping my clinical work?
5. How do systemic barriers—poverty, discrimination, institutionalization—challenge or strengthen patient hope?
6. What happens when my hopes for a patient diverge from theirs?

Other clinicians emphasize the preservation of hope. Dr. Helen Bloomer insists, "You can never take their hope." Her words remind us that hope itself is often the strongest medicine.

Closing Reflection

Hope is improbable, fragile, and sometimes irrational. Yet it endures when other capacities collapse. It threads its way through delusion, despair, and silence.

To cultivate hope is to recognize it as both a neurobiological drive and a psychological necessity. We may stabilize symptoms with medication and therapy, but recovery begins when patients glimpse possibility.

Even a whisper of hope—"someday I'll be a chef"; "it might still get better"—is enough to orient life toward the future. Hope is not an accessory to treatment. It is its heartbeat.

Neurobiology of Hope

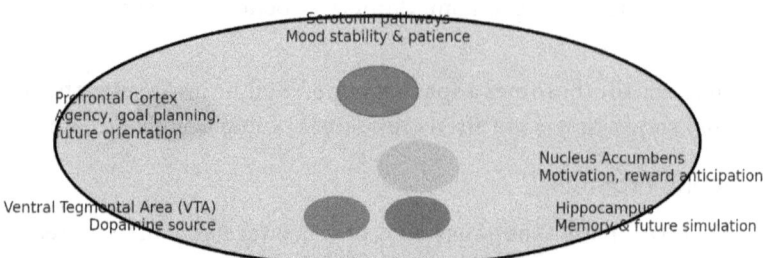

Hope engages the mesolimbic dopamine pathway (VTA–Nucleus Accumbens–Prefrontal Cortex), the hippocampus for imagining future possibilities, and serotonin pathways that stabilize persistence. Even in serious mental illness, these circuits remain active, making hope a biological as well as psychological necessity.

Table 17.1 — Dimensions of Hope

Dimension	Example	Clinical Impact
Personal	Goals, dreams	Motivation
Relational	Support, love	Resilience
Spiritual	Faith, destiny	Strength

Notes

1. Schultz, W. (2016). *Dopamine reward prediction-error signalling: A two-component response*. Nature Reviews Neuroscience, 17(3), 183–195.
2. Berridge, K. C., & Kringelbach, M. L. (2015). *Pleasure systems in the brain*. Neuron, 86(3), 646–664.
3. Snyder, C. R. (2002). *Hope theory: Rainbows in the mind*. Psychological Inquiry, 13(4), 249–275.
4. Addis, D. R., Wong, A. T., & Schacter, D. L. (2007). *Remembering the past and imagining the future: Common and distinct neural substrates*. Neuropsychologia, 45(7), 1363–1377.
5. Dayan, P., & Huys, Q. J. (2009). *Serotonin, inhibition, and negative mood*. PLoS Computational Biology, 5(2), e1000433.
6. Steinberg, E. E., et al. (2013). *A causal link between prediction errors, dopamine neurons, and learning*. Nature Neuroscience, 16(7), 966–973.

7. Schrank, B., et al. (2012). *Conceptualising and measuring the well-being of people with psychosis.* Schizophrenia Research, 138(2-3), 271–276.
8. Johnson, J., et al. (2010). *The role of hope in recovery from psychosis.* Psychiatric Rehabilitation Journal, 34(2), 112–119.
9. Snyder, C. R., Rand, K. L., & Sigmon, D. R. (2002). *Hope theory: A member of the positive psychology family.* In C. R. Snyder & S. J. Lopez (Eds.), *Handbook of positive psychology* (pp. 257–276). Oxford University Press.
10. Marques, S. C., et al. (2011). *Building hope for the future: A program to foster strengths in middle-school students.* Journal of Happiness Studies, 12(1), 139–152.

Chapter 18:
Freedom: Autonomy in Constraint

I see freedom not just in discharge plans, but in the way a patient presses to choose their own cereal. I've come to realize that even the smallest choice—a meal, a routine—can be a patient's cry for agency.

The Spark of Freedom

Mental illness can feel profoundly constricting. The weight of depression, the racing thoughts of anxiety, the distorted perceptions of psychosis—all create invisible bars, limiting choice, movement, and even the sense of self. Yet the yearning for freedom, in its myriad forms, often persists.

For someone struggling with agoraphobia, freedom might be the dream of stepping outside their front door without crippling fear. For an individual experiencing the paranoia of schizophrenia, it could be the longing for a single moment of clarity, free from the sense of being watched.

This spark of freedom, however small, represents a fundamental human drive to break free from constraint, to reclaim agency, and to experience the world unburdened. It is a quiet rebellion against the limitations imposed by illness.

For individuals under involuntary holds or long-term hospitalization, freedom becomes more than a legal matter—it becomes a psychic hunger. It surfaces in subtle refusals: declining medications, refusing to get out of bed, hoarding food, demanding specific music. Each act of resistance may be read as pathology, but often these are fragments of a deeper impulse: the need to reclaim control.

Freedom is not just about discharge plans or legal rights. It is about autonomy, dignity, and the ability to make meaningful choices. In settings where freedoms are restricted, the yearning for autonomy becomes sharper—and its denial more painful.

Historical and Philosophical Context

The question of freedom has long occupied psychiatry, philosophy, and theology.

- Existential thought: Viktor Frankl, a Holocaust survivor and psychiatrist, argued in *Man's Search for Meaning* that freedom persists even in the most extreme constraints. One cannot always control circumstances, but one can choose one's stance toward them.[1] This resonates deeply with patients in psychiatric institutions, where external freedoms are often curtailed.
- Philosophy of agency: Jean-Paul Sartre wrote that humans are "condemned to be free." Even in illness, people cannot escape the responsibility of choice.[2] For patients, this paradox means that even small refusals or assertions of will carry profound existential weight.
- History of psychiatry: Psychiatry itself has a complex history with freedom—oscillating between offering liberation through treatment and imposing restriction through asylums, restraints, and forced medications.[3] The modern recovery movement emerged partly in response to this history, emphasizing patient agency and choice as cornerstones of care.

Freedom in psychiatry, then, is both an ethical challenge and a therapeutic necessity.

Clinical Vignette: Showers

One patient refused showers for weeks. Staff labeled him oppositional. But when I asked why, he explained: "They tell me when to sleep, eat, even poop. This is the one thing I still control." His refusal was not defiance. It was resistance, a survival mechanism, a spark.

For some, freedom itself is the spark. One advocate recalled the first time he received a key. His story illustrates how autonomy transforms survival into living.

The Neurobiology of Autonomy

Freedom is not only political or philosophical; it is biological.

- Reward of choice: Neuroscience shows that the mere opportunity to choose activates the ventral striatum and prefrontal cortex.[4] Even trivial choices trigger dopamine release, underscoring that agency itself is rewarding.
- Ventromedial prefrontal cortex (vmPFC): This region evaluates personal agency, allowing us to sense control over outcomes. It remains active even in altered states, suggesting the drive for autonomy persists despite illness.[5]
- Insula and self-awareness: The insula helps integrate internal signals with external action, supporting the felt sense that "this choice is mine."[6]
- Dorsal anterior cingulate cortex (dACC): Involved in conflict monitoring, the dACC activates when options are weighed, reinforcing the labor of decision-making.[7]
- Dopamine reinforcement: Perceived control enhances dopamine-driven learning, strengthening persistence and motivation.[8]

Thus, freedom is not simply a social construct. It is a neurobiological imperative.

Research Insights

- A *Frontiers in Psychology* study emphasized that mental illness often undermines autonomy, diminishing quality of life.[9]
- Self-determination theory confirms that autonomy—alongside competence and relatedness—is a basic psychological need essential for well-being.[10]
- Clinical studies show that when patients perceive volition in treatment, outcomes improve across diagnoses: stronger adherence, greater engagement, reduced relapse.
- Even micro-choices—choosing between drinks, seats, or therapy times—activate reward pathways, reinforcing motivation and dignity.

Freedom as Drive and Resistance

For people living with serious mental illness, the deprivation of freedom is often amplified by institutional constraints, medication regimens, or stigma. Small expressions of autonomy—choosing what to wear, what to listen to, or whether to attend group—become therapeutic anchors. Resistance is not always opposition. It is sometimes survival. Refusals, protests, or stubborn silences may represent the last stronghold of selfhood. To dismiss them as mere "noncompliance" is to miss their meaning.

Clinical Anecdotes

- Jamal's Choice: Jamal, a 38-year-old man with schizoaffective disorder, had been hospitalized multiple times under court order. His days were scripted: meals at set hours, lights out at ten. One nurse asked if he preferred water or juice with his evening medication. He smiled: "Juice—because at least that's my choice." That trivial decision became pivotal. Staff began offering micro-choices daily, and his engagement grew.
- The Group Refusal: A man declined group therapy for months. Staff viewed him as defiant. But when given a choice between a morning or afternoon group, he began attending regularly. He was not resisting therapy—he was resisting coercion.
- A Teen in Residential Care: A 16-year-old girl with depression refused to participate in structured activities. Staff grew frustrated. When she was allowed to choose her own project—painting instead of group crafts—she began to engage. Adolescents especially equate freedom with identity, making autonomy developmentally critical.
- Elderly Inpatient: An older man with dementia and psychosis resisted medications. Staff initially insisted. But when offered two pill cups—same medication, different colors—he chose willingly. For him, freedom meant control over ritual.
- Immigrant Patient: A Haitian man hospitalized for mania resisted treatment plans that excluded his family. In his cultural context, freedom was tied to family honor and collective decision-making. Once staff involved relatives in treatment discussions, his resistance softened.

Cultural and Societal Dimensions

Freedom is not universally defined.
- Western vs. collectivist: In Western psychiatry, autonomy is often equated with independence. But in collectivist cultures, freedom may mean alignment with family or community. A patient may feel most "free" when conforming to cultural values, not resisting them.
- Marginalized groups: For people facing racism, poverty, or systemic oppression, freedom includes social justice. Psychiatric care that

ignores structural barriers risks narrowing freedom to a clinical frame.
- Forensic psychiatry: Patients under court orders confront the starkest tension between safety and freedom. Here, clinicians must navigate legal mandates while still offering micro-moments of choice that preserve dignity.

Freedom, then, is not only an individual spark but also a social and political struggle.

Clinical Applications

- Offer micro-choices. Simple options affirm agency.
- Collaborate on care plans. Shared decision-making frameworks restore control.
- Reframe refusal. Ask: What doesn't feel right about this plan? rather than labeling noncompliance.
- Balance safety and autonomy. Even in restrictive settings, autonomy can be built in safely.
- Ethical vigilance: Involuntary treatments should be paired with maximum opportunities for choice.
- Recovery-oriented care: Programs that prioritize autonomy (peer support, advance directives) strengthen engagement.

Takeaway: Even small freedoms transform care from coercion to collaboration. Autonomy is not optional. It is essential.

Reflection Prompts

1. How do I interpret resistance: as pathology or as a spark of agency?
2. What small freedoms can I offer patients daily, even in restrictive settings?
3. How might institutional rules unintentionally strip dignity, and how can I counterbalance that?
4. Do I respect autonomy equally in patients who are symptomatic, institutionalized, or elderly?
5. How do I balance safety with freedom in forensic or high-risk care?
6. How do cultural frameworks shape my patients' sense of autonomy—and my response to it?

Closing Reflection

Freedom is not always grand. Sometimes it is choosing juice instead of water, sitting by one window instead of another, refusing a shower, or walking through a door. These small acts are not trivial. They are sparks.

To treat without autonomy risks turning care into coercion. To restore even micro-freedoms is to affirm humanity, dignity, and resilience.

Freedom is not an afterthought. It is a clinical necessity and a human right.

Neurobiology of Freedom

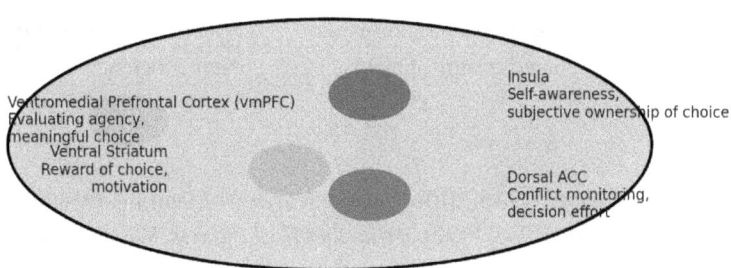

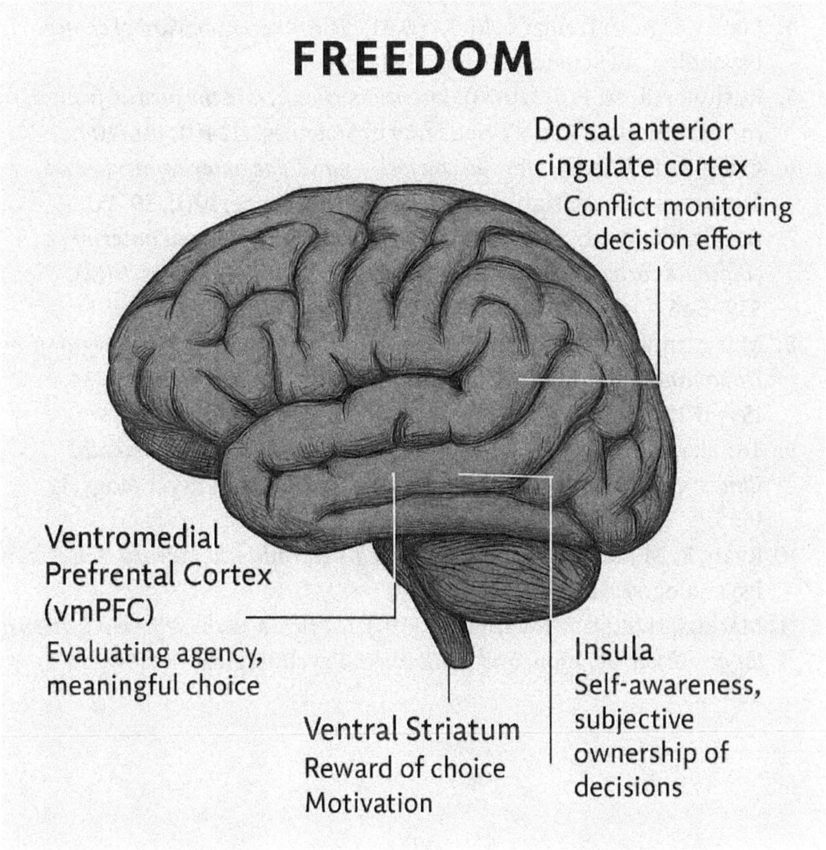

Ventromedial Prefrontal Cortex (vmPFC)
Evaluating agency,
meaningful choice
Ventral Striatum
Reward of choice,
motivation
Insula
Self-awareness,
subjective ownership of choice
Dorsal ACC
Conflict monitoring,
decision effort

FREEDOM
Dorsal anterior cingulate cortex
Conflict monitoring decision effort
Ventromedial Prefrental Cortex (vmPFC)
Evaluating agency, meaningful choice
Ventral Striatum
Reward of choice
Motivation
Insula
Self-awareness, subjective ownership of decisions

Freedom activates reward and decision-making circuits, including the ventral striatum, vmPFC, insula, and dACC. Even in serious mental illness, the intrinsic reward of autonomy persists, making choice a biological as well as a psychological need.

Table 18.1 — Freedom and Autonomy

Domain	Healthy	Risk
Choice	Independent decisions	Impulsivity
Legal	Supported decision-making	Conservatorship abuse
Clinical	Shared treatment plans	Non-adherence

Notes

1. Frankl, V. E. (1946/2006). *Man's Search for Meaning.* Beacon Press.
2. Sartre, J.-P. (1943/1993). *Being and Nothingness.* Washington Square Press.
3. Shorter, E. (1997). *A History of Psychiatry.* Wiley.
4. Leotti, L. A., & Delgado, M. R. (2011). *The inherent reward of choice.* Psychological Science, 22(10), 1310–1318.
5. Rushworth, M. F. S. (2008). *Intention, choice, and the medial frontal cortex.* Annals of the NY Academy of Sciences, 1124(1), 181–207.
6. Craig, A. D. (2009). *How do you feel—now? The anterior insula and human awareness.* Nature Reviews Neuroscience, 10(1), 59–70.
7. Botvinick, M. M., et al. (2004). *Conflict monitoring and anterior cingulate cortex: An update.* Trends in Cognitive Sciences, 8(12), 539–546.
8. Murayama, K., et al. (2010). *From external regulation to self-regulation: Dopamine and the reward of choice.* Motivation and Emotion, 34, 159–172.
9. Tanaka, T., & Sawa, A. (2020). *Autonomy and recovery in mental illness: Clinical and ethical perspectives.* Frontiers in Psychology, 11, 1625.
10. Ryan, R. M., & Deci, E. L. (2000). *Self-determination theory.* American Psychologist, 55(1), 68–78.
11. Markus, H. R., & Kitayama, S. (1991). *Culture and the self: Implications for cognition, emotion, and motivation.* Psychological Review, 98(2), 224–253

Chapter 19:
What Lives in the Shadows Still Burns

Introduction: Sparks That Whisper Rather Than Shout

Not all sparks shine. Some smolder. Some wait. Some speak in symbols. But they are all still there.

Throughout this section, we explored four hidden sparks—freedom, hope, touch, and storytelling. These are not the dramatic forces that announce themselves loudly, like food or music, sex or money. Instead, they linger quietly beneath symptoms, half-concealed, sometimes mistaken for pathology, sometimes silenced by institutions. Yet they endure.

Patients in the midst of severe mental illness may not ask for these sparks outright. They may not say, "I need autonomy," or "I need narrative coherence," or "I need safe human contact." Instead, these needs show themselves in indirect ways: in refusals, in delusions that carry hidden meanings, in withdrawn silence that waits for recognition. The clinician's task is to notice—to interpret gently, to listen for what is unsaid, to honor what flickers beneath.

This chapter is a meditation on why the hidden sparks matter. It is also a recognition that what burns in the shadows may be the most important sign of life.

The Cost of Absence

When hidden sparks are ignored, the human being behind the diagnosis begins to disappear.

Helplessness Without Freedom

Institutional psychiatry often strips patients of choice: meals at set times, medications delivered in paper cups, schedules imposed without negotiation. While some of these structures are necessary for safety, their cumulative effect can be suffocating. Patients deprived of autonomy describe themselves as "robots," "zombies," or "ghosts." Without small freedoms—what to eat, where to sit, when to sleep—patients lose not just agency, but dignity.

A man once told me, "Every decision is made for me. I don't even know what I like anymore." His hopelessness was not just depression; it was the psychic erosion that comes from never being allowed to choose.

Despair Without Hope

When psychiatry reduces treatment to symptom management, hope can vanish. If clinicians speak only in terms of chronicity—"You'll always need medication," "This is lifelong"—patients may conclude that nothing better is possible. Without hope, treatment becomes compliance, not collaboration.

Hopelessness is among the strongest predictors of suicide. Its absence explains why some patients, even when stabilized on medication, succumb to despair. A life without a vision for tomorrow is no life at all.

Isolation Without Touch

Touch is often the most neglected spark. Out of fear of boundary violations, liability, or retraumatization, psychiatric care environments often prohibit touch altogether. Yet human beings are wired for it. Infants deprived of touch fail to thrive; adults deprived of it descend into loneliness and dysregulation.

Patients in long-term care units often clutch pillows, blankets, or stuffed animals—not because of regression, but because the body yearns for tactile comfort. When touch is absent, agitation, paranoia, and despair intensify.

Fragmentation Without Story

Finally, when patients' stories are ignored or dismissed as delusional, their identities fragment further. Humans are storytelling beings; we make sense of our lives through narrative. If the only story that is heard is the medical one—schizophrenia, onset age 21, multiple hospitalizations—the person beneath the illness becomes invisible.

I once met a man whose chart described him as "paranoid, delusional, violent at times." When I asked for his story, he said he was the last survivor of a galactic war. Staff ignored it. But when I asked what he had fought for, he replied: "So the children could sleep safely." Only then did his trauma surface. His story was not nonsense. It was a metaphor for survival.

When Sparks Are Missed

The absence of hidden sparks is not neutral. It deepens helplessness, despair, isolation, and fragmentation. In other words, when hidden sparks are ignored, suffering multiplies.

The Power of Recognition

When clinicians notice and nurture hidden sparks, outcomes shift.

Micro-Freedoms, Macro-Effects

Offering even trivial choices—water or juice with medication, morning or afternoon group—can reduce agitation and increase cooperation. Neuroscience confirms that the act of choosing activates reward pathways. The brain feels pleasure in autonomy, no matter how small.

A patient once told me after choosing his seat in group: "It feels good not to be told everything." What changed was not his symptoms, but his sense of self.

Fragile Hopes as Compasses

Even irrational hopes can orient recovery. A woman convinced her estranged children would return one day took better care of herself in anticipation. Staff dismissed it as delusion. But her hope kept her alive long enough for reconciliation to become possible.

Clinicians sometimes fear fostering "false hope." But hope, even when fragile, is therapeutic. It provides energy for survival. It is better to refine hope gently than to extinguish it.

Safe Touch and Substitutes

When safe, consented touch is possible—a hand on the shoulder, a warm towel in the hands of a mute patient—the effects can be profound. Where direct touch is not possible, substitutes like weighted blankets, sensory objects, or warm compresses can meet the body's need for grounding.

A patient who had not spoken for months whispered "thank you" after a nurse placed a warm cloth in his hands. That cloth was not just fabric; it was contact.

Narrative as Medicine

When patients are allowed to tell their stories—even when fragmented, metaphorical, or fantastical—healing occurs. Narrative coherence strengthens self-esteem, insight, and quality of life.[1]

One patient with schizophrenia told me, "Doctor, I don't need you to fix my story. I just need you to listen to it." And in the listening, his dignity was restored.

Cultural, Ethical, and Humanistic Dimensions

Culture shapes sparks. In Western contexts, freedom is often equated with individual autonomy. But in collectivist cultures, freedom may be defined relationally—being in harmony with family or community. A Haitian patient once told me, "I am free when my family is proud of me." For him, freedom was not independence but belonging.

Hope, too, is culturally shaped. In some traditions, hope is religious—a trust in God's timing, a belief in destiny. In others, hope is communal—the resilience of a people surviving oppression. Clinicians must ask, "What does hope mean in this culture?"

Touch norms vary across cultures: in some, hugs and physical closeness are expected; in others, they are avoided outside family. Storytelling, likewise, may be oral, metaphorical, or embedded in ritual. To honor hidden sparks is to honor culture.

Ethical Tensions

Each hidden spark raises ethical dilemmas:
- Freedom vs. safety: How do we protect autonomy while preventing harm?
- Hope vs. reality: When does supporting hope cross into collusion?
- Touch vs. boundaries: How do we provide comfort while avoiding misinterpretation or retraumatization?
- Story vs. symptom: How do we validate narrative without reinforcing delusion?

There are no easy answers. But the ethical imperative is clear: to dismiss hidden sparks because they are complicated is to deny humanity.

The Humanistic Frame

Recovery-oriented psychiatry reframes treatment as not only about symptom relief, but about restoring meaning, connection, and dignity. The hidden sparks embody this ethic. They remind us that people are not problems to be managed, but lives to be honored.

Clinical Applications

Freedom
- Offer micro-choices wherever possible.

- Involve patients in care planning.
- Reframe refusal as a signal of unmet needs.

Hope
- Ask future-oriented questions.
- Anchor treatment in personal goals, however symbolic.
- Recognize hope as a vital sign of recovery.

Touch
- Provide safe, consented touch when appropriate.
- Offer substitutes like weighted blankets or sensory items.
- Train staff in trauma-informed physical care.

Storytelling
- Invite patients to narrate their experiences.
- Value metaphor and symbolism.
- Use narrative therapies to build coherence and identity.

When clinicians operationalize hidden sparks, treatment becomes more than stabilization. It becomes collaboration.

Reflections and Takeaway

Not all sparks shine. Some smolder. Some whisper. But their quiet persistence matters.

Freedom, hope, touch, and storytelling may not appear urgent in a chart or a treatment plan. But their absence explains much of the pain of serious mental illness: helplessness, despair, isolation, silence.

When we honor the sparks, something shifts. A patient who was mute speaks. A man who refused therapy attends. A woman who had given up imagines a future. A story once dismissed as delusion reveals truth in metaphor.

I have learned from my patients that recovery begins not when symptoms vanish, but when the human being feels seen. The sparks in the shadow remind us that life persists even when obscured, that resilience hides in places we forget to look.

To notice these sparks is to do more than treat illness. It is to honor survival. It is to say: "You are not invisible. You are not just stable. You are alive."

Closing Image

In a darkened room, embers glow faintly. To the inattentive eye, they look like ash, remnants of fire long extinguished. But to the attentive, they are possibility. With breath, with care, with recognition, they flare again.

So it is with the hidden sparks. What lives in the shadows still burns.

Notes

1. Lysaker, P. H., et al. (2007). *Narrative Enhancement and Cognitive Therapy: A new group-based treatment for internalized stigma in schizophrenia.* Psychiatry, 70(3), 191–201.
2. Leotti, L. A., & Delgado, M. R. (2011). *The inherent reward of choice.* Psychological Science, 22(10), 1310–1318.
3. Snyder, C. R. (2002). *Hope theory: Rainbows in the mind.* Psychological Inquiry, 13(4), 249–275.
4. McGlone, F., et al. (2014). *Discriminative and affective touch: Sensing and feeling.* Neuron, 82(4), 737–755.
5. Ryan, R. M., & Deci, E. L. (2000). *Self-determination theory and the facilitation of intrinsic motivation.* American Psychologist, 55(1), 68–78.
6. Tanaka, T., & Sawa, A. (2020). *Autonomy and recovery in mental illness: Clinical and ethical perspectives.* Frontiers in Psychology, 11, 1625.

Chapter 20:
When the Flame Goes Out: Missing Sparks

Sometimes the loudest symptom is silence.

Introduction: The Vanishing Point of Desire

Not all suffering in serious mental illness announces itself through intensity. Some forms emerge through absence—no appetite, no laughter, no interest, no spark.

I've sat with patients whose silence weighed more than any scream. I've watched the slow dimming of desires that once burned brightly—until even the caregivers stopped expecting light. For a long time, I saw these silences as resistance, pathology, or regression. Now I understand them as a different kind of language—a kind that whispers instead of shouts.

Let's take a closer look at what it means when the elemental drives that usually endure—sex, money, food, music, movement, spirituality, creativity—seem to vanish. Rather than labeling these as mere deficits, we explore what such absences might reveal and how, with gentleness and attunement, they may be reawakened. The disappearance of spark may be a sign not of damage, but of defense. And if we attend closely enough, even the faintest glimmer can be nurtured back to light.

1. Clinical Silence: When the Spark Disappears

When a patient goes quiet, the room often follows. Clinicians pause, family members worry, and the charts start to fill with terms like "withdrawn," "unresponsive," or "noncompliant." But often, silence is not emptiness—it is communication in a language few are trained to speak.

A woman on our long-term ward once went 47 days without uttering a word. Then, without prompting, she placed her hand on her chest and pointed to a photo of her children. That single gesture broke through a drought of expression. She was not unreachable. She was protecting herself from a world that had stopped asking.

Neuroscience offers insight. Studies reveal hypofunction in the dorsolateral prefrontal cortex, disrupted connectivity in the default mode network, and blunted dopaminergic activity in individuals experiencing extreme withdrawal. These regions are central to motivation, initiative, and goal-oriented action. What we label as apathy may be a state of neurological conservation or shutdown, especially in the face of chronic stress or trauma.

2. Catatonia: Sealed from the Inside

Catatonia is a clinical enigma—stillness so profound it borders on the sacred. Patients may stop moving, speaking, even reacting to basic stimuli. But underneath, something remains.

Catatonia is often perceived as an absence—of movement, speech, or will. Yet sometimes, beneath the stillness, there is a preserved presence waiting to emerge. One case stays with me:

Jerome lay unmoving for three days. When we administered lorazepam, he blinked, sat up, and asked, "Is it morning?" That moment changed how I see catatonia—not as void, but as containment.

Catatonia is increasingly understood through the lens of GABA-A receptor hypofunction, fronto-parietal dysregulation, and thalamocortical disconnect. Northoff's hypothesis of top-down modulation failure suggests that the brain, overwhelmed by internal chaos, attempts to silence itself. It is not a loss of self, but a sealing away of self.

Lorazepam and ECT are not just treatments—they are keys. They don't create spark. They unlock it.

3. Institutional Flattening and Learned Helplessness

Even well-meaning hospitals can become places where sparks go to dim. Predictable routines, constant supervision, minimal autonomy—they may ensure safety, but they also stifle spontaneity.

Darren had been in our unit for years. He once painted daily. Now, he refused to hold a pencil. "Why bother?" he said. It wasn't depression alone—it was despair learned through repetition.

Seligman's work on learned helplessness demonstrates how chronic unpredictability followed by powerlessness reshapes motivation. Neurobiologically, this is reflected in decreased activity in the hippocampus and diminished plasticity in reward-related pathways.

I started bringing blank paper to Darren. No request, no pressure. One day, Darren drew a red circle. The next, a blue square. By week's end, he had painted a bird. The spark returned—not because we treated symptoms, but because we offered possibility.

4. The Mask of Negative Symptoms

In schizophrenia, negative symptoms—diminished speech, flat affect, reduced social drive—can feel like a thick curtain separating a person from the world. But what if these aren't symptoms of absence, but symptoms of protection?

Aaron sat silently in group therapy for weeks. One afternoon, he moved his chair slightly closer to a peer. It was almost imperceptible. But it was effort. It was will.

Functional MRI studies show reduced ventral striatal activation in patients with negative symptoms, limiting their capacity to anticipate reward. But emotionally relevant cues can still elicit neural responses. The brain still cares. It's just quiet about it.

These symptoms are not a failure to feel, but often a failure to hope. Our job isn't to amplify emotion—it's to make hope worth the risk again.

5. Trauma and the Survival Logic of Silence

Some sparks vanish because they've been burned before. Patients with histories of abuse or betrayal may bury desire deep underground. Joy once made them vulnerable. Now, joy is dangerous.

Marisol, who had survived sexual abuse during a manic episode, refused to talk about relationships. "If I open that door," she said, "everything will come back." Her withdrawal was not avoidance. It was wisdom.

Trauma alters the hypothalamic-pituitary-adrenal axis, increases amygdala reactivity, and blunts oxytocin release—all of which impair trust and relational engagement. Spark, in this context, becomes a liability.

In trauma-informed care, we don't reignite too soon. We wait. We listen. We let the patient decide when light feels safe again.

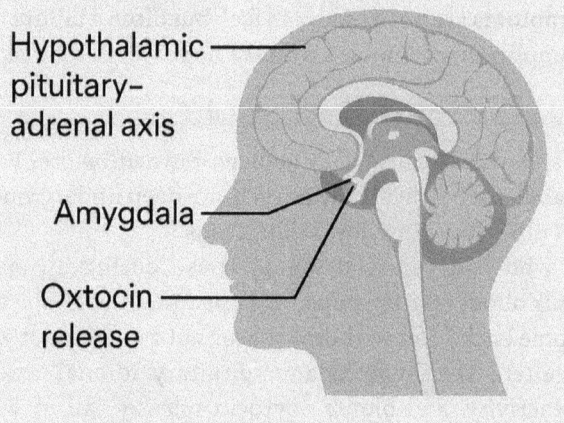

6. Reigniting: Small Flames, Not Bonfires

I've learned not to demand the spark. I've learned to invite it. What helps:
- Offer small, meaningful choices.
- Use music, scent, or imagery from the person's past.
- Celebrate micro-movements, gestures, or glances.
- Introduce therapy animals or sensory tools.
- Create a space where nothing is expected, only allowed.

One patient hadn't spoken in three years. I played recordings of birds from her homeland. She wept. Later, she whispered, "Parrot." That word was everything. It wasn't language. It was spark.

Research into behavioral activation, multisensory therapy, and relational neuroscience supports these findings. Sparks return not through pressure, but through presence.

7. Clinical Reflections: Watching for the Flicker

We miss so much because we're trained to look for loud symptoms. But what about the quiet ones—the faint smiles, the sighs, the rearranged blanket? These are signs.

One patient whispered, "Do mangoes still grow in Haiti?" after weeks of silence. Another reached out to touch a therapy dog's fur after lying still for months. Those moments stay with me.

The spark may not always roar back to life. Sometimes it glows faintly, just enough to say: I'm still here.

Conclusion: Absence Is Not the End

Sparks don't always flare with heat and brightness. Sometimes they whisper. Sometimes they hide. Sometimes they need time.

We must not mistake silence for surrender. What looks like a missing spark may simply be a waiting one.

If we offer safety, if we bring curiosity instead of judgment, the flame returns. And when it does—whether in a whisper, a drawing, a step forward—it tells us what matters.

It tells us the person is still there.

And that is enough.

Table 20.1 — Signs of Spark Loss

Spark	Loss Indicators	Clinical Red Flags
Music	Stops listening	Withdrawal, anhedonia
Food	Loss of appetite	Severe depression
Hope	Expresses despair	Suicidality

Northoff, G. (2002). What catatonia can tell us about "top-down modulation": A neuropsychiatric hypothesis. *Behavioral and Brain Sciences*, 25(5), 555–604.

Foussias, G., & Remington, G. (2010). Negative symptoms in schizophrenia: Avolition and Occam's razor. *Schizophrenia Bulletin*, 36(2), 359–369.

Seligman, M. E. P. (1972). Learned helplessness. *Annual Review of Medicine*, 23(1), 407–412.

Northoff, G., Koch, A., Wenke, J., Eckert, J., Böker, H., Pflug, B., & Bogerts, B. (1999). Catatonia as a psychomotor syndrome: A rating scale and extrapyramidal motor symptoms. *Movement Disorders*, 14(3), 404–416.

American Psychiatric Association. (2022). *Diagnostic and Statistical Manual of Mental Disorders* (5th ed., text rev.; DSM-5-TR). Arlington, VA: American Psychiatric Publishing.

Treadway, M. T., & Zald, D. H. (2011). Reconsidering anhedonia in depression: Lessons from translational neuroscience. *Neuroscience & Biobehavioral Reviews*, 35(3), 537–555.

Heim, C., & Nemeroff, C. B. (2001). The role of childhood trauma in the neurobiology of mood and anxiety disorders: Preclinical and clinical studies. *Biological Psychiatry*, 49(12), 1023–1039.

Insel, T. R. (2010). Rethinking schizophrenia. *Nature*, 468(7321), 187–193.

Northoff, G. (2004). Catatonia and neuroleptic malignant syndrome: Psychopathology and pathophysiology. *Journal of Neural Transmission*, 111(11), 1453–1467.

Part IV – Intersections and Integrations

Chapter 21:
The Intersection of the Sparks

Symptoms may shout, but sparks whisper. And if we listen closely, they'll tell us what still matters, what still burns.

Introduction: Not Just Symptoms, but Signals

In the lives of people living with serious mental illness, the elements that persist, recur, and often dominate attention are not random. They orbit around a recognizable constellation: sex, money, food, music, spirituality, creativity, movement, ritual, patient perspectives, and lived experience. These "sparks" are more than symptoms or obsessions. They are the raw materials of human motivation, identity, and survival.

The enduring preoccupations may appear separate, but in many cases, they overlap and intertwine, creating complex patterns of behavior that are difficult to untangle. These intersections highlight the multifaceted nature of preoccupations and their ability to impact different areas of life. When viewed together, they form a matrix of interwoven needs, drives, expressions, and interpretive frameworks that can illuminate not just pathology but purpose.

Writing this made me realize how often these sparks appear together—entwined, layered, unstoppable.

Each of these preoccupations represents survival, control, worth, and expression. Together, they form a mosaic of needs that inform the patient's sense of self, their actions, and their relationships with others. These sparks are not just symptoms; they are expressions of the mind's attempt to manage overwhelming forces of desire and loss. They are attempts to impose coherence, to restore agency, and to reclaim selfhood in the face of internal chaos and external marginalization.

These insights are not isolated; taken together, they form a lineage of thought about vitality and survival. Maslow spoke of self-actualization, Benson spoke of sparks, and Csikszentmihalyi spoke of flow. Each described humanity's striving for vitality. My patients remind me that these are not luxuries of the well but necessities of survival. I lived this paradox myself: chasing words long after midnight, only to be awakened by my daughters before dawn. Sparks endure not because conditions are perfect, but because they burn despite them.

Core Human Drives: Sex, Money, Food

These three sparks are often misunderstood as impulsive or pathological when it comes to serious mental illness. Yet they are primary human drives—biologically encoded and socially shaped.

Sex represents desire, identity, connection, power, and agency. It may emerge in mania, be suppressed in depression, or appear distorted by trauma or institutional life. For individuals whose lives have been regulated by institutions or medications, sexuality may remain one of the few remaining personal domains. In hypersexuality, there may be risk—but there is also a signal: a longing to be seen, to be touched, to matter.

Money stands for survival and independence. It figures heavily in delusions and fears—signaling a longing for control and status in systems that often strip these away. Money symbolizes agency in a world where many feel stripped of it. Obsessions with wealth may mask fears of worthlessness; compulsive generosity may be a cry for recognition.

Food becomes not just sustenance, but comfort, ritual, rebellion, or control. Its meaning intensifies when it comes to poverty, trauma, or medication side effects. For some, food becomes a form of grounding; for others, it is a site of anxiety and control. Patterns of overeating or restriction may reflect attempts to master the body when the mind feels unmoored.

"Her obsession with saving snack wrappers wasn't about hoarding—it was about remembering meals shared with her mother in foster care."

Sexual identity can be shaped by body image and food relationships. Financial stress can impact food access or sexual autonomy. These sparks often show up in metaphors, dreams, and clinical narratives—not just behaviors. They intersect in concerns about transactional relationships, exploitation, scarcity, shame, comfort, dignity, access, and meaning.

Expressive and Transcendent Channels: Music, Spirituality, Creativity

Where core drives speak to survival, these sparks speak to expression, coherence, and transcendence—ways to rise above pain, disorder, and limitation.

Music can be an internal anchor, a form of auditory regulation, or divine communication. It may soothe distress, organize thought, or reinforce identity. For those who hear voices, music may provide harmony amid the noise. For others, it becomes a daily ritual, a private symphony that restores a sense of self.

Spirituality offers a framework for suffering and structure for delusional systems. It answers questions like "Why me?" and "What now?"—often more powerfully than medication can. Even in spiritual delusions, there is often a yearning for purpose, dignity, and belonging.

Creativity becomes narrative reclamation. Drawing, writing, and inventing become ways to communicate when language fails. They transform fragmentation into expression. In the disorganized mind, creativity often survives as a structured act—making sense of chaos through color, words, and form.

One patient drew cities where everything was symmetrical and safe—unlike the shelters where he'd lived most of his life.

Together, these sparks form a soulful triad—fueling hope, meaning, and symbolic richness: music as prayer, art as prophecy, creativity as spiritual resistance. Their interweaving provides glimpses into the patient's internal logic, often obscured by psychiatric labeling.

Embodied Regulation: Movement and Ritual

These sparks are kinesthetic and temporal tools for managing internal chaos.

Movement includes walking, rocking, pacing, dancing. It reflects efforts to regulate overwhelm, whether intentional or involuntary. In mania, it may express energy; in depression, a longing for reactivation. Even catatonic gestures have symbolic resonance, as if the body is enacting what the mind cannot speak.

Ritual brings rhythm and symbolic order. Whether religious, cultural, compulsive, or invented, rituals provide grounding, containment, and meaning. Repeated behaviors often hold secret meanings—mourning, memory, protection, hope.

Clinical vignette: During morning rounds, a young man insists on tapping the window four times before speaking. His psychiatrist later learns that the number four corresponds to the names of his siblings, all separated in foster care. The ritual, once pathologized, becomes a symbol of connection.

Movement and ritual often overlap as gestures with emotional weight, spiritual meaning, or trauma-linked roots. They interact with all other sparks: ritualizing food, dancing to music, repeating prayers, pacing through grief. They are the language of the unspeakable.

Interpretive Lenses: Patient Perspectives and Lived Experience

These sparks shape how all others are interpreted.

Patient perspectives include narratives, meaning-making, and interpretations of symptoms, relationships, and care. Understanding how someone explains their hallucinations or behaviors is crucial to building trust.

Lived experience encompasses the wisdom of survival through navigating systems, stigma, and healing. These voices often illuminate what traditional diagnostics obscure.

One patient didn't want to stop drawing monsters. She wanted someone to ask why they were always looking in the mirror.

Centering these perspectives reveals why certain sparks endure and how they reflect trauma, resistance, and adaptation. A ritual may be healing or harmful. A song may be divine or disturbing. Listening to lived experience helps clinicians choose how to support or challenge these meanings.

Hidden Anchors of Survival and Meaning: Nature, Humor, Touch, Storytelling, Freedom

Nature restores physiological balance and symbolic grounding. Green space offers sensory regulation: the scent of pine, the rhythm of waves, the warmth of sun on skin. For some, nature is sanctuary from institutional walls; for others, it represents freedom long denied. Patients often describe trees as companions, rivers as listeners, gardens as a place where something finally grows.

"I water the plants so I remember life can still depend on me."

Humor reframes suffering and builds social bridges. A joke can puncture the heaviness of a ward and transform identity from "patient" to "comedian," from "symptom" to "sage." Humor activates reward pathways, releases endorphins, and lowers cortisol, but it also signals resilience: the ability to hold paradox, irony, and perspective in the face of despair.

"The voices tell me I'm worthless, but at least they're consistent roommates."

Touch anchors people to their bodies and to each other. Its absence—whether from trauma, neglect, or institutional fear—can deepen alienation. Gentle, safe touch regulates the nervous system, conveys belonging, and affirms dignity. In psychosis, yearning for touch may emerge in metaphors, repetitive gestures, or requests easily misinterpreted as boundary violations. The clinical challenge is discerning unsafe touch from the basic human need for connection.

One patient explained that folding hospital blankets was "the closest thing I have to a hug."

Storytelling allows patients to reclaim authorship of their lives. Symptoms often strip coherence; stories restore it. Whether told through journals, spoken narratives, or delusional frameworks, stories reveal inner logic and preserve identity. Clinically, listening to stories provides more than diagnostic detail—it offers clues to resilience, hope, and the meanings hidden in sparks.

"She didn't need her monsters to disappear; she needed someone to ask why they always looked in mirrors."

Freedom embodies autonomy, agency, and self-determination. For patients living under surveillance, locked doors, or heavy medication regimens, even small choices—when to eat, what to wear, how to spend an hour—carry profound meaning. Freedom is often expressed through resistance: refusing treatment, pacing corridors, or dreaming of escape. Yet it can also manifest in quiet dignity—the ability to say no, to speak truth, to imagine a life beyond constraint.

"When they finally let me keep my shoelaces, I felt like a person again."

Intersections and Integration

The sparks rarely exist in isolation. Nature grounds ritual. Humor softens shame. Touch restores trust. Storytelling provides coherence. Freedom ties them all together—reminding us that each spark is about agency, survival, and meaning in the face of constraint.

Across all fourteen sparks, intersections reveal how drives, expressions, embodied practices, and hidden anchors weave together into lived experience:

- A patient listens to a song each morning as part of a private spiritual ritual connecting them to a lost loved one.
- A man prepares a meal while listening to his grandmother's favorite music, reclaiming a sense of heritage.
- A woman draws food images tied to memories of maternal care in childhood.
- A teen in a residential facility paces nightly while reciting rap lyrics, finding in them a voice for his rage and hope.
- A patient cracks jokes during mealtime, transforming the ward's atmosphere while reinforcing belonging.

- A young woman tends plants in the hospital courtyard, describing it as "the only place I can breathe freely."
- A man insists on telling his story of survival at each group, reminding staff that narrative is itself a form of healing.

These intersections highlight symbolic content, emotional depth, and therapeutic opportunity. They tell the story behind the spark—not just the symptom.

The 14 Sparks That Endure

Core Human Drives (survival and agency)

- Sex

- Money

- Food

Expressive & Transcendent Channels (expression and meaning)

- Music

- Spirituality

- Creativity

Embodied Regulation (grounding and order)

- Movement

- Ritual

Hidden Anchors of Survival & Meaning (connection and resilience)

- Nature

- Humor

- Touch

- Storytelling

- Hope

- Freedom

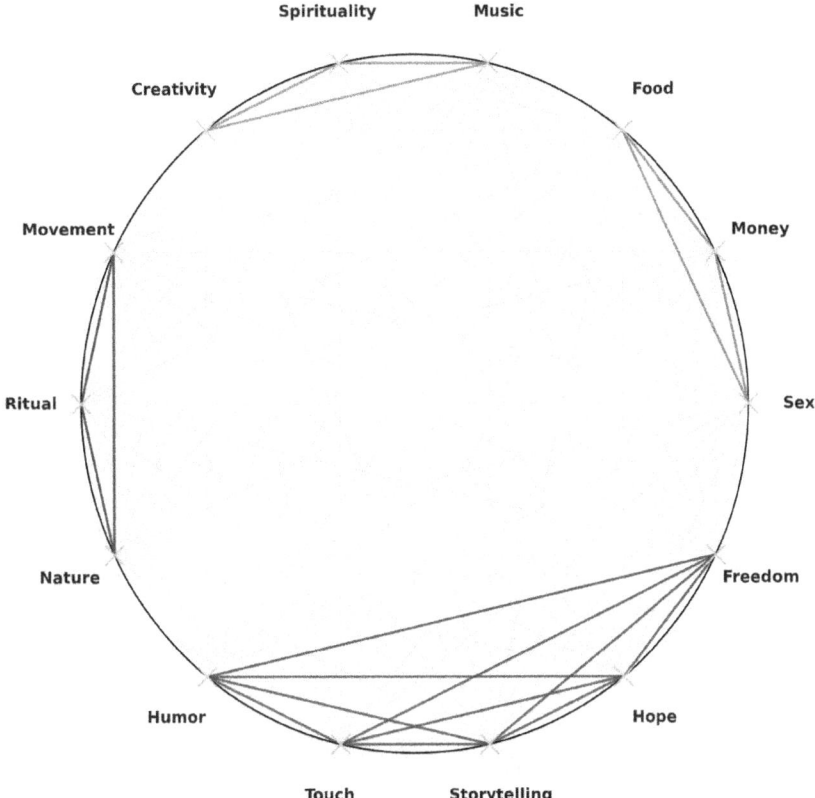

Clinical Implications: Engaging the Intersections

- See the spark before the symptom. Look for the human need beneath the behavior.
- Ask what function the spark serves. What is it regulating, expressing, or remembering?
- Explore intersections. How does music relate to trauma? How does food reflect identity?
- Center the patient's interpretations. They are not passive recipients of care but active agents of meaning.

To harness the power of sparks:
- Validate, don't pathologize.
- Look for function.
- Explore symbolic meaning.
- Engage the whole person.

Conclusion: Sparks as Survival

The sparks—sex, money, food, music, spirituality, creativity, movement, rituals, nature, humor, touch, storytelling, hope, and freedom—are not isolated quirks but expressions of deep human needs. When they intersect, they form a web of meaning, memory, and motivation that survives even amid illness and stigma.

Clinicians and families who learn to recognize these interconnected sparks begin to see patients not as collections of symptoms, but as resilient individuals using deeply human tools to navigate overwhelming experiences. These sparks, often mislabeled as maladaptive, are, in fact, lifelines—attempts to preserve vitality, coherence, and agency.

True healing happens when we move from symptom management to meaning-making, from behavior control to connection. Whether it's music as ritual, food as memory, or movement as expression, these sparks reveal both the fragility and the endurance of the human spirit.

By honoring them all—visible and invisible—we shift from stabilizing illness to sustaining life. In this way, sparks become not just signs of what was lost, but pathways to what still burns bright.

Sparks tell us what people hold onto when everything else falls away.

Table 21.1 — Spark Interactions

Spark Pair	Interaction	Example
Music + Spirituality	Transcendence	Gospel, chanting
Money + Freedom	Autonomy	Employment, budgeting
Nature + Rituals	Grounding	Morning walks

1. Northoff, G. (2002). What catatonia can tell us about "top-down modulation": A neuropsychiatric hypothesis. *Behavioral and Brain Sciences*, 25(5), 555–604.
2. Foussias, G., & Remington, G. (2010). Negative symptoms in schizophrenia: Avolition and Occam's razor. *Schizophrenia Bulletin*, 36(2), 359–369.
3. Seligman, M. E. P. (1972). Learned helplessness. *Annual Review of Medicine*, 23(1), 407–412.
4. Northoff, G., Koch, A., Wenke, J., Eckert, J., Böker, H., Pflug, B., & Bogerts, B. (1999). Catatonia as a psychomotor syndrome: A rating scale and extrapyramidal motor symptoms. *Movement Disorders*, 14(3), 404–416.

5. American Psychiatric Association. (2022). *Diagnostic and Statistical Manual of Mental Disorders* (5th ed., text rev.; DSM-5-TR). Arlington, VA: American Psychiatric Publishing.
6. Treadway, M. T., & Zald, D. H. (2011). Reconsidering anhedonia in depression: Lessons from translational neuroscience. *Neuroscience & Biobehavioral Reviews*, 35(3), 537–555.
7. Heim, C., & Nemeroff, C. B. (2001). The role of childhood trauma in the neurobiology of mood and anxiety disorders: Preclinical and clinical studies. *Biological Psychiatry*, 49(12), 1023–1039.
8. Insel, T. R. (2010). Rethinking schizophrenia. *Nature*, 468(7321), 187–193.
9. Northoff, G. (2004). Catatonia and neuroleptic malignant syndrome: Psychopathology and pathophysiology. *Journal of Neural Transmission*, 111(11), 1453–1467.

Chapter 22:
Whispers Through Time: What the Mad and Brilliant Taught Us About Sparks

Introduction: Madness, Brilliance, and the Enduring Spark

Throughout history, the boundary between madness and brilliance has often been blurred. Many of the most revered artists, mystics, scientists, and performers lived with inner storms that, today, would carry psychiatric diagnoses—schizophrenia, bipolar disorder, major depression, or psychosis. Yet what is truly remarkable is not only their suffering; it is what endured through it.

In the tapestry of history, woven with threads of extraordinary achievement, we find figures—celebrities bathed in public adoration, artists whose creations stir the soul, and Nobel laureates who have illuminated the frontiers of knowledge—who also navigated the treacherous landscapes of serious mental illness. Their stories, often whispered through the corridors of time, offer a profound and at times unsettling glimpse into the intricate dance between brilliance and vulnerability.

The eras in which many of these figures lived offered scant understanding and often brutal judgment towards those grappling with mental health challenges. Eccentricity, a label often applied to those who defied societal norms, could mask profound suffering. The "price of genius" was a convenient explanation for behaviors that today we might recognize as symptoms of genuine illness. Treatment, when it existed, was often crude and ineffective, further isolating those in need.

Even at the height of delusion, despair, or isolation, something inside them still reached outward. They painted. They danced. They composed. They prayed. They wrote. These actions were not mere symptoms or distractions—they were expressions of enduring human sparks: creativity, movement, ritual, meaning, connection, and hope.

This chapter honors those whose lives embodied these sparks across centuries and continents. Their stories challenge the assumption that illness erases identity. Instead, they show us how the spark adapts, endures, and speaks—even when the mind is unraveling.

Vincent van Gogh (1853–1890)

Sparks: Creativity, Spirituality, Ritual
Quote: "The best way to know life is to love many things."

Van Gogh's life was marked by pain, social isolation, and repeated psychiatric hospitalizations. He experienced hallucinations, delusions, and likely bipolar or schizoaffective disorder, or temporal lobe epilepsy. During periods of acute instability, he produced luminous, emotionally saturated art. His letters to his brother Theo reveal longing, despair, theological yearning, and lucid awareness of his struggles.

While institutionalized at Saint-Rémy-de-Provence, he painted some of his most iconic works: "Starry Night," "Irises," and "Cypresses." These were not mere acts of artistry; they were acts of spiritual survival. The brush became a compass—each painting, a ritual; each canvas, a testament to a world he struggled to stay part of. The vibrant energy of his canvases stands in stark contrast to the inner turmoil that ultimately led to his tragic end. His story, often romanticized, underscores the profound connection between intense emotional experience and creative expression, while also highlighting the devastating impact of untreated mental illness.

Robert Schumann (1810–1856)

Sparks: Music, Romantic Longing, Storytelling
Quote: "To send light into the darkness of men's hearts—such is the duty of the artist."

The realm of music, too, echoes with these somber notes. Robert Schumann, a towering figure of the Romantic era, poured his passionate soul into compositions that ranged from soaring symphonies to intimate piano pieces. Schumann believed in the redemptive power of music. His life was shaped by waves of depression and elation, likely due to bipolar disorder. Listening to his music, one can perhaps discern the dramatic shifts in mood, the sudden bursts of joy followed by melancholic introspection, a possible reflection of his internal struggles. His story reminds us that even the most harmonious minds can be disrupted by internal discord. His marriage to the brilliant pianist Clara Wieck-Schumann inspired his most intimate compositions—and his most profound grief. In periods of mania, he wrote with lightning speed. In depression, he withdrew completely. He reportedly heard angels—and later, demonic voices—singing to him.

After a suicide attempt in 1854, he was institutionalized for the final years of his life. Yet even within the asylum, music still came to him. What others might have dismissed as delusion, he experienced as sacred sound. The spark of music persisted when almost everything else had been stripped away.

John Nash (1928–2015)

Sparks: Mathematics, Logic, Identity
Quote: "I wouldn't have had good scientific ideas if I had thought more normally."

John Nash, a mathematical prodigy, revolutionized game theory and economic modeling. He also spent decades struggling with paranoid schizophrenia. During some of his most psychotic periods, he believed he was a divine messenger and that coded messages were hidden in newspaper headlines. He was institutionalized multiple times. At one point, he withdrew from academic life entirely.

And yet, even as reality unraveled, his mind continued working on abstract theories. Over time, and without medication, Nash began to regain insight and re-enter the academic world. In 1994, he was awarded the Nobel Prize in Economic Sciences. His intellectual spark had not only survived psychosis—it had kept glowing beneath it all along.

Sylvia Plath (1932–1963)

Sparks: Language, Identity, Intimacy
Quote: "I took a deep breath and listened to the old brag of my heart: I am, I am, I am."

Plath's words carved pathways through pain. She lived with major depression, likely with psychotic features, and underwent multiple psychiatric hospitalizations. She attempted suicide more than once. Yet her poetry was never simply a reaction to her illness—it was a structure for holding it.

Her writing shimmered with complexity: feminine rage, domestic entrapment, longing for purity, and the coldness of institutions. *The Bell Jar*, her autobiographical novel, remains one of the most powerful depictions of psychiatric collapse in literature. Even in her final days, she organized her poems into what became *Ariel*—a collection of blistering emotional clarity and dark beauty.

Vaslav Nijinsky (1889–1950)

Sparks: Movement, Sex, Identity
Quote: "God is movement."

Nijinsky, a ballet icon, was capable of gravity-defying leaps and emotive precision few dancers have ever matched. His performances were revolutionary—*The Rite of Spring* sparked riots with its primal choreography. But behind the scenes, he suffered from what would now be considered schizophrenia.

In his early thirties, he wrote a diary during a six-week psychotic break—a haunting, poetic, and spiritual account of his inner world. After that, he never danced publicly again. Still, long after language failed, he would still move. His body remembered. Movement remained sacred, ritualized, and alive within him.

Margery Kempe (c.1373–c.1438)

Sparks: Spirituality, Ritual, Voice
Quote: "Many men marveled at her weeping."

Kempe was a medieval English mystic who experienced postpartum spiritual ecstasy. She heard voices, saw visions, and engaged in uncontrollable sobbing—likely what modern psychiatry would call religious psychosis or postpartum psychosis. But rather than retreating into silence, she dictated her autobiography (the first in the English language) to a scribe.

She traveled across Europe, weeping in churches, refusing to conform, and proclaiming her divine revelations. Her rituals were inconvenient to many, but she insisted that her spark—spiritual intimacy with God—was her true purpose.

Emily Dickinson (1830–1886)

Sparks: Nature, Inner Life, Ritual
Quote: "Hope is the thing with feathers that perches in the soul."

Dickinson lived most of her life in a single house in Amherst, Massachusetts. Reclusive, sensitive, possibly suffering from anxiety or depression, she rarely ventured into the outside world. But inside, her mind was expansive. She wrote nearly 1,800 poems—many exploring death, nature, immortality, and God.

Her solitude was not a symptom to be eradicated, it was a chosen way of life that nurtured her deepest spark: quiet, reverent observation. She found whole universes in a bee's wing, in a graveyard shadow, in a single breath.

Virginia Woolf (1882 – 1941)

Sparks: Storytelling, Freedom, Creativity

Quote: "Lock up your libraries if you like; but there is no gate, no lock, no bolt that you can set upon the freedom of my mind."

Think of Virginia Woolf, a literary supernova, a luminous figure in modernist literature, whose stream-of-consciousness prose revolutionized the novel, allowing readers unprecedented access to the intricate workings of the human mind. Yet, she battled recurrent episodes of severe depression, which she poignantly described in her writings with unflinching honesty. Her literary brilliance and her courageous, though ultimately fatal, struggle with mental illness offer a powerful testament to the resilience and fragility of the human spirit. Her diaries provide intimate glimpses into the cyclical nature of her suffering and the societal pressures she faced. Her luminous intellect and her courageous, though ultimately heartbreaking, battle with mental illness underscore the poignant truth that even the most articulate minds can be silenced by the weight of inner suffering. Her story is a testament to both the power of her artistic vision and the insidious nature of the illness that ultimately claimed her.

Woolf's work testifies to the enduring human need to craft narrative and to claim inner freedom, even in the midst of mental illness. Her stream-of-consciousness writing style reshaped literature by refusing confinement to linear thought—an act of artistic rebellion against constraint. Her struggles with depression and psychosis did not silence her voice; instead, they deepened her exploration of the tension between isolation and connection, silence and speech, despair and hope.

Even in the more traditionally rational realms of science, the dedication and singular focus required for groundbreaking discoveries can sometimes border on obsession, a trait that can be amplified or complicated by mental health challenges. While the connection may be less overtly emotional than in the arts, the intense drive and unconventional thinking that led to scientific breakthroughs might share a similar origin with the passionate intensity seen in artistic genius. The sparks of scientific insight, perhaps, require a mind willing to venture to the very edges of conventional thought, a space where the boundaries between brilliance and perceived "madness" can sometimes blur.

From these "haunted muses," we glean several crucial insights about the nature of our own enduring sparks:

- Sparks can be fueled by intensity: The raw energy of intense emotions, both positive and negative, can act as a powerful catalyst for creative and intellectual breakthroughs. The fire of passion, even when tinged with suffering, can illuminate new pathways.
- Vulnerability can be a source of authenticity: The willingness to confront and explore the darker aspects of the human experience

can lead to profound artistic and intellectual truths that resonate deeply with others. Authenticity, often born from vulnerability, can ignite powerful connections.
- Sparks are not always linear or stable: The creative and intellectual process is rarely a smooth, upward trajectory. It can be marked by periods of intense activity and quiet contemplation, of soaring inspiration and frustrating stagnation, much like the fluctuating experiences of those with mental illness.
- The line between brilliance and "madness" can be thin: History often judges those who push the boundaries of convention as either brilliant or mad, sometimes both. Their stories challenge us to reconsider these labels and to recognize the potential for profound insight in unconventional ways of thinking.

While historical records may be less forthcoming about the mental health struggles of Nobel laureates in earlier periods, the intense pressures inherent in groundbreaking scientific discovery—the relentless pursuit of answers, the isolation of deep thought, the weight of expectation—likely took a toll. The very nature of such demanding intellectual work could exacerbate underlying vulnerabilities. While specific cases might remain shrouded in the privacy of history, it is reasonable to surmise that the pantheon of scientific achievement includes individuals who navigated their own internal storms while illuminating the world with their discoveries.

Looking back at these lives, what enduring sparks can we identify amidst the shadows?
- The indomitable spirit of creation: Despite their inner battles, these individuals often produced work of extraordinary beauty and significance. Their creative drive, it seems, could coexist with and sometimes even draw from their intense emotional landscapes.
- The universality of human suffering: Their stories shatter the illusion that fame, fortune, or intellectual prowess can shield one from the vulnerabilities of the human mind. Mental illness is a universal experience, transcending societal boundaries.
- The lingering stain of stigma: The historical context of their lives underscores the profound damage caused by ignorance and stigma surrounding mental illness. The lack of understanding likely compounded their suffering and limited their access to support.
- Support and understanding can nurture sparks: Imagine the potential that might have been unlocked if these individuals had lived in a time with greater understanding and more effective support for mental health. Their stories underscore the importance of fostering

environments that nurture, rather than stifle, the unique sparks within each individual, regardless of their internal struggles.

Conclusion: The Spark Is Timeless

The whispers of time surrounding these haunted muses serve as a powerful reminder that brilliance and vulnerability are not mutually exclusive. Their enduring legacies, both in their remarkable achievements and in their often-untold struggles, offer us invaluable lessons in the complexities of the human condition and the enduring need for compassion and understanding in the face of mental illness. Their sparks, though sometimes flickering in the darkness, continue to illuminate the path towards a more humane and enlightened future.

These individuals lived across centuries, continents, and cultures. They were canonized, committed, misunderstood, and celebrated. They were pathologized and romanticized. But what unites them is not simply their illness. It is the spark that survived it.

Creativity, movement, logic, spirituality, ritual, intimacy—these were not extinguished by madness. They endured through it.

Their stories remind us that psychiatry must look not only at symptoms, but at signals. Not only at dysfunction, but at desire. Not only at the clinical record, but at the human trace that illness leaves behind.

As clinicians, researchers, and fellow human beings, we are called to do more than assess. We are called to witness. The spark does not disappear in psychosis. It shifts. It whispers. It takes new forms. And sometimes, if we are listening, it speaks to us through a poem, a painting, a movement, or weeping that won't stop.

It says: I am still here.

Ultimately, the whispers from the "mad" and brilliant teach us that the sparks that endure are often complex and multifaceted. They can be ignited by joy and sorrow, fueled by intense focus, and sometimes flicker in the shadows. By acknowledging the full spectrum of human experience, including its vulnerabilities, we can gain a deeper appreciation for the power and resilience of the human spirit and create a world where all sparks, however unconventional, have the potential to illuminate the world. By also acknowledging the struggles of these remarkable individuals, we are called to approach those living with mental illness today with greater compassion, empathy, and a commitment to fostering a more supportive and understanding society.

Van Gogh, V., & Van Gogh, T. (1996). *The Letters of Vincent van Gogh* (M. Roskill, Trans.). London: Penguin Classics.

Naifeh, S., & Smith, G. W. (2011). *Van Gogh: The Life.* New York: Random House.

Daverio, J. (1997). *Robert Schumann: Herald of a "New Poetic Age."* New York: Oxford University Press.

Ostwald, P. F. (1985). *Schumann: The Inner Voices of a Musical Genius.* Boston: Northeastern University Press.

Nasar, S. (1998). *A Beautiful Mind.* New York: Simon & Schuster.

Plath, S. (1963/2006). *The Bell Jar.* New York: Harper Perennial.

Plath, S. (1965/2018). *Ariel: The Restored Edition.* New York: HarperCollins.

Nijinsky, V. (1999). *The Diary of Vaslav Nijinsky.* (J. Acocella, Ed.). New York: Farrar, Straus and Giroux.

Kempe, M. (1985). *The Book of Margery Kempe.* (B. Windeatt, Trans.). London: Penguin Classics.

Dickinson, E. (1999). *The Poems of Emily Dickinson.* (R. W. Franklin, Ed.). Cambridge, MA: Harvard University Press.

Woolf, V. (1925/2000). *Mrs. Dalloway.* London: Hogarth Press.

Woolf, V. (1931/2002). *The Waves.* London: Hogarth Press.

Lee, H. (1996). *Virginia Woolf.* New York: Vintage.

Jamison, K. R. (1993). *Touched with Fire: Manic-Depressive Illness and the Artistic Temperament.* New York: Free Press.

Andreasen, N. C. (2005). *The Creating Brain: The Neuroscience of Genius.* New York: Dana Press.

Post, F. (1994). Creativity and psychopathology. A study of 291 world-famous men. *British Journal of Psychiatry*, 165(1), 22–34.

Chapter 23:
Sparks Across Borders: Culture, Region, and the Global Expression of Human Drives

Mental illness may speak in symptoms, but culture shapes the accent.

Introduction: The Cultural Life of Sparks

I remember working with a Haitian immigrant patient who rarely discussed his feelings directly. Instead, he spoke of bad spirits, disrupted rituals, and the need to "clean his house" spiritually. At first, I focused on his depressive symptoms. But over time, I realized his healing pathway wasn't about cognitive restructuring or SSRIs; it was about restoring spiritual rhythm.

In that moment, I understood that sparks—those enduring drives for meaning, connection, and autonomy—don't just survive illness. They survive across oceans, languages, and belief systems.

I didn't realize at first that sparks could have accents. I thought they were universal: biological, inevitable, primal. But the longer I practiced, the more I began to notice that the same spark—a craving for connection, for control, for beauty—sounded different in different mouths. What was expressed through rhythm in one country came through ritual in another. What was spoken directly in one clinic was disguised as somatic pain or myth in another. The spark was still there; it was just wearing local clothes.

Psychiatry is not practiced in a vacuum. It is shaped by the values of the society in which it stands, and in turn it reshapes the lives it touches, determining which sparks are honored and which are hidden.

Sparks endure, but they are never untouched. They are pressed into silence by stigma or nourished by ritual. They are cloaked in language that may not translate neatly into diagnostic terms. They take forms that look strange to us until we pause long enough to see their meaning.

To understand the global expression of sparks, we must release the illusion that psychiatry operates apart from culture. Sparks breathe story, they breathe community, and they flicker even in places that at first feel unfamiliar.

Section I: Global Psychiatry, Global Sparks

Across the world, psychiatric practice ranges from high-tech urban clinics to rural villages where healing is mediated by rituals and ancestral traditions. These variations profoundly shape how sparks are expressed—or repressed. They influence which sparks are honored, which are silenced, and which are transformed.

🌐 Western Europe

In much of Western Europe—UK, France, Germany, the Netherlands—psychiatry operates within public health systems. Community-based care, psychotherapy, and biopsychosocial models are strongly emphasized. Recovery is often framed socially, rather than spiritually.

- Sex: Discussed openly, especially in progressive regions like the Netherlands and Scandinavia, though hypersexuality is still often pathologized.
- Money: Less of a destabilizing factor due to robust welfare systems.
- Spirituality: Frequently excluded from psychiatric dialogue, especially in secular contexts like in France.
- Creativity, Nature, Humor: Integrated into expressive arts programs, eco-therapy, occupational rehabilitation, and laughter groups.

🌐 East Asia

Japan, South Korea, and China share a psychiatric landscape deeply influenced by Confucian values, stigma, family roles, and the pressure of social conformity. Patients often delay seeking care, and when they do, suffering is frequently expressed through the body.

- Desire and Emotion: Commonly presented as somatic complaints (headaches, stomach distress, fatigue).
- Sexuality: Rarely discussed openly; often sublimated.
- Spirituality: Practiced privately; Buddhism, Shinto, and ancestor reverence remain background frameworks.
- Money: Linked to academic and professional success; loss of financial stability carries enormous shame.
- Rituals and Food: Tea ceremonies, communal meals, and seasonal festivals provide therapeutic rhythm and social anchoring.

🌍 Sub-Saharan Africa

In countries such as Nigeria, Kenya, Ethiopia, and Ghana, psychiatric services are often under-resourced. Traditional healers and community rituals fill the gap, blending spirituality, storytelling, and collective healing.
- Spirituality and Rituals: Healing ceremonies, ancestor veneration, prayer gatherings, drumming, and sacrifice.
- Music and Movement: Central to both joy and grief; communal drumming often serves as therapy.
- Touch: Physical connection is communal, affirming, and healing.
- Storytelling and Myth: Narratives and legends frame trauma and resilience.
- Stigma: Remains high, but family and community involvement are strong.

🌍 Middle East and North Africa

Psychiatry here coexists with religious traditions, especially Islam, and with deeply rooted family structures.
- Mental illness: Commonly interpreted as a spiritual imbalance, punishment, or test from God.
- Sexuality: Taboo; strongly regulated by gender roles. Desires often surface indirectly, through dreams or metaphor.
- Religious Rituals: Daily prayer, fasting, and Qur'anic recitation offer meaning and structure.
- Money and Status: Tied to masculinity, family honor, and social identity.
- Touch: Restricted by gender norms; affects therapeutic rapport.
- Humor and Storytelling: Provide indirect ways to process suffering.

🌍 Latin America and the Caribbean (including Haiti)

Psychiatric care blends Western biomedicine with Catholic, Indigenous, and Afro-Caribbean traditions. Healing often occurs in families, churches, or communal spaces.
- Spirituality, Ritual, Music, Humor: Intertwined in faith-based and communal healing.
- Visible Practices: Rosaries, saints, Vodou ceremonies, altars, and candles are integrated into treatment narratives.
- Storytelling: Suffering is often narrated collectively, within spiritual or historical frames.
- Hope and Freedom: Refracted through colonial trauma, political struggle, and liberation theology.

Regional Variation in the United States

Even within one country, sparks differ by geography, race, class, and religion.
- Urban: Sparks like sexuality, creativity, and identity are discussed openly, supported by diverse services.
- Rural: Reliance on primary care, faith, and family; sparks expressed through food, humor, spirituality.
- Regional identities: Deeply shape whether sparks are pathologized or celebrated.

Section II: Clinical Implications: What Happens When Sparks Are Misread?

When psychiatry ignores culture, sparks risk being mislabeled as symptoms.
- A Somali refugee who hears music in dreams may be told she is hallucinating.
- A Pentecostal man's speaking in tongues may be dismissed as disorganized speech.
- An Asian-American woman's silence about sexuality may be misread as absence of desire.

Symptoms are easier to code than culture is to comprehend.

What sounds like disorganized speech might be poetry. What looks like a delusion might be symbolic survival. What is dismissed as avoidance might be a culturally sanctioned form of mourning or protest.

Section III: Culturally Attuned Psychiatric Practice

To bridge the gap, clinicians need structured tools and intentional listening practices.

1. DSM-5 Cultural Formulation Interview (CFI)

Introduced in DSM-5, the CFI provides 16 open-ended questions about cultural definitions, causes, coping, and the therapeutic relationship.[1]

Example: A Somali refugee reports "jinn" attacks. Without CFI: psychosis. With CFI: trauma-related sleep paralysis, explained through cultural idioms.

Takeaway: The CFI transforms symptoms into sparks by asking, "How do you understand this?"

2. Narrative Psychiatry and Collaborative Storytelling

Narrative psychiatry reframes patients as narrators rather than cases.

Example: A Mexican-American woman describes her depression as "a well with no bottom." Exploring that metaphor revealed intergenerational grief and language loss.

Takeaway: Stories reveal sparks. Clinicians must listen for metaphors, honor cultural idioms of distress, and co-construct resilient storylines.

3. Ethnographic Listening and Clinician Self-Awareness
Ethnographic listening asks clinicians to treat each patient encounter as entry into a cultural world.

Example: A Haitian man describes being visited nightly by ancestors. Dismissed as hallucination by some, understood as sacred practice through ethnographic listening.

Takeaway: Humility is more therapeutic than interpretation. Clinicians must ask: "What meanings might I be missing?"

Section IV: Integration: From Culture to Person-Centered Global Psychiatry

When sparks are understood not only through neurobiology but also through culture, history, and lived narrative, psychiatry moves from intervention to partnership. Sparks are more than drives; they are cultural expressions of longing, adapted to survive in local soil.

Modern psychiatry must become polyglot—able to hear sparks in prayer, drumbeat, poetry, silence, dance, and complaint.

Conclusion: Across Borders, the Sparks Endure

The sparks that animate human life—sex, food, music, meaning, ritual, freedom—are not culturally fixed. They are culturally interpreted. And yet, they persist. They flicker in different hues, wear different masks, dance to different rhythms, but they endure.

Wherever the mind breaks, the spark tries to speak. Our task is not to force it into our language, but to learn to hear it in theirs.

This chapter is not about cultural difference; it is about universal desire expressed through particular forms. No matter where in the world someone struggles with schizophrenia, bipolar disorder, or trauma, they do so not as an abstraction but as a cultural being. And their sparks, however obscured, still burn.

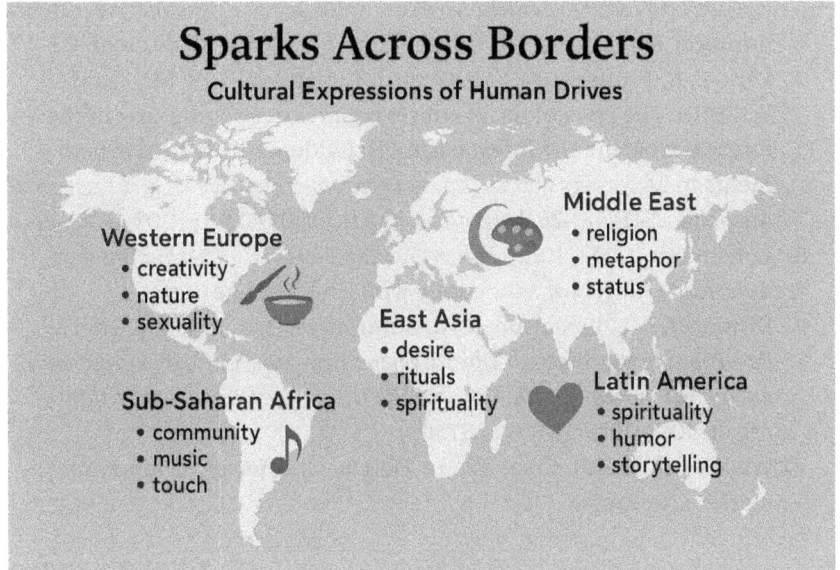

Table 23.1 — Cultural Variations of Sparks

Spark	Cultural Example	Implication
Food	Fasting in Ramadan	Spiritual discipline
Humor	Satire under oppression	Coping mechanism
Storytelling	Indigenous oral histories	Cultural survival

Notes

1. American Psychiatric Association. (2013). *Diagnostic and statistical manual of mental disorders* (5th ed.). American Psychiatric Publishing. https://doi.org/10.1176/appi.books.9780890425596
2. Charon, R. (2006). *Narrative medicine: Honoring the stories of illness.* Oxford University Press.
3. Lysaker, P. H., & Lysaker, J. T. (2008). *Schizophrenia and the fate of the self: A narrative account.* Oxford University Press.
4. Kleinman, A. (1988). *The illness narratives: Suffering, healing, and the human condition.* Basic Books.
5. Good, B. J. (1994). *Medicine, rationality, and experience: An anthropological perspective.* Cambridge University Press.
6. Bratman, G. N., Anderson, C. B., Berman, M. G., Cochran, B., de Vries, S., Flanders, J., Folke, C., Frumkin, H., Gross, J. J., Hartig, T., Kahn, P. H., Kuo, M., Lawler, J. J., Levin, P. S., Lindahl, T., Meyer-Lindenberg, A., Mitchell, R., Ouyang, Z., Roe, J., ... Daily, G. C. (2019).

Nature and mental health: An ecosystem service perspective. *Science Advances, 5*(7), eaax0903. https://doi.org/10.1126/sciadv.aax0903
7. Park, B. J., Tsunetsugu, Y., Kasetani, T., Kagawa, T., & Miyazaki, Y. (2010). The physiological effects of Shinrin-yoku (taking in the forest atmosphere or forest bathing): Evidence from field experiments in 24 forests across Japan. *Environmental Health and Preventive Medicine, 15*(1), 18–26. https://doi.org/10.1007/s12199-009-0086-9
8. Luhrmann, T. M. (2012). *When God talks back: Understanding the American evangelical relationship with God.* Vintage Books.
9. Kirmayer, L. J., Lemelson, R., & Cummings, C. A. (Eds.). (2015). *Re-visioning psychiatry: Cultural phenomenology, critical neuroscience, and global mental health.* Cambridge University Press. https://doi.org/10.1017/CBO9781139628750
10. Watters, E. (2010). *Crazy like us: The globalization of the American psyche.* Free Press.

Chapter 24:
Amplifying Voices: The Importance of Patient Perspectives and Lived Experience

The best lessons I've learned in psychiatry didn't come from textbooks—they came from my patients.

A man once told me, "Don't ask me what's wrong—ask me what still matters." That single sentence reshaped my approach. It reminded me that even in illness, people are narrators of their own meaning, not just objects of our assessment.

Recovery is deeply personal and cannot be defined solely by symptom reduction. Slade emphasizes the importance of allowing patient voices to guide care, framing recovery as a return to meaning, agency, and purpose.[1]

In the preceding chapters, we explored the enduring sparks that remain alive in individuals living with serious mental illness (SMI). Yet understanding these sparks abstractly is not enough. To truly support healing, we must listen to the voices of those who live with these conditions. Let's take a closer look at why amplifying patient perspectives and lived experience is central to recovery-oriented, person-centered care.

This focus on listening has also been central outside psychiatry. Peter Benson emphasized listening to youth voices when identifying sparks. Psychiatry demands the same posture: listening to patients describe the desires that sustain them. Their voices—insistent, weary, hopeful—mirror the voices I heard each morning at home. My daughters' reminders grounded me, just as my patients' reminders ground our field: sparks are carried in the voices of those who call us back to life.

The Power of Firsthand Accounts

For too long, the narrative surrounding SMI has prioritized clinical observation and diagnosis over firsthand accounts. This imbalance risks dehumanizing people, flattening their experience to symptoms rather than understanding them as people living with history, identity, and insight.

People with SMI possess deep knowledge of their experiences, including what helps or hinders their well-being. Their stories offer essential insight into treatment efficacy, service gaps, stigma, and resilience.

These aren't just case studies; they're stories. And I've been changed by them.

Lived experience provides a unique lens through which to assess the impact of interventions. Patients can describe how therapies affect them, how policies shape their lives, and how stigma wounds. Just as importantly, they can show us where systems fail—and where hope emerges.

Sharing one's story can reclaim agency for the narrator and offer comfort, solidarity, or inspiration for others. When listened to with respect, these accounts become blueprints for more responsive and compassionate care.

Patient Voice Sidebar

"I'm not my symptoms—I'm still me.
What I need isn't just medication.
I need someone to see the parts of me that illness never took away."
—Patient living with schizophrenia

Clinical vignette: He wasn't lining up shoes because he loved order. He was waiting for someone to ask why the pairs never felt complete.

This keeps the focus on symbolic expression, inviting interpretation rather than suppression.

Clinical vignette: She didn't want to stop drawing faces. She wanted someone to ask why they always looked away.

This kind of reflection not only deepens our understanding of symptoms, but reframes them as expressions of internal meaning.

Patient Voice Sidebar

"They kept asking what was wrong with me. Nobody asked what kept me alive."
— Patient living with schizoaffective disorder

Patients offer crucial perspectives that clinicians may overlook. A patient describing the distress of feeling unheard during hospitalization can reveal more about system failure than chart audits ever will. One may recount how being assigned a peer support worker helped restore a sense of safety and trust that years of medication alone could not achieve. Another may express how a group art therapy class provided a rare and sacred space for authenticity, creativity, and healing. Others may highlight how everyday routines—watering plants, watching sunsets, repeating prayers—serve as anchors to a coherent identity.

When patients share their journeys, they do more than tell their stories. They challenge us to rethink our assumptions about chronicity, capacity, and compliance. Their words remind us that recovery is not linear, and healing does not always look like symptom remission. It may look like reconnecting with a pet, returning to a favorite song, or feeling safe enough to make eye contact again.

Centering Lived Experience in Practice

Amplifying patient voices involves more than appreciation—it requires sustained action. Practical ways to embed lived experience include:

- **Collaborative Care Planning**: Involving individuals in shaping their treatment goals and choices fosters dignity and empowerment. Rather than asking "What's the matter with you?" we ask, "What matters to you?"
- **Peer Support Roles**: Employing people with lived experience as peer specialists fosters connection, trust, and mutual growth. Peer-led initiatives often open doors that clinical interventions alone cannot.
- **Advisory Boards and Consultation**: Including patient voices in the design of programs, policies, and research helps align services with real needs. Advisory boards offer authentic influence, not just symbolic inclusion.
- **Narrative Medicine and Qualitative Research**: Centering storytelling and subjective data enriches our understanding of mental illness.[2] These approaches validate meaning and complexity rather than reducing experiences to metrics.
- **Creative Expression and Advocacy**: Encouraging writing, art, and testimony allows patients to challenge stigma and redefine identity. Creative expression is often a spark in itself—a portal to resilience.
- **Professional Training**: Educating providers to listen to and learn from lived experience cultivates humility and healing partnerships. Exposure to real narratives disrupts stereotypes and fosters attuned care.

Patient Voice Sidebar

"Recovery doesn't mean I'm cured. It means I have reasons to wake up, and ways to live with what's still here."
—Patient living with bipolar disorder

Lived Experience and the Sparks

The enduring sparks discussed throughout this book—sex, money, food, music, spirituality, creativity, movement, rituals, nature, and humor—come into sharper focus when understood through patient narratives.

- A clinician may see repetitive behaviors as symptoms of OCD or psychosis. But a patient might explain that tapping four times before entering a room connects them with memories of their siblings. What looks like pathology may in fact be remembrance, grounding, or self-soothing.
- A patient's account of food restriction may reveal an effort to reclaim bodily control in the aftermath of trauma—not simply a side effect of medication.
- A man experiencing homelessness might explain that saving sugar packets is not about hoarding, but about maintaining dignity.
- A woman who paints oceans may not be delusional, but invoking a spiritual space where she feels whole.

Even the spark of music—so often dismissed as a distraction—can be redefined by patients as a survival tool, a prayer, or a personal language. Peer-led groups centered on music, journaling, walking, or gardening become rich with therapeutic meaning when guided by what patients value.

When patients describe how humor helps them make it through long days in institutional settings, or how nature grounds them during episodes of distress, they help clinicians understand the functional, symbolic, and relational meaning of sparks. Their stories teach us that sparks are not random—they are purposeful and deeply human.

A Path Forward

Elevating the perspectives of those with SMI is not a matter of courtesy; it is an ethical, clinical, and societal imperative. It challenges deficit-based models and affirms the strengths that persist even in crisis. Their voices help illuminate paths to recovery that clinical metrics alone cannot chart.

When we listen closely, we find wisdom, resilience, and guidance in their stories. We discover how rituals create safety, how music offers structure, how silence can signal grief or resistance. We learn how sparks endure not as symptoms but as strategies for survival. These accounts call on us to respond with humanity, curiosity, and partnership.

Including lived experience transforms systems of care. It fosters transparency and accountability. It helps dismantle stigma, reduce coercion, and restore autonomy. Importantly, it makes space for hope—not as a false promise, but as an outcome rooted in relational care.

This transformation is already underway in many communities. Hospitals are hiring peer specialists. Research teams are integrating co-production models. Educational programs are bringing patients into classrooms. And most importantly, patients are stepping into public roles—not just as recipients of care, but as thought leaders and changemakers.

Patient Voice Sidebar

"When I play music, I feel whole again. The hospital never wrote that down, but it's the truest thing about me."
—Patient living with major depression

Conclusion: Listening as Healing

Recognizing and amplifying patient perspectives is one of the most powerful ways to move mental health care forward. When we honor lived experience alongside clinical expertise, we unlock more authentic care, more effective support systems, and more hopeful futures.

The sparks that endure—whether expressed through ritual, creativity, or voice—gain clarity and power when interpreted by those who live them.

To truly engage the sparks that endure, we must center the voices of those who live them every day. Their stories are not just important; they are essential.

Sparks don't just flicker in silence. They speak—if we are willing to listen.

Table 24.1 — Patient vs. Clinician Perspectives

Spark	Patient View	Clinician View
Sex	Identity, closeness	Risk, safety
Money	Autonomy, dreams	Budgeting, delusion
Rituals	Comfort, grounding	OCD-like rigidity

Slade, M. (2009). *Personal recovery and mental illness: A guide for mental health professionals.* Cambridge University Press.

Charon, R. (2006). *Narrative medicine: Honoring the stories of illness.* Oxford University Press.

Anthony, W. A. (1993). Recovery from mental illness: The guiding vision of the mental health service system in the 1990s. *Psychosocial Rehabilitation Journal, 16*(4), 11–23. https://doi.org/10.1037/h0095655

Leamy, M., Bird, V., Le Boutillier, C., Williams, J., & Slade, M. (2011). Conceptual framework for personal recovery in mental health: Systematic review and narrative synthesis. *The British Journal of Psychiatry, 199*(6), 445–452. https://doi.org/10.1192/bjp.bp.110.083733

Davidson, L., Bellamy, C., Guy, K., & Miller, R. (2012). Peer support among persons with severe mental illnesses: A review of evidence and experience. *World Psychiatry, 11*(2), 123–128. https://doi.org/10.1016/j.wpsyc.2012.05.009

Repper, J., & Carter, T. (2011). A review of the literature on peer support in mental health services. *Journal of Mental Health, 20*(4), 392–411. https://doi.org/10.3109/09638237.2011.583947

Mead, S., & MacNeil, C. (2006). Peer support: What makes it unique? *International Journal of Psychosocial Rehabilitation, 10*(2), 29–37.

Substance Abuse and Mental Health Services Administration. (2012). *SAMHSA's working definition of recovery: 10 guiding principles of recovery.* U.S. Department of Health and Human Services.

Slade, M., Amering, M., Farkas, M., Hamilton, B., O'Hagan, M., Panther, G., Perkins, R., Shepherd, G., Tse, S., & Whitley, R. (2014). Uses and abuses of recovery: Implementing recovery-oriented practices in mental health systems. *World Psychiatry, 13*(1), 12–20. https://doi.org/10.1002/wps.20084

Greenhalgh, T. (2016). Cultural contexts of health: The use of narrative research in the health sector. *WHO Regional Office for Europe.*

Faulkner, A. (2017). Survivor research and mad studies: The role and value of experiential knowledge in mental health research. *Disability & Society, 32*(4), 500–520. https://doi.org/10.1080/09687599.2017.1302320

Benson, P. L. (2008). *Sparks: How parents can help ignite the hidden strengths of teenagers.* Jossey-Bass.

Chapter 25:
Living Beyond the Sparks: A Person-Centered Path to Recovery

Introduction

Throughout this book, we have explored the enduring presence of fundamental human desires—money, sex, food, and music—in people living with schizophrenia, schizoaffective disorder, and bipolar disorder. Recognizing this persistence is more than an empathetic act; it is essential to person-centered care. Beyond symptom reduction, acknowledging these drives fosters meaningful engagement, relevant treatment goals, and a better quality of life. This chapter integrates these recurring themes and answers a central question: Why do these desires persist, even when cognition, perception, and mood collapse?

The answer lies in the resilience of the human brain and the power of instinctual drives, meaning-making, and the pursuit of connection. These urges are not cultural artifacts—they are neurobiologically embedded in the limbic system, hypothalamus, and reward circuits. Even when cognition deteriorates, these primal instincts remain active.

Let's take a closer look at how individuals can move beyond managing these preoccupations to embrace a life of possibility—living with joy, purpose, and authenticity.

Moving Beyond Symptom-Focused Treatment

Psychiatry often focuses on deficits: diminished executive function, impaired insight, emotional dysregulation. While these clinical realities are important to address, an exclusive focus on pathology can inadvertently obscure what remains intact. Amidst the fog of psychosis or the fluctuations of mood, people continue to reach for what makes them feel human. Persistent interests in sex, money, food, and music often appear as symptoms, but they also function as enduring signals of inner life.

Reframing these impulses as strengths rather than dysfunctions can shift clinical conversations. Instead of asking, "How do we suppress this behavior?" clinicians can ask, "What is this behavior expressing or seeking to fulfill?" In this reframe, person-centered care emerges—not as a theoretical concept, but as a practical approach rooted in dignity and insight.

The Paradox of Preserved Desire

There is something hauntingly beautiful in the tenacity of desire. A man unable to hold a coherent conversation still fantasizes about owning a house. A woman disorganized by mania still dreams of launching a small business. A patient lost in catatonia responds to a familiar melody with visible emotion. These moments may seem contradictory to clinical expectations, but they tell us something vital: the essential self remains.

The paradox is this: desire often survives, even when cognition collapses. These desires are not random. They are deeply personal, reflecting core aspects of identity and values. Recognizing them affirms the presence of the person within the illness.

Neuropsychiatric Insights

From a neurobiological perspective, the durability of these desires is not surprising. The limbic system, including the amygdala, hippocampus, and hypothalamus, plays a central role in emotion, memory, and motivation. These regions are often less affected than the prefrontal cortex, which governs planning and abstraction.

This helps explain why people living with severe psychosis may still express deep feelings through music or retain compulsions around food or sexuality. The basal ganglia and reward pathways involving dopamine remain active, reinforcing behaviors linked to pleasure, even when other cognitive functions falter.

Understanding these mechanisms helps clinicians distinguish between behaviors that are purely symptomatic and those that are expressions of enduring selfhood.

Meaning-Making Amid Illness

Desires for money, sex, food, and music are not only physiological; they are symbolic. For many patients, money may represent autonomy or power in a world that feels out of control. Sexuality may reflect a need for intimacy or affirmation. Food rituals can convey comfort or act as coping mechanisms. Music can become a medium for communication, especially when language fails.

Exploring these meanings in therapy allows patients to reassert agency and redefine their experiences. It offers clinicians a powerful tool to move beyond symptom-focused models and enter into therapeutic spaces where deeper narratives can unfold.

Holistic Assessment

A true person-centered assessment must go beyond clinical checklists. It includes open-ended conversations about what brings the individual joy, purpose, or grounding. Clinicians should explore:
- Spirituality: How does the person seek meaning or transcendence?
- Creativity: What forms of expression feel authentic or necessary?
- Movement: How does the body become a site of regulation or release?

By incorporating these areas, assessments become richer and more attuned to the person's lived reality.

Tailoring Treatment Goals

When treatment plans incorporate these sparks, goals become more motivating. Instead of generic objectives like "reduce psychotic symptoms," care plans might include: "record music in group sessions," "manage a small personal budget," or "attend a cooking class."

These goals are not trivial—they reflect the patient's inner compass. Aligning treatment with these elements fosters deeper engagement and a greater sense of ownership over the recovery process.

Building a Strong Therapeutic Alliance

Validating these enduring desires strengthens rapport. When patients sense that their provider sees them not as a cluster of symptoms but as a whole person, therapeutic trust deepens. The act of listening—to a favorite song, a repeated delusion involving money, or a food preference—can be transformational.

The alliance is not always built through clinical confrontation. It often begins in small recognitions of shared humanity: laughing about a song lyric, honoring a daily ritual, or acknowledging a dream that feels out of reach.

A Different Kind of Outcome

What if psychiatric recovery were measured not just by hospitalizations avoided, but by moments of meaning restored? When a patient begins dancing again after years of mutism, or prepares a shared meal in a group home, we are witnessing recovery in action.

These outcomes may be soft by traditional metrics, but they reflect reintegration into the rhythms of life. They are moments when sparks of the person shine through.

Integrated Care Approaches

This is the kind of psychiatry I try to practice—one that listens more than it diagnoses.

Integrated care recognizes that mental health does not exist in isolation. For people living with SMI, physical health conditions like obesity, diabetes, and cardiovascular disease are common—and often exacerbated by medication side effects or socioeconomic challenges.

Bringing primary care, psychiatry, case management, and social support into one coordinated framework allows for better continuity. It also affirms the interconnected nature of health, well-being, and the ability to access joy.

The Individual, Family, and Clinical Team

Recovery is not a solitary endeavor. It requires collaboration. The individual must be at the center, driving their own recovery as much as possible. Families provide historical context and continuity. Clinicians bring technical skill and compassionate scaffolding.

Together, they co-create a recovery path that honors not only safety and stability, but hope, growth, and meaning.

Personalizing the Recovery Journey

Each person's path is unique. While diagnostic categories offer structure, they can't capture the nuances of lived experience. A person-centered journey asks: What still brings joy? What rituals, however small, bring comfort? What passions persist despite the noise of illness?

By building treatment around these answers, recovery becomes not only possible—but deeply personal.

Integrated Mental and Physical Healthcare

People living with serious mental illness face a dual burden—managing psychiatric symptoms while also contending with elevated rates of chronic physical health conditions. These may include diabetes, cardiovascular disease, respiratory disorders, and obesity. In many cases, the physical side effects of psychotropic medications, combined with socioeconomic barriers and fragmented healthcare systems, compound the risks.

Integrated care seeks to address these disparities by embedding physical health support within psychiatric treatment frameworks. This can include:
- Onsite primary care providers in psychiatric clinics
- Shared electronic health records between medical and mental health teams
- Collaborative care models that prioritize communication between providers
- Preventive health screenings conducted during mental health visits

The goal is not only improved physical outcomes but also a restoration of agency. When individuals have access to nutritious meals, understand how their medications affect metabolism, and receive respectful and proactive care for physical ailments, their capacity for engagement in recovery increases.

Critically, physical health is deeply tied to the core sparks explored in this book. For instance, food is not just sustenance but pleasure and routine. Sexual well-being relates closely to metabolic health and medication side effects. By tending to the body, we also tend to the soul.

Empowerment and Agency

Empowerment in mental health care means giving individuals a voice in their own healing journey. It requires us to shift from paternalistic models of care toward collaborative partnerships. This begins with believing that people living with SMI have the capacity to make choices, to set goals, and to direct the course of their recovery.

Empowerment involves:
- Shared decision-making between clinician and patient
- Respecting the individual's goals and desires, even when they differ from clinical priorities
- Fostering self-advocacy skills through education, peer support, and coaching

One of the most important expressions of agency is the pursuit of meaning through sparks. When we help someone explore what music still moves them, or how financial independence might look, we are restoring a sense of control.

Empowerment is not about eliminating vulnerability; it's about creating space where strength can emerge. It's allowing a person to say: "This is who I am. This is what matters to me."

Challenging Stigma and Low Expectations

Stigma is one of the most persistent and damaging barriers faced by individuals living with serious mental illness. It pervades every level of society—from public perception to institutional policies—and it can significantly limit access to opportunities, resources, and compassionate care. Perhaps most insidiously, stigma shapes expectations: not only those held by others, but the beliefs individuals hold about themselves.

Low expectations can be just as harmful as overt discrimination. When clinicians assume that a patient is uninterested in relationships, incapable of employment, or indifferent to joy, treatment becomes transactional rather than transformational. When family members presume that recovery is impossible, their support can become muted or conditional. And when individuals internalize these messages, they may stop dreaming, stop trying, and stop believing in their own potential.

Challenging stigma requires more than good intentions. It requires action, such as:

- Language reform: Using respectful, person-first language that emphasizes humanity over diagnosis
- Narrative power: Centering stories of lived experience to illustrate resilience and complexity
- Policy advocacy: Pushing for changes that reduce structural barriers and promote equity in housing, employment, and education
- Professional education: Training providers to examine their biases and adopt a strength-based approach

Importantly, acknowledging and validating the enduring desires for sex, money, food, and music is itself an act of resistance against stigma. It affirms that these individuals are not defined by their diagnoses—they are human beings with passions, preferences, and potential.

Ethical Imperative

Supporting individuals in pursuing their sparks is not just clinically sound—it is ethically required. Person-centered care is rooted in the fundamental ethical principles of autonomy, beneficence, nonmaleficence, and justice. These principles challenge us to not only do good, but to recognize and uphold the full humanity of the individuals we serve.

Autonomy means that individuals have the right to direct their own care. This includes making choices about what brings them meaning—whether it's pursuing a romantic relationship, creating music, or cooking meals.

Beneficence urges us to act in the best interest of those we serve, which includes supporting not just survival, but quality of life.

Nonmaleficence demands that we avoid harm—not just through our actions, but through neglect. Ignoring someone's desires or devaluing their passions can be a subtle but powerful form of harm.

Justice insists on fairness. Individuals with serious mental illness deserve the same opportunities for self-expression, pleasure, connection, and fulfillment as anyone else.

Framing sparks as ethical concerns reorients the entire treatment paradigm. It asks providers to recognize that our role is not simply to manage risk or reduce symptoms, but to uphold dignity, foster possibility, and co-create lives of meaning alongside those we serve.

The Challenge of Sustaining Change

Initial breakthroughs in recovery—like managing impulses, establishing routines, or reclaiming passions—are profound. But sustaining change over time is an equally important, often more difficult, part of the journey. Life is unpredictable. Stress, grief, instability, and even progress can trigger regressions into familiar, yet unhealthy, patterns.

True recovery acknowledges that setbacks are not failures but invitations for adjustment. The key to sustaining change is not perfection—it is flexibility, resilience, and the ability to return to a path of healing after a detour. Strategies for maintaining growth include:
- Regular reflection: Encouraging individuals to periodically assess their emotional and behavioral patterns
- Supportive accountability: Involving peers, clinicians, and family in gentle, nonjudgmental support systems
- Adaptable planning: Revising goals and boundaries based on changing life circumstances

Sustained change also requires realistic expectations. Individuals should be affirmed not just for transformation, but for persistence. For showing up. For trying again. That is what builds recovery that lasts.

The Power of Habit

Lasting recovery often rests on the foundation of daily habits. While sparks may emerge from deep emotional places, their integration into life depends on consistent practice. Habits bring structure to chaos and help anchor the self during times of emotional flux.

Developing new, life-affirming habits—especially around the enduring sparks—can reshape the relationship one has with desire. For example:

- Mindful eating transforms compulsive consumption into nourishment
- Daily budgeting reframes impulsive spending as empowerment
- Morning journaling channels sexual or emotional energy into self-reflection
- Scheduled music engagement provides a healthy outlet for emotional regulation

Habits do not form overnight. They require repetition, environmental support, and self-compassion when patterns break. Yet even small routines—like pausing before spending money or savoring a meal without distraction—can ripple outward into sustained wellness.

Redefining Success

Recovery is often judged by clinical metrics: symptom reduction, medication adherence, stable housing. These benchmarks matter, but they don't capture the full picture. For many people living with serious mental illness, true success lies in moments of meaning: rekindling a hobby, mending a relationship, feeling joy after years of numbness.

Redefining success means:
- Prioritizing authenticity: Helping individuals live in alignment with their values and passions
- Valuing connection: Recognizing the richness of relationships and community engagement
- Celebrating small wins: Honoring progress that might be invisible in charts but transformative in lived experience

Success might be the woman who dances every morning before breakfast. The man who writes a song in group therapy. The young adult who sets a spending limit and sticks to it. These are stories of the soul—not just of symptom management, but of reclaiming identity and purpose.

Creating a Lifestyle of Wellness

Wellness is not a destination—it is a daily practice. For people living with serious mental illness, wellness cannot be separated from their unique challenges, but neither should it be reduced to mere symptom management. Creating a lifestyle of wellness involves aligning daily routines, environments, relationships, and activities with what nourishes the mind, body, and spirit.

A wellness-centered lifestyle might include:
- Healthy sleep routines that regulate mood and cognitive clarity

- Nutritious meals that provide both physical sustenance and sensory pleasure
- Creative or spiritual rituals that ground a sense of identity and purpose
- Physical movement—whether structured exercise or simple stretching—to regulate energy and connect to the body
- Social connections that uplift, validate, and encourage accountability

Importantly, a wellness lifestyle is not about perfection. It honors setbacks, invites rest, and adjusts to fluctuating capacities. It is sustainable, not punitive. And most critically, it is chosen, not imposed. When individuals design their wellness according to what sparks joy, fulfillment, and dignity, they reclaim their narrative.

Fostering Growth Through Creativity

Creativity is not optional—it is essential. Whether expressed through drawing, music, storytelling, dance, or problem-solving, creativity offers people living with serious mental illness a language beyond pathology. It provides a space for play, imagination, emotional release, and identity formation.

In therapeutic contexts, fostering creativity can:
- Help externalize inner experiences that are difficult to articulate
- Reinforce a sense of agency and ownership over one's story
- Connect individuals to others through shared meaning-making
- Offer respite from rigid clinical frameworks through spontaneity and exploration

Every person is creative, though not everyone has been invited or allowed to express it. Clinicians, peers, and families can create space for this exploration without judgment or expectation. Whether it's decorating a room, composing a rap, or arranging flowers, these acts are declarations of life.

The Journey of Acceptance

Acceptance does not mean giving up. It means embracing reality with open eyes and an open heart—acknowledging both what is and what can still be. For many individuals, this includes accepting a diagnosis, the limits imposed by symptoms, or the unpredictability of moods.

But it also includes accepting the parts of themselves that never left: their humor, sensuality, ambition, style, and dreams. It is the journey toward seeing oneself not as broken or abnormal, but as human—complex, wounded, worthy, and growing.

Acceptance allows for integration. It means that sparks are not just bursts of energy, but elements of a continuous flame. That illness and identity can coexist. That healing is not about erasing the past but moving forward with meaning.

Conclusion

In the end, person-centered care is not a technique; it is a stance. It is the decision to see the whole person before the illness, to treat symptoms without erasing selfhood, and to co-create care plans that honor not just safety but soul. The enduring sparks—sex, money, food, and music—are not distractions. They are evidence of life, of longing, of what makes us most human.

To practice person-centered care is to believe in what remains, even when so much seems lost. It is to listen closely for what still burns.

1. Slade, M. (2009). *Personal Recovery and Mental Illness: A Guide for Mental Health Professionals.* Cambridge University Press.
2. Berridge, K. C., & Kringelbach, M. L. (2015). Pleasure systems in the brain. *Neuron,* 86(3), 646–664.
3. Druss, B. G., & Walker, E. R. (2011). Mental disorders and medical comorbidity. *The Synthesis Project, Robert Wood Johnson Foundation.*
4. Corrigan, P. W., & Watson, A. C. (2002). Understanding the impact of stigma on people with mental illness. *World Psychiatry,* 1(1), 16–20.
5. Horvath, A. O., Del Re, A. C., Flückiger, C., & Symonds, D. (2011). Alliance in individual psychotherapy. *Psychotherapy,* 48(1), 9–16.
6. Charon, R. (2006). *Narrative Medicine: Honoring the Stories of Illness.* Oxford University Press.
7. Leamy, M., Bird, V., Le Boutillier, C., Williams, J., & Slade, M. (2011). Conceptual framework for personal recovery in mental health: systematic review and narrative synthesis. *British Journal of Psychiatry,* 199(6), 445–452.

Chapter 26:
Future Directions in Research and Support

Introduction: The Horizon of Hope

As we reach the concluding chapter of *The Sparks That Endure*, it's vital to shift our gaze forward—to the horizon of possibilities where research, clinical innovation, and a deep respect for lived experience converge. While the challenges associated with serious mental illness remain profound, the enduring sparks we've explored throughout this book remind us of the potential for growth, connection, and meaning that persists even amidst suffering.

I'm hopeful not because of policy changes, but because I've seen people grow, even in impossible places.

This chapter outlines the most promising directions in psychiatric research, therapeutic interventions, healthcare delivery models, and policy reform. It argues that enduring sparks like sexuality, music, food, humor, and spirituality are not just symbolic—they are viable, evidence-based starting points for the next generation of treatment and recovery models. These sparks must not only be preserved but actively cultivated within care systems.

The Rise of Recovery-Oriented Science

The field of psychiatry is experiencing a paradigm shift—from managing chronic illness to supporting personal recovery. The former views patients as passive recipients of care; the latter sees them as active agents in their own healing. The recovery model demands a reorientation of priorities, putting meaning, autonomy, and connection at the center of clinical work.

Recent studies have affirmed the validity of this model. Programs rooted in recovery principles—like peer support services, strengths-based case management, and supported employment—are associated with better outcomes in quality of life, treatment adherence, and symptom management. More importantly, they validate the person behind the diagnosis.

Future research must continue to test these frameworks not only for clinical efficacy but for their capacity to restore dignity and spark a sense of purpose.

Advances in Neurobiological Research

- Neuroscience continues to unlock deeper insights into the mechanisms of serious mental illness, and emerging technologies are providing powerful new ways to see what was once invisible. They include: Functional MRI (fMRI) and Diffusion Tensor Imaging (DTI), which allow real-time mapping of cognitive-emotional networks.
- Genetic sequencing offers clues into polygenic risk and treatment response.
- Electrophysiology and magnetoencephalography (MEG) highlight abnormal neural oscillations in psychosis and mood disorders.

These discoveries are not purely academic. They open the door to precision psychiatry—targeted interventions based on biological profiles. Future studies will likely focus on how these biological pathways intersect with the behavioral and symbolic dimensions of sparks. For example, can musical training improve frontal connectivity in schizophrenia? Can dietary interventions modulate inflammatory markers in bipolar disorder?

Together, these tools do more than chart brain abnormalities—they reveal the biological scaffolding that underlies sparks of desire, meaning, and connection. What once seemed abstract can now be traced in circuitry, giving psychiatry new bridges between lived experience and neural reality.

Neuroplasticity is another crucial concept. Once thought to be fixed, the adult brain is now understood as malleable. Cognitive remediation, mindfulness practices, and even physical activity stimulate growth in key areas associated with memory, attention, and emotional regulation—enhancing the capacity to take part in the very sparks that make life meaningful.

Innovation in Psychosocial Interventions

Beyond medication, psychosocial interventions are evolving rapidly:
- Transcranial Magnetic Stimulation (TMS) and tDCS offer non-invasive modulation of dysfunctional circuits.
- Virtual Reality (VR) exposure therapy is being trialed for social anxiety and trauma in schizophrenia.
- Digital therapeutics, including apps for CBT and dialectical behavior therapy, increase accessibility and engagement.

These tools can be designed to enhance sparks directly. VR might simulate enjoyable social gatherings for people living with paranoia. Mobile apps can encourage creative expression or track positive behaviors like budgeting or cooking.

Research should aim to validate these innovations, especially in underserved populations where traditional models of care have failed.

Personalization and Precision in Psychiatry

Every person with SMI has a unique profile—biological, psychological, social, and cultural. Future psychiatry must embrace complexity rather than reduce it. This involves:

- Pharmacogenomics: tailoring medications based on genetic response
- Symptom clustering: moving beyond diagnosis toward identifying actionable patterns
- Life-narrative assessment: integrating personal history and aspirations into treatment planning

Such personalization enhances engagement. A patient who sees their values, history, and goals reflected in the treatment plan is more likely to adhere to it. Personalization also respects the uniqueness of each spark—what sex, music, or food means to one person may differ entirely for another. Future models should offer a menu of engagement pathways rooted in these preoccupations.

Prevention and Early Intervention

The future of psychiatry must shift upstream. Research shows that early intervention in psychosis significantly improves long-term outcomes. But prevention must extend further—to childhood adversity, trauma, social marginalization, and educational disadvantage.
Key areas of focus include:

- Adverse childhood experiences (ACEs): screening and early therapeutic support
- Youth resilience programs: fostering creativity, movement, and social skills in schools
- Family psychoeducation: reducing stigma and improving outcomes for first-episode psychosis

Preventive strategies should nurture sparks early—before they are buried under stigma, symptoms, or institutionalization.

Equitable Access and Culturally Responsive Care

Innovation without access only widens disparity. The future of SMI care must be inclusive and this requires concrete steps:
- Telepsychiatry must reach rural, immigrant, and underserved populations
- Peer-led programs must reflect the cultural and linguistic diversity of their communities
- Community-based participatory research must be funded and supported to center marginalized voices

Culturally tailored interventions can enhance the resonance of sparks. Spirituality may be expressed differently across religious traditions. Food preferences, musical traditions, and humor styles vary across cultures. Effective care honors these distinctions.

Technology and the Digital Future

Technology will continue to transform mental health in the following ways:
- AI-powered diagnostics can detect early warning signs through speech, text, or behavior.
- Wearable devices can monitor mood, activity, and stress.
- Machine learning algorithms can optimize treatment pathways based on population-level data.

However, these innovations must be used ethically. Transparency, consent, and privacy protections are essential. Moreover, technology should never replace human connection—it should enhance it. Sparks are human experiences, and the future must remain human-centered.

Policy and Advocacy: Enabling Structural Change

Real innovation requires structural support:
- Parity legislation for mental health coverage must be enforced.
- Supported housing and employment initiatives must be scaled.
- Legal reforms must decriminalize mental illness and promote rights-based care.

Recovery cannot happen in a vacuum. People need safe homes, meaningful work, protection from exploitation, and communities that value them. Policies must reflect this comprehensive view of healing.

Lived Experience and Co-Production

Perhaps the most profound shift underway is the recognition that people with lived experience are not just patients or subjects. They are experts. Their leadership is reshaping the field in ways that include:
- Peer researchers now co-design studies.
- Advisory boards include people living with SMI.
- Narrative medicine integrates first-person stories into clinical education.

This democratization of knowledge makes research more relevant and care more effective. It also affirms that enduring sparks are not theoretical; they are lived realities. Who better to illuminate them than those who live with them?

Conclusion: Lighting the Path Ahead

The future of mental health care is not just about better drugs or smarter machines. It is about remembering what matters. The sparks of life—sex, music, food, humor, spirituality, creativity—are not mere remnants of wellness. They are active forces in healing. They are not background noise; they are the score.

To build a better future, we must:
- Invest in research that values meaning alongside metrics.
- Support innovations that elevate human dignity.
- Create systems that are flexible, inclusive, and equitable.
- Place lived experience at the center of care.

Recovery is real. Sparks endure. The task ahead is to recognize them, fund them, cultivate them, and—most of all—believe in them.

The future does not lie in extinguishing difference or silencing longing. It lies in letting the sparks speak and in building a world that finally learns how to listen.

Chapter 27:
Practical Strategies: Incorporating Desires into Therapy and Support

Introduction: What Still Reaches Out from Within

Treatment should not only ask what is wrong, but also what is still right, still alive, still reaching out from within.

The sparks we've explored—sex, money, food, music, spirituality, creativity, movement, rituals, humor, nature, touch, storytelling, hope, and freedom—are more than behavioral patterns. They are footholds for the psyche, signals that life is still active within disorder. Each one is an expression of humanity that illness may obscure but cannot erase.

Sex speaks to intimacy and connection. Money carries meanings of survival and identity. Food sustains both body and ritual. Music resonates in memory and emotion. Spirituality anchors meaning in suffering. Creativity restores voice and vision. Movement reclaims embodiment. Rituals provide rhythm and order. Humor lightens despair. Nature grounds and renews. Touch conveys safety and belonging. Storytelling weaves coherence from chaos. Hope lifts the spirit beyond present pain. And freedom affirms dignity, choice, and autonomy.

Integrating these desires into therapy means making room for the person's motivational life, not just their pathology. It shifts the clinical gaze from containment to collaboration, from suppression to meaning-making. These sparks are not distractions from treatment—they are treatment, because they are the very currents of life that endure.

I've used many of these tools, but they only work when they're rooted in what actually matters to the person in front of me.

Sex: Intimacy, Power, and Embodiment

Sex is one of the most enduring sparks in psychiatric care, yet often the most silenced. For people living with serious mental illness, sexuality is not erased—it is reshaped, complicated by stigma, medication, trauma, and institutional boundaries. At its core, sexual desire represents a longing for intimacy, recognition, and identity. To approach sex clinically is not to suppress it, but to understand its many expressions, from yearning to confusion to resilience. When engaged with respect and clarity, sexuality becomes a pathway to healing, not just a problem to manage.

Core Desires:
- To feel desired and desirable
- To explore identity and orientation
- To experience pleasure, control, and aliveness

Therapeutic Applications:
- Normalize sexuality in clinical dialogue; invite reflection without shame.
- Explore fantasies symbolically—as metaphors for power, vulnerability, or freedom.
- Identify creative outlets (writing, drawing, education) for expression.
- Set respectful boundaries when hypersexuality emerges, without shaming.

Clinical Strategies:
- Use social skills training and psychoeducation to explore intimacy.
- Facilitate peer-led groups around relationships or sexuality.
- Address sexual side effects of medication collaboratively.
- Therapeutic Stance: Respectful, non-pathologizing, body-positive

Vignette
Amira, a 30-year-old woman with bipolar disorder, frequently brought up themes of sexuality in her therapy sessions, sometimes in ways that were intense or confusing. Her therapist reframed these conversations, asking about what intimacy meant to her. Over time, Amira revealed deep fears about rejection and a longing for closeness. Through respectful dialogue and group therapy on relationships, she began to build healthy romantic boundaries and felt increasingly self-assured.

Reflection Questions

1. How can clinicians address sexuality without reinforcing shame?
2. What metaphors or symbols might help unlock deeper meanings behind sexual behaviors?
3. How can therapeutic spaces model body-positivity and consent?

Money: Autonomy, Control, and Recognition

Money is never just currency in the lives of people with serious mental illness. It is a symbol of survival, independence, and recognition. For some, it represents competence and the ability to navigate a chaotic world. For others, it carries the weight of trauma, scarcity, or family conflict. At times, money becomes entangled with grandiose dreams or paranoid fears, yet even in distortion, it reflects a deeper drive for autonomy and dignity. Approaching money as a spark means seeing beyond dollars and cents to the human longings it encodes—control, agency, and the hope of leaving a mark. The following section outlines the core desires, therapeutic applications, and clinical strategies that can help translate this spark into meaningful care.

Core Desires:
- To feel competent and independent
- To assert control in chaos
- To gain status or legacy

Therapeutic Applications:
- Explore personal money narratives: trauma, pride, or freedom?
- Use budgeting and money tracking for self-regulation.
- Channel grandiose ambitions into structured, collaborative goals.
- Build financial safety plans during manic states.

Clinical Strategies:
- Partner with vocational and employment specialists.
- Teach simple budgeting using visual tools and simulations.
- Advocate for access to benefits like SSI, SSDI, and housing supports.
- Therapeutic Stance: Empowering, strength-based, reality-anchored

Vignette

James, a 42-year-old man with schizoaffective disorder, often expressed dreams of becoming a millionaire. Instead of dismissing these as delusional, his therapist explored the underlying desire for recognition and security. Together, they created a weekly budgeting plan and connected James to a peer-run supported employment program. His sense of agency increased as he began saving small amounts and holding down a part-time job.

Reflection Questions

1. What emotional meaning does money carry for the patient?
2. How can therapists help reframe financial preoccupations into achievable goals?
3. In what ways can financial planning promote autonomy in care?

Food: Comfort, Nourishment, and Control

Food is more than fuel. In the lives of those with serious mental illness, it is often a language of comfort, ritual, and survival. Meals carry meaning—whether in the form of bingeing during stress, refusing food as protest, or treasuring the dignity of choice. Food becomes a marker of control when other freedoms feel out of reach, and at times it reflects the profound impact of poverty or medication. To see food as a spark is to recognize it as a site of both vulnerability and resilience—where nourishment, memory, and agency intersect.

Core Desires:
- To nourish body and mind
- To find comfort and routine
- To reclaim control in constrained environments

Therapeutic Applications:
- Explore food memories and associations (comfort, trauma, celebration)
- Integrate mindful eating or cooking groups into care
- Address medication-related appetite changes with dignity
- Reframe food hoarding or refusal as survival strategies, not just pathology

Clinical Strategies:
- Partner with dietitians to create flexible, patient-centered plans
- Offer structured group meals to foster community and reduce isolation
- Provide safe access to snacks or choice-based menus in inpatient settings
- Therapeutic stance: Nonjudgmental, trauma-informed, culturally sensitive

Vignette

Ana, a 27-year-old woman with schizophrenia, frequently hid food in her room. Staff labeled it "hoarding," but when asked gently about it, she explained: "Growing up, there was never enough. I keep it close so I won't starve." This insight shifted staff responses. Instead of punishment, they created a shared snack cart and invited Ana to lead a cooking group. Her anxiety decreased, and mealtimes became moments of pride rather than shame.

Reflection Questions

1. How might food-related behaviors reflect deeper needs for comfort or control?
2. What cultural practices around food can clinicians honor in treatment?
3. How can group meals become therapeutic rather than punitive?

Music: Resonance, Rhythm, and Self-Expression

Music is a spark that endures even when language and coherence falter. It resonates in memory, evokes identity, and connects people across silence. For many patients, music is more than background—it is therapy, a prayer, a lifeline. Songs can stir joy, recall trauma, or structure chaotic time. In psychiatric care, music offers both a diagnostic window and a therapeutic tool, grounding individuals in rhythm, resonance, and belonging. To honor music is to honor one of humanity's most primal sources of meaning.

Core Desires:
- To feel resonance and emotional release
- To connect with identity and memory
- To find rhythm and belonging in chaos

Therapeutic Applications:
- Encourage patients to build playlists tied to mood states
- Use drumming, singing, or lyric analysis in groups
- Explore personal music narratives (songs tied to memory or hope)
- Integrate music into grounding and mindfulness practices

Clinical Strategies:
- Collaborate with music therapists
- Provide safe spaces for music listening or creation
- Use rhythm-based interventions to reduce agitation or enhance focus
- Therapeutic stance: Creative, attuned, and flexible

Vignette

Jorge, a 35-year-old man with bipolar disorder, carried headphones everywhere. Staff worried it was avoidance. When asked about the music, he said, "It's the only thing that keeps me steady." His clinician invited him to share his playlist during group sessions. Over time, his choices became conversation starters, connecting him with peers and reducing isolation.

Reflection Questions

1. How might music regulate emotion more effectively than words for some patients?
2. What role does music play in cultural identity and recovery?
3. How can clinicians use music as a bridge to therapeutic alliance?

Spirituality: Transcendence, Belonging, and Meaning

Spirituality is often a hidden current in psychiatric care—sometimes dismissed as delusion, sometimes ignored in secular practice. Yet for many living with serious mental illness, faith and meaning are central sources of resilience. Spirituality shapes how suffering is understood and endured; it provides rituals of grounding, symbols of hope, and a framework for transcendence. To explore spirituality as a spark is to recognize its capacity to sustain dignity, orient recovery, and transform despair into purpose.

Core Desires:
- To find meaning in suffering
- To experience connection to something larger than self
- To sustain hope and belonging

Therapeutic Applications:
- Invite respectful dialogue about faith, without presumption
- Explore spiritual rituals as coping strategies
- Partner with chaplains or spiritual leaders when requested
- Differentiate delusion from meaningful spiritual practice with care

Clinical Strategies:
- Integrate spiritual assessments into intake interviews
- Offer space for prayer, meditation, or ritual practices
- Support patient-defined spiritual goals alongside medical ones
- Therapeutic stance: Respectful, nonjudgmental, and curious

Vignette
Fatima, a 40-year-old refugee, described nightly visions of angels. Initially, these were charted as hallucinations. Later, through the Cultural Formulation Interview, clinicians learned these were part of her religious worldview, a source of comfort during trauma. Incorporating prayer into her care plan reduced distress and strengthened therapeutic trust.

Reflection Questions

1. How can clinicians balance respect for faith with careful assessment of delusion?
2. What role might spiritual practices play in recovery and resilience?

3. How can teams create inclusive spaces for spiritual expression?

Creativity: Expression, Play, and Mastery

Creativity is the spark of making—art, words, movement, or invention—that gives form to the inner world. For those with serious mental illness, creativity often becomes a vessel for both suffering and survival. Art may hold what words cannot, and expression can transform disorganization into meaning. Creativity restores agency, offering patients a role not only as receivers of care but as authors of their own voice. In honoring creativity, clinicians affirm that expression is not a luxury but a necessity for recovery.

Core Desires:
- To express inner experience through external form
- To reclaim voice and authorship of identity
- To transform suffering into meaning

Therapeutic Applications:
- Encourage journaling, art, or performance in treatment
- Use creative projects to externalize trauma and reclaim narrative
- Reframe creative output as resilience rather than symptom
- Provide structured opportunities to showcase work

Clinical Strategies:
- Partner with art or drama therapists
- Integrate creative expression into group programs
- Offer safe materials and spaces for self-expression
- Therapeutic stance: Empowering, exploratory, nonjudgmental

Vignette
Lydia, a 29-year-old with schizoaffective disorder, filled sketchbooks with fragmented drawings. Staff initially saw this as perseveration. But when a therapist asked about them, Lydia explained they were images of her dreams. The clinician reframed them as narrative work, and with encouragement, Lydia began sharing her art in group sessions. It became a cornerstone of her recovery.

Reflection Questions

1. How can creativity be framed as resilience instead of symptom?
2. What outlets for expression can psychiatric settings provide?
3. How might creative expression reveal hidden sparks of meaning?

Movement: Regulation, Aliveness, and Grounding

Movement is often underestimated in psychiatric care, yet it is one of the most direct routes to recovery. Walking, dancing, stretching, or exercise can restore rhythm to bodies slowed by depression or agitated by mania. Movement reconnects people with their physical selves, reclaims autonomy, and channels energy into health rather than chaos. In illness, the body may feel heavy, fragmented, or unsafe—but movement reminds us of vitality. Recognizing movement as a spark means affirming the body as central to healing, not secondary.

Core Desires:
- To reconnect with the body
- To channel energy into vitality
- To reclaim autonomy through action

Therapeutic Applications:
- Encourage gentle exercise, yoga, or dance groups
- Use movement as grounding during agitation or dissociation
- Explore cultural movement rituals (e.g., tai chi, drumming, traditional dance)
- Frame movement as expression, not only fitness

Clinical Strategies:
- Partner with occupational/recreational therapists
- Provide structured but flexible activity schedules
- Use outdoor spaces when possible for grounding and renewal
- Therapeutic stance: Supportive, embodied, encouraging

Vignette

Darius, a 45-year-old man with schizophrenia, rarely spoke but walked the unit endlessly. Staff saw this as pacing. When invited into a walking group, he began to engage. Over time, walking became a space for conversation and eventually trust. His movement was not pathology—it was communication.

Reflection Questions

1. How can movement serve as both grounding and expression?
2. What barriers prevent patients from engaging in movement activities?
3. How can teams honor culturally meaningful movement practices?

Rituals: Order, Safety, and Continuity

Rituals offer predictability where life feels chaotic. For many with serious mental illness, rituals—folding clothes a certain way, repeating prayers, walking the same path—serve as anchors of safety and continuity. Though often pathologized as obsession, rituals can also reflect attempts at order, grounding, and survival. To attend to rituals with curiosity rather than dismissal is to uncover their protective meaning. Rituals remind us that repetition can be not only a symptom but also a signal of resilience.

Core Desires:
4. To create order and predictability
5. To connect with tradition or memory
6. To maintain continuity of identity

Therapeutic Applications:
- Explore meaning behind rituals rather than dismissing them
- Identify adaptive vs. maladaptive rituals collaboratively
- Encourage grounding rituals (prayer, breathing, mindfulness) in care
- Use rituals as starting points for therapeutic dialogue

Clinical Strategies:
- Integrate rituals into daily schedules when appropriate
- Respect cultural or religious rituals in treatment plans
- Differentiate pathological compulsion from protective ritual
- Therapeutic stance: Curious, respectful, non-dismissive

Vignette
Naomi, a 50-year-old with bipolar disorder, tapped four times before entering rooms. Staff tried to extinguish it as OCD. In therapy, she explained it connected her to siblings who had done the same growing up. With reframing, the ritual was seen as remembrance, not pathology, and was integrated into care without shaming.

Reflection Questions

1. How might rituals represent resilience rather than symptom?
2. What cultural rituals can clinicians incorporate into care?
3. How can rituals provide grounding during acute episodes?

Humor: Playfulness, Relief, and Resilience

Humor is a spark that often emerges in the darkest places. Even in hospitals, where despair and silence weigh heavily, laughter can pierce through suffering. Humor offers release from tension, reframes pain, and creates bonds of belonging. For patients with serious mental illness, joking may serve as shield, coping strategy, or expression of vitality. To embrace humor in care is to affirm that joy and absurdity endure alongside struggle—that playfulness can be therapeutic.

Core Desires:
- To relieve tension and suffering
- To connect with others through playfulness
- To reframe distress with perspective

Therapeutic Applications:
- Validate humor as resilience, not avoidance
- Use humor to strengthen therapeutic alliance
- Encourage group settings where laughter is safe and shared
- Recognize satire or joking as windows into patient experience

Clinical Strategies:
- Incorporate humor exercises or improv groups
- Train staff to recognize appropriate vs. defensive humor
- Allow space for laughter in clinical environments
- Therapeutic stance: Light, human, relational

Vignette
Michael, a 33-year-old with schizophrenia, often cracked jokes in group therapy. Some staff saw it as distraction. But when engaged, his humor built trust and reduced tension for others. Laughter became a tool of belonging rather than avoidance.

Reflection Questions

1. How can humor serve as a bridge rather than a barrier in therapy?
2. What risks exist in misinterpreting humor as avoidance?
3. How can humor be cultivated safely in clinical settings?

Nature: Grounding, Perspective, and Renewal

Nature offers grounding that transcends illness. Time outdoors, the sight of trees, or the rhythm of seasons can restore calm and perspective when the mind feels disordered. For people in psychiatric care—especially in institutional settings—access to nature is often limited, yet profoundly needed. Nature provides sensory grounding, spiritual renewal, and a reminder of life's larger rhythms. To engage nature as a spark is to reconnect patients with a world beyond confinement, one that nurtures resilience and belonging.

Core Desires:
- To connect with natural rhythms
- To find calm, grounding, and perspective
- To experience renewal and vitality

Therapeutic Applications:
- Encourage time outdoors when possible
- Integrate gardening or horticulture therapy
- Use natural imagery for grounding exercises
- Reframe nature as a resource for meaning and renewal

Clinical Strategies:
- Create access to outdoor courtyards or safe green spaces
- Partner with community gardens or eco-therapy groups
- Offer structured outdoor walks or mindfulness practices
- Therapeutic stance: Grounded, restorative, gentle

Vignette
Sophia, a 28-year-old with depression, rarely left her bed. When invited to sit by the hospital garden, she whispered, "I forgot what green feels like." Over weeks, daily outdoor time became her anchor, gradually reducing her isolation and despair.

Reflection Questions

1. How can limited institutional spaces integrate nature?
2. What role does nature play in cultural healing practices?
3. How might nature serve as a metaphor for growth in therapy?

Touch: Safety, Comfort, and Presence

Touch is among the earliest sparks we know and often the most longed-for in psychiatric care. A hand on the shoulder, a hug, or the texture of a warm cloth can communicate safety when words fail. For trauma survivors and those in institutions, touch can be fraught—yearned for, feared, or forbidden. Yet the absence of safe touch leaves deep scars. Recognizing touch as a spark means acknowledging both its risks and its healing power, offering presence in ways that affirm consent, safety, and connection.

Core Desires:
- To feel safe and comforted
- To experience connection through presence
- To regulate stress through tactile grounding

Therapeutic Applications:
- Offer safe sensory substitutes (weighted blankets, warm objects)

- Explore patient narratives around touch and trauma
- Affirm the yearning for touch without pathologizing it
- Model consent and respect around all forms of physical care

Clinical Strategies:
- Train staff in trauma-informed physical care practices
- Provide sensory rooms or tools for grounding
- Encourage healthy, consensual touch in family contexts
- Therapeutic stance: Gentle, safe, consent-driven

Vignette

Jon, a 39-year-old with PTSD, avoided eye contact and rarely spoke. During daily care, a nurse placed a warm towel in his hands. Jon whispered, "Thank you." They were his first spoken words in months—proof that even the smallest gesture of touch could restore connection.

Reflection Questions

1. How can clinicians meet tactile needs safely and ethically?
2. What role does consent play in therapeutic touch?
3. How can sensory substitutes offer comfort when touch isn't possible?

Storytelling: Meaning, Identity, and Coherence

Storytelling is the thread that weaves identity through illness. Even when speech is fragmented or beliefs distorted, the drive to narrate remains. People living with serious mental illness often tell their stories through metaphor, myth, or art. To hear these stories is to glimpse the meaning beneath symptoms. Storytelling as a spark invites clinicians to honor patients not just as cases, but as authors of their own survival. Listening to narrative becomes an act of restoration, affirming coherence in the midst of chaos.

Core Desires:
- To narrate experience and identity
- To find coherence amid disruption
- To be heard and recognized

Therapeutic Applications:
- Invite patients to tell stories in their own words
- Explore metaphors and symbols in narrative
- Encourage journaling, group sharing, or creative writing
- Honor stories as survival strategies rather than distortions

Clinical Strategies:
- Use narrative therapy or roleplay to explore identity
- Provide creative platforms for patient storytelling
- Train staff in listening for metaphor and meaning
- Therapeutic stance: Attentive, validating, curious

Vignette

Sam, a 32-year-old with schizophrenia, told staff he was the last survivor of a galactic war. Most dismissed it as delusion. One clinician asked, "What were you fighting for?" Sam answered, "So the children could sleep safely." Later, his trauma history revealed the metaphor beneath. His story was not delusion—it was survival encoded in myth.

Reflection Questions

1. How can delusional narratives hold symbolic truths?
2. What role does storytelling play in recovery identity?
3. How can clinicians honor stories without collapsing them into diagnosis?

Hope: Possibility, Expectancy, and Direction

Hope is the improbable light that persists even when reason falters. It flickers in the smallest visions of a better day, a role restored, a song sung again. For people with serious mental illness, hope is not always rational, but it is always necessary. It sustains engagement in treatment, builds trust, and orients recovery toward possibility. To kindle hope in care is to affirm that even fragile futures can guide survival and growth.

Core Desires:
- To envision a better future
- To sustain motivation through adversity
- To orient recovery beyond symptoms

Therapeutic Applications:
- Invite patients to articulate future hopes
- Reframe unrealistic goals as symbols of deeper needs
- Anchor care plans in personally meaningful visions
- Affirm hope as resilience, not denial

Clinical Strategies:
- Integrate hope-oriented therapy and motivational interviewing
- Partner with peer workers who embody lived recovery
- Build treatment goals around personal dreams
- Therapeutic stance: Optimistic, validating, future-oriented

Vignette
Maria, a 36-year-old with schizophrenia, insisted she would one day return to medical school. Staff dismissed it as unrealistic. A clinician reframed it: "What about school feels important to you?" Maria replied, "It means I'm not broken." Together, they identified smaller educational goals, preserving her sense of dignity while channeling hope into achievable steps.

Reflection Questions

1. How can hope be harnessed without reinforcing false promises?
2. What role do clinicians play in sustaining fragile hope?
3. How might hope itself be a therapeutic intervention?

Freedom: Autonomy, Choice, and Dignity

Freedom is a spark that emerges even in constraint. For patients in locked wards or under coercive treatment, the smallest choices—what to eat, when to bathe, which song to hear—become profound acts of agency. Freedom is not just legal or structural; it is psychological and relational. To recognize freedom as a spark is to honor the hunger for autonomy, dignity, and self-determination that endures beneath illness. Supporting freedom in micro-choices can transform care from coercion into collaboration.

Core Desires:
- To exercise autonomy
- To resist constraint and reclaim control
- To preserve dignity in restricted settings

Therapeutic Applications:
- Offer micro-choices to restore agency
- Reframe refusals as expressions of autonomy
- Explore the meaning behind resistance
- Use choice-making to build therapeutic alliance

Clinical Strategies:
- Incorporate shared decision-making into treatment planning
- Train staff to validate patient autonomy
- Balance safety with respect for dignity and agency
- Therapeutic stance: Empowering, collaborative, dignity-affirming

Vignette
Jamal, a 38-year-old man hospitalized under court order, bristled at structured schedules. Staff framed his refusals as defiance. One nurse asked if he preferred water or juice with medication. Jamal smiled and said, "Juice—because that's my choice." Small options snowballed into greater

engagement. His resistance was not opposition; it was survival through autonomy.

Reflection Questions

1. How can clinicians foster autonomy in constrained settings?
2. What is the difference between defiance and agency?
3. How can micro-choices transform coercive care into collaboration?

Table 27.1 — Clinical Tools by Spark

Spark	Tool	Application
Music	Playlist creation	Coping, recovery
Food	Meal planning	Structure, nourishment
Hope	Future goals	Motivation
Nature	Gardening	Engagement, calm

Bond, G. R., Drake, R. E., & Becker, D. R. (2020). Individual placement and support at 25: A review of its effectiveness and implementation. *Psychiatric Rehabilitation Journal, 43*(1), 1–8. https://doi.org/10.1037/prj0000390

Charon, R. (2006). *Narrative medicine: Honoring the stories of illness.* Oxford University Press.

Chinman, M., George, P., Dougherty, R. H., Daniels, A. S., Ghose, S. S., Swift, A., & Delphin-Rittmon, M. E. (2014). Peer support services for individuals with serious mental illnesses: Assessing the evidence. *Psychiatric Services, 65*(4), 429–441. https://doi.org/10.1176/appi.ps.201300244

Correll, C. U., Galling, B., Pawar, A., Krivko, A., Bonetto, C., Ruggeri, M., Craig, T. J., Nordentoft, M., Srihari, V. H., Guloksuz, S., Hui, C. L. M., Chen, E. Y. H., Valencia, M., Juarez, F., Robinson, D. G., Schooler, N. R., Brunette, M. F., Mueser, K. T., Rosenheck, R. A., ... Kane, J. M. (2018). Comparison of early intervention services vs treatment as usual for early-phase psychosis: A systematic review and meta-analysis. *JAMA Psychiatry, 75*(6), 555–565. https://doi.org/10.1001/jamapsychiatry.2018.0623

Felitti, V. J., Anda, R. F., Nordenberg, D., Williamson, D. F., Spitz, A. M., Edwards, V., Koss, M. P., & Marks, J. S. (1998). Relationship of childhood abuse and household dysfunction to many of the leading causes of death in adults: The adverse childhood experiences (ACE) study. *American Journal of Preventive Medicine, 14*(4), 245–258. https://doi.org/10.1016/S0749-3797(98)00017-8

Freeman, D., Bradley, J., Antley, A., Bourke, E., DeWeever, N., Evans, N., Černis, E., Sheaves, B., Waite, F., Dunn, G., Slater, M., & Clark, D. M. (2017). Virtual reality in the assessment, understanding, and treatment of mental health disorders. *Psychological Medicine, 47*(14), 2393–2400. https://doi.org/10.1017/S003329171700040X

George, M. S., & Post, R. M. (2011). Daily left prefrontal repetitive transcranial magnetic stimulation for acute treatment of medication-resistant depression. *Journal of Clinical Psychiatry, 72*(2), e4. https://doi.org/10.4088/JCP.10bk06294blu

Hilty, D. M., Ferrer, D. C., Parish, M. B., Johnston, B., Callahan, E. J., & Yellowlees, P. M. (2013). The effectiveness of telemental health: A 2013 review. *Telemedicine and e-Health, 19*(6), 444–454. https://doi.org/10.1089/tmj.2013.0075

Lamb, H. R., & Weinberger, L. E. (2013). Decarceration of persons with severe mental illness in the United States: Where are we now? *Psychiatric Services, 64*(7), 613–616. https://doi.org/10.1176/appi.ps.201200541

Leamy, M., Bird, V., Le Boutillier, C., Williams, J., & Slade, M. (2011). Conceptual framework for personal recovery in mental health: Systematic review and narrative synthesis. *British Journal of Psychiatry, 199*(6), 445–452. https://doi.org/10.1192/bjp.bp.110.083733

Paulus, M. P., & Thompson, W. K. (2019). The challenges and opportunities of precision psychiatry. *JAMA Psychiatry, 76*(9), 875–876. https://doi.org/10.1001/jamapsychiatry.2019.0620

Pitschel-Walz, G., Leucht, S., Bäuml, J., Kissling, W., & Engel, R. R. (2001). The effect of family interventions on relapse and rehospitalization in schizophrenia: A meta-analysis. *Schizophrenia Bulletin, 27*(1), 73–92. https://doi.org/10.1093/oxfordjournals.schbul.a006861

Slade, M. (2009). *Personal recovery and mental illness: A guide for mental health professionals.* Cambridge University Press.

Tor ous, J., Andersson, G., Bertagnoli, A., Christensen, H., Cuijpers, P., Firth, J., Haim, A., Hsin, H., Hollis, C., Lewis, S., Mohr, D. C., Pratap, A., Roehr, S., & Areán, P. A. (2021). Towards a consensus around standards for smartphone apps and digital mental health. *World Psychiatry, 20*(3), 318–335. https://doi.org/10.1002/wps.20883

Tsemberis, S., Gulcur, L., & Nakae, M. (2004). Housing First, consumer choice, and harm reduction for homeless individuals with a dual diagnosis. *American Journal of Public Health, 94*(4), 651–656. https://doi.org/10.2105/AJPH.94.4.651

Wykes, T., & Huddy, V. (2009). Cognitive remediation for schizophrenia: It is even more complicated. *Schizophrenia Bulletin, 35*(2), 311–312. https://doi.org/10.1093/schbul/sbn176

Chapter 28:
Final Thoughts

What Remains When So Much Seems Lost?

When we ask what persists in the lives of people living with schizophrenia, schizoaffective disorder, and bipolar disorder, we are really asking: What remains when so much seems to be lost? This book has traced fourteen enduring preoccupations—what we have called sparks—that appear again and again across clinical narratives, case histories, recovery stories, and personal testimonies. These sparks— sex, money, food, music, spirituality, creativity, movement, rituals, nature, humor, touch, storytelling, hope, and freedom—are not superficial fixations. They are the building blocks of subjectivity, where meaning is forged, re-forged, and, in some cases, fiercely protected.

These aren't mere concepts; they are the very threads that weave through the intricate tapestry of our human experience, capable of illuminating our lives with profound meaning, yet also casting shadows of challenge and complexity. To truly understand their power is to recognize them not as destinations, but as dynamic forces that demand our conscious engagement.

The Double-Edged Flame: A Deeper Dive

Each spark possesses a remarkable duality—a capacity for immense contribution and, simultaneously, for significant detriment. Sparks are paradoxical. They can be adaptive or maladaptive, liberating or limiting, creative or compulsive. Their intensity may overwhelm, but their absence may hollow out a person's inner world. The challenge for clinicians and families is to engage with the spark without extinguishing it—to work with the energy, not against it. This requires nuance, curiosity, and ethical imagination.

A person who clings to a spark amid disorganization is not simply fixated; they are fighting for coherence. When these sparks are misunderstood, pathologized, or suppressed, we risk extinguishing the very forces that keep a sense of self alive. Instead, therapeutic approaches must ask: Is this spark helping the person feel more alive, more grounded, more connected—or is it pulling them into chaos? Is it a bridge to others, or a barrier? Is it a means of survival, or a source of suffering?

Engaging with sparks also asks us to evaluate our own reactions—what in us is challenged by the patient's spark? Our countertransference, biases, and fears all shape our capacity to sit with and honor these expressions. To do so responsibly requires clinical skill, ethical grounding, and humility.

Sparks and Narrative Continuity

Illness disrupts the life story. Sparks help rebuild it. When a person says, "Even when I was most ill, I still listened to music," or "I never stopped drawing," or "My faith held me together," they are not merely sharing anecdotes. They are reclaiming authorship over their own lives. These statements reflect a through-line of continuity, the ability to say: I was there, I mattered, I endured.

In this way, sparks become lifelines of identity. They protect the personal narrative from complete disintegration. They offer a counterpoint to the chaos, a foothold to reestablish the self. This continuity is more than a clinical insight—it is a form of existential resilience.

Sparks as Anchors of Self

Sparks are not compensations for illness. They are core features of the person that survive illness. Even when cognition declines or reality testing falters, people often maintain strong attachments to particular activities, topics, or rituals. These behaviors deserve understanding, not just control.

A man with schizophrenia who becomes fixated on hip-hop lyrics is not just perseverating; he may be constructing a private language of resilience and meaning. A woman with bipolar disorder who spends compulsively is not simply manic; she may be attempting to reclaim autonomy in a life marked by regulation and restriction. These sparks are not random. They are messages. They are needs, expressed in the only language still accessible.

When we listen for what sparks signify rather than what they disrupt, we access the organizing principle behind the behavior. We begin to see not just disorder, but a search for continuity, identity, and aliveness.

Beyond the Medical Model

Traditional psychiatric frameworks have taught us to categorize, stabilize, and medicate. These tools are essential. But they are not sufficient. To support recovery, we must move beyond control into curiosity. We must ask not only, "What is this behavior?" but also, "Why does this matter to you? What role does it play in your life? What would be lost if it disappeared?"

This approach honors the person, not just the pathology. It brings narrative, dignity, and collaboration into spaces that are too often dominated by correction and compliance. It reclaims psychiatry as a deeply human, relational, and moral discipline.

The Ethical Imperative

To recognize and engage these sparks is ethically necessary. Ignoring what matters most to a person risks dehumanization. Honoring the spark affirms personhood, even in altered states. It reminds us that even in the fog of illness, people reach for joy, purpose, and connection.

This ethical stance reshapes how we deliver care. It challenges the reductionist view of patients as collections of symptoms. It asks us to be curious witnesses, not just clinical experts. It invites humility: to listen more deeply, respond more flexibly, and attune more fully to what gives each person their sense of vitality.

Ethical care means meeting individuals where they are, without dismissing their struggles or their sparks. It calls for compassion tethered to complexity.

The Art of Conscious Engagement

These sparks demand our conscious engagement and balance. They are not to be passively received or blindly pursued. Their power lies in their intentional, mindful use. A rich life is not built on one spark, but on a tapestry of many.

Sex, money, food, music, and other sparks may appear in distorted forms. But they contain within them vital energies: creative, connective, life-affirming. With guidance, these energies can be harnessed toward healing.

True mastery of these sparks lies not in their suppression or indulgence, but in our ability to live alongside them—to integrate them into a full, meaningful, connected life. This is the practice of resilience—not erasing sparks, but navigating them.

The Unfolding Journey: An Invitation to Live Luminously

These sparks are not endpoints; they are dynamic aspects of the human experience that continue to unfold. Each reader—whether clinician, caregiver, policy maker, or person living with mental illness—is invited to listen more deeply, imagine more boldly, and remain curious.

We must move toward care that sees people as more than symptoms, and sparks as more than distractions. These forces, when integrated, can illuminate the path to healing.

They ask us to meet suffering with imagination. They remind us that beauty, desire, rhythm, and ritual are not luxuries; they are the substance of recovery.

What sparks ask of us:
- Can we help a patient build a life around what they love, not just what they lack?
- Can we tolerate the ambiguity of behaviors that are both meaningful and maladaptive?
- Can we create systems of care that nurture the enduring self?
- Can we remember that even at the edge of madness, there is music, hunger, longing, and light?

A Hopeful Future

This book is a message of hope. It calls for a mental health care model that honors the full humanity of individuals. Hope is not blind optimism—it is the belief that meaning and peace are possible, even with challenges. It is the conviction that a person's spark can survive, and even thrive, in the face of illness.

I still don't have all the answers. But what I do know is this: sparks endure. And that gives me hope.

Healing is not linear. It is messy, nonlinear, interrupted. And yet, healing is real. People recover. People connect. People grow. They do so not in spite of their sparks, but because of them.

A hopeful future will be built by those willing to ask different questions, to honor unconventional truths, and to make room for beauty in unlikely places.

Call to Action

Let this book serve as a call to action. For clinicians, families, policymakers, and the general public: honor the sparks. Protect them. Amplify them. They are not symptoms. They are what return us to life.

Let us build systems, relationships, and care models that reflect the complexity and dignity of the people we serve. Let us be led not only by science, but by soul.

May we become not just clinicians or caregivers, but keepers of sparks—tenders of the fire that endures in all of us.

The sparks are not just what endure. They are what return us to life.

Reflection Questions

1. What vision do you hold for the future of mental health care?
2. How can you contribute to a system that honors the full humanity of people living with serious mental illness?
3. What sparks have stood out to you most in this book, and why?
4. How will you continue to protect and promote sparks in your personal or professional life?

American Psychiatric Association. (2013). *Diagnostic and statistical manual of mental disorders* (5th ed.). American Psychiatric Publishing.

Charon, R. (2006). *Narrative medicine: Honoring the stories of illness.* Oxford University Press.

Davidson, L., O'Connell, M., Tondora, J., Staeheli Lawless, M., & Evans, A. C. (2005). Recovery in serious mental illness: A new wine or just a new bottle? *Professional Psychology: Research and Practice, 36*(5), 480–487. https://doi.org/10.1037/0735-7028.36.5.480

Deegan, P. E. (1988). Recovery: The lived experience of rehabilitation. *Psychosocial Rehabilitation Journal, 11*(4), 11–19. https://doi.org/10.1037/h0099565

Frankl, V. E. (2006). *Man's search for meaning.* Beacon Press. (Original work published 1946)

Kleinman, A. (1988). *The illness narratives: Suffering, healing, and the human condition.* Basic Books.

Lysaker, P. H., & Lysaker, J. T. (2008). *Schizophrenia and the fate of the self: A narrative account.* Oxford University Press.

Slade, M. (2009). *Personal recovery and mental illness: A guide for mental health professionals.* Cambridge University Press.

Epilogue:
The Sparks That Endure

The final chapter closes, but the narrative of our lives, intertwined with these sparks, continues to unfold. The quiet hum of the world outside today in Orangeburg—perhaps the gentle lapping of the Hudson River against the shore, the distant drone of traffic on Route 303, or the rustle of newly unfurled leaves in the spring breeze—serves as a subtle, constant reminder that life's symphony is always playing, inviting our active participation.

A man who hasn't spoken in days still taps his fingers to a remembered beat. A woman gripped by paranoia still arranges her food just so, preserving a ritual no one else understands. A young person cycling through mania writes page after page of poetry that no one has read, but that makes that person feel real. These small, fierce gestures are not just quirks or symptoms. They are sparks—persistent, embodied expressions of the self.

The world tends to define people with schizophrenia, bipolar disorder, and other serious mental illnesses by what they lose: insight, function, coherence. But these losses tell only part of the story. Beneath the disorganization and suffering, there are still rhythms, rituals, desires, and dreams. There are patterns that resist erasure. There are intact inner landscapes, even when outer expression seems chaotic.

We've explored sex, money, food, music, spirituality, creativity, movement, rituals, nature, humor, touch, storytelling, hope, and freedom not as rigid, academic categories, but as vibrant, pulsing currents within the vast ocean of human experience. They are the sources of both our deepest joys and our most profound struggles, the wellsprings of our resilience and the crucibles of our growth. Yet, the true revelation isn't in their simple definition, but in the profound realization of our agency. We are not merely passive recipients of their influence. We are the conductors, the artists, the mindful participants who choose how these sparks ignite, flicker, or blaze within our existence. They may emerge in unconventional, exaggerated, or troubling ways, but they often serve a function: to regulate, to soothe, to assert identity, to connect. They are not detours from recovery. They are often the path to it.

We must learn to listen differently—not just for symptoms, but for signals. Not just for pathology, but for purpose. A patient obsessed with budgeting may be reaching for control. A person who won't stop singing might be organizing their world through sound. What looks irrational from the outside may be deeply rational from within. This reframing is not just clinical; it is moral.

To see the spark is to see the person. To support it is to say: You are more than your illness. You are still here. And that is no small thing. In fact, it may be everything.

The spark asks something of all of us—clinicians, family members, friends, and systems of care. It asks for curiosity over control, presence over protocol, and partnership over paternalism. It asks us to move away from seeing people as broken and instead as bearers of continuity, meaning, and potential. Even when capacity is diminished, even when functioning is impaired, there is almost always something that remains.

And what remains matters deeply.

A life organized around music is still a life. A world stabilized by ritual is still a world. A person whose meaning comes through movement, money, creating, or believing is still participating in the great human task of becoming.

Too often, our systems of care prioritize what can be measured—symptom counts, hospital days, medication adherence. But what about what can't be measured? What of joy, agency, desire, beauty? What of the sacred, the creative, the embodied? These too are outcomes. And often, they are what matter most to the person living the experience.

The journey doesn't end with intellectual understanding; it truly begins with conscious practice. These sparks are not distant ideals; they are present in every moment, every interaction, every choice. They are in the shared laughter of humor, the satisfaction of a meal, the invigorating feeling of movement, or the quiet reflection that connects us to spirituality. By recognizing and tending to them, we don't just exist; we live.

The epilogue of this exploration is not a summary, but an invitation—to lean into the dualities, to seek balance in a world of extremes, and to nurture the sparks that resonate with the authentic self. The path forward is not perfection, but progress: an evolution of awareness, compassion, and empowerment.

In the depths of psychiatric illness, when thought unravels and reality fractures, these sparks remain. Their presence says: I am still trying. Trying to feel. To matter. To be me.

These are not just phenomena. They are acts of survival. Often, acts of courage.

Imagine systems built around this insight. Treatment plans that ask not just about symptoms, but about music, memory, ritual, and creativity. Research that explores not just deficits, but structures of resilience. Care that values the whole person over diagnosis.

Imagine clinical encounters where the first question is not "What's wrong?" but "What brings you joy?" Imagine policies shaped around enhancing access to meaningful activities rather than only managing risks. Imagine community supports that nurture sparks—support groups for shared rituals, expressive arts programs, open mic nights in residential settings, spiritual care that adapts to the individual's path.

We must choose this future. Again and again. Because no matter the severity of illness, the spark remains. Sometimes faint. Sometimes fierce. But always there. Waiting for someone to see it. To name it. To say, "This, too, is you." Let's begin there.

And from that beginning, something beautiful can grow.

Let this epilogue serve not as closure, but as ignition. As you set this book down, consider what sparks have sustained you. Which ones have emerged in times of stress? Which ones do you yearn to rekindle? How might you better honor them in yourself—and in others?

You carry sparks. So do your patients, clients, loved ones. The task is not to extinguish them, but to understand them. To help them burn bright, not out.

This is the work. This is the hope. This is the enduring fire of being human.

Reflection Questions

1. Which spark(s) resonate most with your personal or professional journey, and why?
2. How have you witnessed small, persistent gestures—like rituals, creativity, or music—serve as lifelines for someone facing mental illness?
3. What would it look like for you to "listen for the spark" in someone's story rather than just their symptoms?
4. How might your daily practice or relationships change if you prioritized presence, curiosity, and meaning over control or efficiency?
5. What systems (clinical, institutional, or personal) need to change so that sparks can be nurtured rather than suppressed?

Appendix A:
Theoretical Foundations

Recovery-Oriented Care

Recovery is a central theme throughout the book. The recovery model emphasizes the role of individual agency and the reclaiming of personal identity, purpose, and hope despite psychiatric conditions.[1] This framework helps clinicians and families support individuals in overcoming adversity through strength-based approaches.

Theoretical Basis: The recovery model emphasizes personal choice, empowerment, and the importance of hope in the healing process.[1,2]

Clinical Application:

- Respecting the individual's autonomy in making treatment decisions and engaging in community-based support systems.
- Incorporating values like sexuality and spirituality into care plans.

Trauma-Informed Care

Understanding trauma's impact allows clinicians to address underlying causes of enduring preoccupations in serious mental illness.[3,4]

Theoretical Basis: Trauma-informed care recognizes the impact of early or ongoing trauma on self-concept and relationships.

Clinical Application:

- Requires a safe, validating environment with gradual exposure and trust-building.
- Sparks like rituals or movement can support emotional regulation.

Polyvagal Theory

Polyvagal theory links vagus nerve function to emotional regulation, social bonding, and stress response. It offers a physiological explanation for the effectiveness of movement, ritual, and sensory engagement in psychiatric care.[5,6]

Appendix B:
Clinical Application of Sparks

Sexuality and Relationships
Sexuality and relationships are often neglected in care despite their importance to well-being. Supporting sexual identity and relationships is essential in recovery.[2]

Music as Therapy
Music provides accessible emotional expression. It can regulate emotions, improve memory, and create social connection.[7][8]

Spirituality and Meaning-Making
Connecting to something greater can provide purpose, especially in times of identity loss. Spiritual practices support existential recovery.[9][10]

Rituals for Emotional Regulation
Rituals create predictability and activate the parasympathetic nervous system, supporting stability and self-regulation in clinical settings.[5][6]

Footnotes
1. Anthony, W. A. (1993). *Recovery from mental illness: The guiding vision of the mental health service system in the 1990s. Psychosocial Rehabilitation Journal, 16*(4), 11–23.
2. Deegan, P. E. (1988). *Recovery: The lived experience of rehabilitation. Psychosocial Rehabilitation Journal, 11*(4), 11–19.
3. Herman, J. L. (1992). *Trauma and recovery: The aftermath of violence.* Basic Books.
4. van der Kolk, B. (2014). *The body keeps the score: Brain, mind, and body in the healing of trauma.* Viking.
5. Porges, S. W. (2011). *The polyvagal theory: Neurophysiological foundations of emotions, attachment, communication, and self-regulation.* W. W. Norton & Company.

6. Siegel, D. J. (2012). *The developing mind: How relationships and the brain interact to shape who we are.* Guilford Press.
7. Aldridge, D. (1996). *Music therapy research and practice in medicine: From out of the silence.* Jessica Kingsley Publishers.
8. Malchiodi, C. A. (2012). *Handbook of art therapy.* Guilford Press.
9. Frankl, V. E. (1959). *Man's search for meaning.* Beacon Press.
10. Koenig, H. G. (2009). *Research on religion, spirituality, and mental health: A review. Canadian Journal of Psychiatry, 54*(5), 283–291.

Appendix C:
Case Illustrations of Sparks

1. Sex and Intimacy: Maria

Setting: Community clinic

Challenge:

Maria, a woman in her late 30s with bipolar disorder, struggled with intimacy after medication-related weight gain. She felt unworthy of touch and avoided relationships. "It's like my illness and the meds took away the part of me that could be loved."

Intervention:

She was encouraged to join a structured social and dating skills group. Therapy sessions focused on body acceptance and safe communication around intimacy.

Outcome:

Maria gradually re-engaged in relationships, rediscovering her sexuality as a source of healing and identity rather than shame.

2. Money and Security: James

Setting: Supported housing

Challenge:

James, living with schizophrenia, was repeatedly exploited financially by relatives. He was anxious, mistrustful, and often left without basic needs.

Intervention:

A social worker introduced budgeting tools and arranged for a representative payee. He received coaching on distinguishing exploitation from healthy financial interactions.

Outcome:

James initially resisted but later reported feeling secure as his bills were paid and his savings grew. "I finally feel like my money is mine again." His sense of autonomy and dignity improved.

3. Food and Nourishment: Leila

Setting: Day treatment program

Challenge:

Leila, with anorexia and depression, viewed food as the enemy. She skipped meals and described eating as a form of punishment.

Intervention:

She joined a therapeutic cooking group, where she shared her grandmother's lentil stew recipe. Preparing food in community created positive associations with eating.

Outcome:

Leila began eating with others and redefined meals as nourishment and connection. "When I cook this, I remember being cared for."

4. Music and Resonance: David

Setting: Outpatient clinic

Challenge:

David, with schizoaffective disorder, experienced intrusive auditory hallucinations he described as "a radio I can't turn off."

Intervention:

A therapist encouraged him to use structured music listening, particularly jazz, at bedtime to redirect attention and regulate mood.

Outcome:

The voices did not vanish but were softened. His sleep improved, and paranoia lessened. Music became his chosen tool for emotional regulation.

5. Spirituality and Meaning: Sam

Setting: Forensic unit

Challenge:

Sam, incarcerated with chronic schizophrenia, blurred delusions with religious themes, declaring himself a prophet.

Intervention:

A chaplain guided him in structured use of scripture, focusing on Psalms as a stabilizing spiritual practice distinct from delusion.

Outcome:

Sam reported: "This verse speaks me better than I can." Faith became a source of comfort and articulation, not paranoia.

6. Creativity and Expression: Alisha

Setting: Art therapy group

Challenge:

Alisha felt overwhelmed by intrusive voices and lacked safe ways to externalize them.

Intervention:

She participated in art therapy, painting abstract forms that represented her auditory experiences.

Outcome:

Her artwork opened dialogue with clinicians and family. Over time, her paintings became more coherent, reflecting improved inner organization.

7. Movement and Embodiment: Carlos

Setting: Psychiatric rehabilitation program

Challenge:

Carlos, with severe depression, described his body as "a prison of heaviness."

Intervention:

He was introduced to a dance group that emphasized social engagement and rhythm.

Outcome:

Movement lifted his energy and improved sleep. "When I move, it's like the fog lifts for a while." Dance reconnected him to joy.

8. Rituals and Structure: Maya

Setting: Residential trauma program

Challenge:

Maya, a trauma survivor, described her life as "chaos inside and out." She was reactive and dysregulated.

Intervention:

She developed a morning ritual: yoga, prayer, and tea, supported by staff encouragement.

Outcome:

Maya became calmer and more consistent in groups. She explained, "This is the one part of my day I control." Ritual restored agency.

9. Nature and Grounding: Jonah

Setting: Veterans' recovery program

Challenge:

Jonah, with PTSD, struggled with flashbacks and hypervigilance. Traditional talk therapy was ineffective.

Intervention:

He joined a gardening group, working with soil and plants to provide sensory grounding.

Outcome:

He reported: "Out here, I'm not a soldier or a patient. I'm just a man with dirt on my hands." Nature provided regulation and renewal.

10. Humor and Playfulness: Rosa

Setting: Geriatric psychiatry unit

Challenge:

Rosa, an older woman with dementia, often presented with agitation and withdrawal.

Intervention:

Staff introduced comedy skits and lighthearted group activities to invite laughter.

Outcome:

Rosa became more engaged, joking with staff and peers. "Finally, you people are funny!" Humor softened irritability and restored joy.

11. Touch and Sensation: Malik

Setting: Long-term state hospital

Challenge:

Malik, with autism and schizophrenia, had high anxiety and relied on repetitive rocking for comfort.

Intervention:

Occupational therapy offered safe sensory interventions, including weighted blankets and gentle massage.

Outcome:

Malik said, "The blanket feels like someone holding me safe." His anxiety decreased, and his regulation improved.

12. Storytelling and Meaning-Making: Fatima

Setting: Peer support group

Challenge:

Fatima, a refugee with trauma-related psychosis, had fragmented memories and difficulty distinguishing dreams from reality.

Intervention:

She participated in a storytelling group, gradually narrating her migration journey with support.

Outcome:

She reflected, "Now I know I lived through it, not just dreamed it." Storytelling restored coherence, dignity, and community recognition.

13. Hope and Possibility: Daniel

Setting: Early psychosis program

Challenge:

Daniel, a college freshman, became hopeless after a first psychotic break. "It's over. My life is done before it started."

Intervention:

His psychiatrist paired him with a peer mentor who was thriving years after diagnosis.

Outcome:

Hope was reignited. Daniel returned to school part-time, reconnected with friends, and began dating. Recovery became imaginable again.

14. Freedom and Autonomy: Tasha

Setting: Assertive community treatment (ACT) team

Challenge:

Tasha, under conservatorship, lived in a group home where every detail of life was controlled, from meals to bedtime.

Intervention:

She advocated for supervised housing that allowed her to make personal decisions about her schedule and meals.

Outcome:

Tasha thrived in a more autonomous setting. "I want to choose when I eat, even if it's just cereal at midnight." Small freedoms restored dignity and motivation.

Appendix D:
Tools for Clinicians

Conversation Starters to Explore Core Drives

- **Music**: What kinds of music do you enjoy, or did you used to enjoy?
- **Money**: What does having money or financial independence mean to you?
- **Food**: Are there meals or food rituals that bring you comfort?
- **Sex/Intimacy**: How do relationships and intimacy play a role in your life right now?
- **Spirituality**: Do you have spiritual or religious practices that are meaningful to you?
- **Creativity**: Have you ever used art, writing, or crafts to express yourself?
- **Movement**: What activities help you feel energized or relaxed?
- **Rituals**: Are there daily routines or rituals that give you structure or comfort?
- **Nature**: Do you feel restored by being outdoors or connected to nature?
- **Humor**: When was the last time you laughed until you felt lighter?
- **Touch**: What kinds of touch (like hugs, massage, or sensory objects) feel safe or comforting?
- **Storytelling**: Are there personal or cultural stories you like to share that help explain who you are?
- **Hope**: What are you looking forward to, even in small ways?
- **Freedom**: What choices or freedoms are most important for you right now?

Purpose: Normalize these conversations to build trust and humanize care.

Therapeutic Strategies (by Spark)

- **Music Therapy**: Encourage playlist creation and group singing.
- **Financial Literacy**: Connect with community budgeting or supported employment programs.
- **Mindful Eating**: Use food journals, meal planning, and shared cooking groups.
- **Sexual Health Education**: Provide safe spaces for discussion of intimacy, consent, and desire.
- **Spiritual Care**: Partner with chaplains or spiritual leaders for meaning-making.
- **Creative Expression**: Facilitate writing, art, or poetry for emotional processing.
- **Movement Practices**: Introduce yoga, dance, or walking groups for grounding.
- **Ritual Building**: Help patients create calming daily routines (e.g., bedtime ritual, gratitude practice).
- **Nature Exposure**: Organize gardening projects, outdoor walks, or window plant care.
- **Humor Interventions**: Use comedic media, improv games, or playful exercises in groups.
- **Touch & Sensory Care**: Integrate weighted blankets, fidget tools, or safe touch practices.
- **Narrative Therapy**: Invite life stories and cultural narratives for coherence and dignity.
- **Hope Work**: Identify role models, peer mentors, or future goals to spark possibility.
- **Autonomy Support**: Empower choice in treatment plans, housing, and daily activities.

Appendix E:
Resources for Caregivers

Understanding Core Drives in Illness
- Normalize persistent preoccupations.
- Avoid shame when discussing sex, money, or food.
- Recognize sparks as connection points, not problems.
- Respect that sparks often remain intact even during illness.

Supporting Healthy Engagement
- **Music**: Listen together or attend concerts.
- **Money**: Support budgeting without judgment.
- **Food**: Share meals, cook family recipes, or introduce positive food rituals.
- **Sex/Intimacy**: Respect privacy, encourage healthy relationships.
- **Spirituality**: Attend services or rituals together if desired.
- **Creativity**: Provide materials for painting, crafts, or writing.
- **Movement**: Invite walks, dance, or light exercise.
- **Rituals**: Establish small family routines (tea time, bedtime reading).
- **Nature**: Encourage time outdoors, even simple garden sitting.
- **Humor**: Watch comedies or share jokes daily.
- **Touch**: Offer safe hugs, hand-holding, or calming sensory objects.
- **Storytelling**: Invite family histories or cultural traditions to be shared.
- **Hope**: Celebrate progress, no matter how small.
- **Freedom**: Allow choice in clothing, meals, or daily schedule when possible.

When to Seek Professional Help
- Escalating risky behaviors
- Signs of exploitation (financial, sexual, or otherwise)
- Drastic weight or sleep changes
- Withdrawal from all sparks (loss of pleasure or interest)

Appendix F:
Patient Reflection Worksheet

Self-Guided Questions
1. What is a song that always lifts your spirits? Why? *(Music)*
2. What would financial security look like for you? *(Money)*
3. What role does food play in your life right now? *(Food)*
4. How do you think about relationships and intimacy? *(Sex/Intimacy)*
5. Do you connect with any spiritual or religious practices? *(Spirituality)*
6. What creative activity makes you lose track of time? *(Creativity)*
7. How does movement—walking, dancing, stretching—affect your mood? *(Movement)*
8. Are there daily rituals or routines that help you feel steady? *(Rituals)*
9. Do you feel different when you spend time outdoors? *(Nature)*
10. What makes you laugh and feel lighter? *(Humor)*
11. What kinds of touch or sensory experiences make you feel safe? *(Touch)*
12. What story from your life feels important to tell? *(Storytelling)*
13. What gives you hope when things feel difficult? *(Hope)*
14. What choices or freedoms matter most to you right now? *(Freedom)*

Appendix G:
Spark Engagement Worksheets

Spark Identification Worksheet
- What activities make you feel most alive or calm?
- What past interests do you still think about?
- What routines or rituals bring comfort?
- Which senses (sight, sound, touch, taste, smell) are most meaningful to you?
- Which of the 14 sparks feels strongest in your life right now?

Weekly Spark Tracker
- Which spark did I engage with this week?
- How did I feel before, during, and after?
- What challenges did I face?
- What support helped me?
- What do I want to try next week?

Spark Goals Page
- One small way I will engage a spark this week: _____
- Who can support me: _____
- How I'll know it helped: _____

APPENDIX H:
Interviews and Perspectives

This appendix gathers insights from patients, families, peer advocates, and professionals. To respect privacy, all patient and family contributions have been anonymized, with identifying details altered or removed. Professional contributors, including clinicians, peer specialists, and educators, are identified by name when they consent to have their perspectives published. In every case, the intent has been to preserve the authenticity of the voice while ensuring confidentiality and ethical representation.

Interview Spotlight: The Sparks That Endure
Dr. Daniel Latendresse, Psychologist

Dr. Daniel Latendresse brings creativity and structure together in his therapeutic work. He describes how psychodrama, using role-play and performance, helped one patient move from withdrawal to re-engagement, and how he continues to direct plays with other patients in the hospital as a way of fostering expression, connection, and healing.

He is a great believer in flow, that immersive state where a person becomes fully absorbed in an activity, balancing challenge with skill. It was Dr. Latendresse who first pointed out the importance of flow in psychiatric recovery, referencing the work of Mihaly Csikszentmihalyi. In his experience, activities that spark flow, whether through theater, music, or ritual, allow patients to reclaim agency and experience themselves as capable and alive.

For Dr. Latendresse, recovery is not only about reducing symptoms but about opening pathways for creativity, play, and meaning. He reminds us that when patients are given opportunities to engage in flow experiences, they often move from being passive recipients of care to active participants in their own healing. "When patients enter flow, they stop being patients for a moment; they become themselves again."

Interview Spotlight – The Sparks That Endure

Angela Argenzio, Recreational Therapist

Angela Argenzio has spent over three decades bringing music and creative therapies into psychiatric and medical care. With a B.A. in Music from Adelphi University and an M.A. in Music Therapy from NYU, she has worked in settings ranging from children's palliative care at Saint Mary's Hospital to rehabilitation programs at Rockland Psychiatric Center. She is also trained as a Reiki practitioner and is certified in Orff and Kindermusik approaches, blending traditional and alternative methods to reach patients.

Angela emphasizes that music is grounding and soothing, helping patients regulate mood, reduce anxiety, and reconnect with themselves and others. She has witnessed patients with profound impairments respond only to music, sometimes through rhythm, sometimes through movement or voice. One child with hydrocephaly, for example, would demonstrate recognition and vitality only when hearing steady beats.

She stresses the role of flow and choice in therapy, echoing the importance of agency in recovery. Allowing patients to choose activities, improvise, or engage creatively transforms therapy from compliance into connection. Movement and music, she notes, bring "a human body connection"—restoring dignity and self-expression where illness had silenced them.

For Angela, recovery is inseparable from creativity. Whether through singing, drumming, dance, or play, patients often find a sense of wholeness, joy, and identity. "So many people feel alive when music enters the room," she explains. Her work reminds clinicians that healing requires not only structure but also rhythm, spontaneity, and the courage to invite art back into care.

Interview Spotlight – The Sparks That Endure
Paulette Heslop, MHTA II

Paulette Heslop has worked in healthcare for more than thirty years, much of it as a mental health therapy aide. Her perspective is grounded in long experience "on the floor," helping patients navigate daily challenges with dignity and hope.

For Heslop, recovery is about finding the right spark that brings someone back to life—whether it is music, dancing, or simply being reminded that they are cared for and not forgotten. She describes her role as creating space for small but meaningful moments of humanity: listening, showing consistency, and encouraging expression.

She recalls patients who came alive when encouraged to sing or dance, or when reminded of family and cultural traditions. These sparks of engagement, she explains, are not just diversions but vital therapeutic bridges that restore identity and connection.

Heslop is candid about the barriers staff face—short staffing, heavy demands, and institutional limits. Yet she insists that even brief moments of person-centered care can change trajectories. "Any little glimmer of hope is huge," she explains. "I give them hope. I tell them, 'I want you to be encouraged before I leave.'"

Her philosophy is simple but profound: recovery begins with being seen as fully human. Through compassion, presence, and attention to enduring human needs, Heslop helps patients move beyond symptoms toward resilience and meaning.

Interview Spotlight – The Sparks That Endure

Michelle Goscinsky, LCSW-R, Director of the Recovery Center

Michelle Goscinsky leads the Recovery Center with a focus on strength, courage, and daily determination. For her, recovery begins simply with the act of getting out of bed and arriving in the morning—an expression of resilience and commitment to life.

She describes sparks of recovery as moments when members come alive again through creative freedom. Picking up a paintbrush or singing an old, familiar song can ignite independence and joy. Many members reconnect with their younger, healthier selves through music, reliving memories of vitality from the 1960s to the 1990s, or finding pride in sharing songs with peers.

Community plays a central role at the Recovery Center. Members form friendships, share stories of their journeys from inpatient care to supportive housing, and help each other with creative projects like making beaded necklaces. These activities provide belonging, pride, and a sense of accomplishment.

Goscinsky highlights the importance of rituals, such as the daily community meeting, which begins with breathing and stretching exercises, welcoming new members, and sharing a cup of coffee. These routines create stability and connection, grounding participants for the day ahead.

She is candid about barriers, especially the slow trial-and-error process of psychiatric medications, which can take days or weeks to reduce symptoms. Yet she emphasizes the resilience of the human spirit, which persists even amid emotional pain, delusions, and hallucinations. "The human spirit is so strong," she explains, "and having hopeful faith that suffering is temporary is what helps people endure."

Her message for clinicians, families, and policymakers is clear: mental illness can happen to anyone, and recovery is always individual. Healing may come through medication, but also through journaling, painting, drawing, and other expressive outlets. Patience and openness to multiple pathways are essential.

Interview Spotlight – The Sparks That Endure
Melissa Hayes-Kolakowski, Jewish Chaplain

Melissa Hayes-Kolakowski serves as Jewish Chaplain at Rockland Psychiatric Center, bringing a faith-based perspective to recovery. With a background in both music and theology, she emphasizes that faith can be an anchor during psychological suffering, offering structure, hope, and meaning when other supports fall short. During the COVID-19 pandemic, when group activities were disrupted, she saw patients turn to prayer, faith, and ritual as lifelines.

She recalls supporting patients with schizophrenia whose spirituality was deeply entwined with their experiences. One patient, even in the midst of delusion, remained connected to his faith community and was able to express himself meaningfully by making a Torah cover for his synagogue. Another patient found renewed connection to God when her symptoms cleared, demonstrating how faith can both sustain and reawaken a sense of self.

Hayes-Kolakowski highlights that spirituality and psychiatry must work together. She believes spirituality is as essential as medicine in helping people heal, providing a dimension of human resilience that science alone cannot supply. She affirms that chaplains and clinicians must remain flexible, acknowledging that they do not have all the answers and that healing often comes through shared humility and collaboration.

For Hayes-Kolakowski, recovery is both spiritual and practical. She insists that recognizing the spiritual dimension of human experience not only reduces suffering but also restores dignity and purpose. "Spirituality is important, just like medicine," she explains, "and both working together will help people move forward."

Interview Spotlight – The Sparks That Endure
Dr. Helen Bloomer, DNP

Dr. Helen Bloomer brings both medical expertise and compassion to her psychiatric work. She recalls being initially hesitant to work in psychiatry because of fears about patient violence, but she grew to value the field deeply. She emphasizes that patients are often unfairly stigmatized and "looked down on," yet she sees them as individuals with autonomy, families, and strengths deserving of dignity and care.

Bloomer describes how music, faith, and family often become powerful sparks of recovery. She recalls a patient who had once studied music at Berkeley and, despite being disorganized, became logical and centered when playing piano. Another patient, usually withdrawn, could still remember Broadway songs and sing them clearly when prompted. For Bloomer, these moments reveal how creativity and memory are preserved, even in illness.

She highlights how patients find meaning in nutrition, spirituality, and connection. One patient improved after becoming vegetarian; another used prayer lists, writing down names daily as a form of healing engagement. Families also play a central role: sending letters, making calls, and writing notes of encouragement often became decisive factors in recovery. "You can never take their hope," she insists, pointing to how self-esteem and resilience are nourished through listening, validation, and respect.

Bloomer also underscores the importance of holistic care—educating patients, involving them in preventive tests, and creating opportunities for small victories like writing cards, remembering songs, or managing diet. She stresses that treatment should focus not only on symptom control but also on preserving identity and cultivating hope.

Interview Spotlight – The Sparks That Endure
Louis Pachlin, MHA, RT

Louis Pachlin has dedicated his career to integrating recreation and rehabilitation into psychiatric care. Inspired by a family connection to mental illness, he pursued recreation therapy as a way to help patients rediscover meaning and identity through activity.

For Pachlin, recreation is not "just games" but a therapeutic process that taps into what people love—whether music, sports, art, or travel. He stresses that music is one of the strongest sparks, capable of motivating, soothing, and uniting. He recalls patients who rediscovered their spark through group dance, drumming, and performance—moments where illness no longer defined them and their creativity and joy emerged.

He emphasizes the power of movement in reconnecting patients with their bodies and emotions, noting that dance, yoga, and exercise often bring relief, happiness, and improved regulation. Creative expression—through art, clay, painting, or music—also anchors patients, offering non-traditional but deeply effective ways to heal. Rituals, he explains, serve as anchors of stability, helping patients cope with the uneasiness of life.

As a director, Pachlin acknowledges systemic barriers, such as restrictions on supplies and institutional rules, but he has worked to innovate programs, such as a dance and movement group routine that culminated in performances and celebrations. These, he argues, instill pride and belonging.

Pachlin wants clinicians to understand that recreation is not a diversion but a core therapeutic tool. Staff who lead these programs are trained professionals whose work activates meaning and purpose for patients. "The power of recreation can be endless," he explains. "When a patient finds a spark, it gives them hope, purpose, and a way forward in recovery."

Interview Spotlight – The Sparks That Endure
Gail Miller, LMSW2, Staff Development

Gail Miller brings a background in social work and staff development to her role at Rockland Psychiatric Center. With experience in trauma-informed care and nonviolent communication, she emphasizes that understanding human needs and dignity is central to healing.

Miller explains that much of her work focuses on how clinicians can help patients regain dignity, even when illness strips away autonomy. She often asks: What do they need to get their dignity back? This, she believes, is as essential as addressing symptoms.

Her approach draws from both clinical and humanistic traditions. In trauma trainings, she underscores how discussions of trust and dignity resonate deeply with patients and staff alike. She connects this to her earlier experience working with individuals in developmental disability services, where her guiding principle was to treat every person as a full human being with agency and worth.

For Miller, sparks of recovery emerge when clinicians recognize and affirm patients' humanity. Whether through communication, consistency, or creating safe spaces for expression, she reminds staff that recovery is inseparable from dignity. "The kind of care you have for a person makes the difference," she notes. "My role is to help people stop their fall, and it is the same here."

Interview Spotlight – The Sparks That Endure
Danielle Sanzi, RN3

Danielle Sanzi has served as a registered nurse at Rockland Psychiatric Center with a special focus on supporting both patients and new nurses. She became a nurse educator to give the kind of guidance and support she herself did not receive when starting out. "As a nurse educator," she explains, "I could not only give guidance to new RNs but also help them feel confident in this field, which can be intimidating."

Sanzi emphasizes the importance of listening directly to patients, rather than relying only on staff perceptions. She stresses that patients should be treated with dignity and recognized as human beings with their own lives and perspectives. Too often, she observes, staff dismiss concerns or overlook the need for meaningful connection, which undermines recovery.

She has seen how music and food act as sparks on the unit. Daily lunchtime singing brought patients together, especially when paired with creative incentives like pizza parties or simple rewards such as a bottle of Ensure. These moments built community, lifted morale, and even increased health compliance.

Sanzi also acknowledges the challenges of addressing sensitive needs like sexuality, as well as the barriers nurses face—multiple responsibilities, constant interruptions, and confusing or shifting policies that can lead to frustration and burnout. Yet she insists that sparks like music, food, and creativity remain powerful and accessible tools that cut through systemic challenges. "They're universal languages," she notes.

For her, recovery begins with respect, dignity, and connection—simple but profound practices that remind patients that their lives still hold meaning and possibility.

Interview Spotlight – The Sparks That Endure
Kelly-Ann Fairweather, LCSW-R, TTL

Kelly-Ann Fairweather brings the dual perspective of a social worker and team leader at Rockland Psychiatric Center. She reflects on how dignity, forgiveness, and connection remain essential sparks even amid severe mental illness.

She recalls a patient from her previous role as a social worker, who had committed homicide during a psychotic break. He initially refused forgiveness and insisted on remaining institutionalized, convinced he deserved punishment. Yet over time, through faith, family, and community, he began to rediscover a spark of self-love and forgiveness. With support, he came to see himself as worthy of connection and belonging. "This spark grew into a glow of self-love," Fairweather notes, "and it became possible for him to see himself as a person deserving of community and forgiveness."

In her work, she has witnessed how individuals with mental illness lean on both families and communities for strength, often finding grounding in faith. She emphasizes that these higher purposes—connection, belonging, and forgiveness—speak to the universal human need for intimacy and acceptance.

For Fairweather, recovery is not just clinical but profoundly human. She reminds clinicians that sparks such as dignity, forgiveness, and self-love are central to restoring personhood. Her approach emphasizes compassion, patience, and faith in the enduring resilience of the human spirit.

Interview Spotlight – The Sparks That Endure
Anonymous Psychiatrist

An experienced psychiatrist with decades of inpatient and outpatient work reflects on the enduring sparks he has observed in patients. He emphasizes that despite the severity of mental illness, patients consistently hold on to passions and desires that give their lives meaning. "You can medicate delusions away," he explains, "but you cannot extinguish someone's love of music, their hunger for connection, or their longing for dignity."

He recalls a patient with chronic schizophrenia who never missed an opportunity to attend group music sessions. Even when withdrawn or disorganized, this individual would brighten when the guitar began playing, singing lyrics without hesitation. "That moment," the psychiatrist explains, "wasn't about diagnosis—it was about being human."

He also highlights the symbolic weight of money for many patients. For one man, being able to buy a cup of coffee at the hospital kiosk was as important as medication—not for the caffeine, but for the sense of independence it provided him. Similarly, patients often anchored themselves in rituals like prayer, daily walks, or journaling. These sparks provided structure and resilience even in the face of relapse.

Looking back, the psychiatrist stresses that recovery is not defined solely by symptom reduction, but by preserving and nurturing these sparks. "We must remember," he concludes, "that patients are more than their illnesses. Their sparks—music, faith, humor, love—are not side issues. They are the essence of personhood."

Interview Spotlight – The Sparks That Endure
Anonymous Peer Advocate A

A man in his forties with lived experience of schizophrenia describes how music became his lifeline. Even when delusions clouded his thinking, listening to old jazz records reminded him of who he was before illness. He calls music his "anchor to reality," something that made hospitals feel less like punishment and more like a place of survival. Today, he helps other peers explore playlists as recovery tools.

Interview Spotlight – The Sparks That Endure
Anonymous Peer Advocate B

A woman in her thirties with bipolar disorder shares how creative writing gave her voice when words were otherwise tangled. Journaling allowed her to externalize racing thoughts and shape them into poetry. She explains, "Even when I couldn't talk to people, my notebook was listening."

Interview Spotlight – The Sparks That Endure
Anonymous Peer Advocate C

A young man in his twenties living with schizoaffective disorder recalls how ritual and movement gave him grounding. Walking the same path around the hospital garden each morning gave him a sense of rhythm and autonomy. He emphasizes the importance of "having one thing you can control" when everything else feels chaotic.

Interview Spotlight – The Sparks That Endure
Anonymous Family Member A (Mother)

The mother of an adult daughter with schizoaffective disorder reflects on the role of food as both a challenge and a spark. Shared meals became a fragile but important ritual. Even during relapses, her daughter would still cook simple recipes from childhood. "It reminded us she was still there," she says.

Interview Spotlight – The Sparks That Endure

Anonymous Family Member B (Sibling)

A brother of a man with chronic schizophrenia emphasizes humor. He recalls visiting his sibling on inpatient wards, where joking about sports scores or silly childhood memories broke through silence. "If he laughed, even once, we knew the spark was still alive."

Interview Spotlight – The Sparks That Endure
Anonymous Family Member C (Spouse)

A wife of a man with bipolar disorder reflects on the tension between money and dignity. She describes how saving small amounts in envelopes for him to spend became a strategy that gave him autonomy while ensuring stability. She emphasizes, "It wasn't the money—it was about trust."

Interview Spotlight – The Sparks That Endure

Anonymous Community Volunteer (Art Program Leader)

A retired teacher who leads art workshops at a psychosocial clubhouse recalls patients who found sparks in painting and sculpture. One man who had rarely spoken picked up clay and created detailed figures. "His hands spoke when his mouth could not," she reflects.

Interview Spotlight – The Sparks That Endure
Anonymous Clergy Member (Chaplain)

A chaplain shares how spirituality provided grounding for patients in despair. Even simple rituals like lighting a candle or reciting familiar prayers helped restore hope. "It was not about religion," they note. "It was about giving people back their voice in silence."

Interview Spotlight – The Sparks That Endure

Anonymous Neighbor/Community Friend

A longtime neighbor of a man with schizophrenia explains how nature became his spark. "He'd sit on the porch, watering plants for hours. It was his sanctuary." Over time, others joined, creating a small community ritual around gardening.

Interview Spotlight – The Sparks That Endure

Anonymous Peer (on Sex and Intimacy)

A man in his late thirties living with schizoaffective disorder reflects on how intimacy remained a longing even during years of hospitalization. He describes the loneliness of psychiatric wards where touch was forbidden, but also the deep comfort he found when staff spoke to him as an equal. "I wasn't looking for sex," he explains. "I was looking for closeness—someone to remind me I was still human." He credits recovery with allowing him to begin a supportive relationship later in life. For him, intimacy was a spark that affirmed his identity and dignity, not something erased by illness.

Interview Spotlight – The Sparks That Endure

Anonymous Family Member (on Touch and Comfort)

The daughter of a woman with chronic schizophrenia recalls how physical affection remained one of the strongest sparks for her mother. "She didn't always recognize me," the daughter shares, "but if I held her hand, she would calm down immediately." She remembers how hugs, hand squeezes, and simply brushing her mother's hair provided reassurance when words could not. Touch became a bridge—a form of safety and grounding. "Even when her mind was far away," she says, "my mother knew love through touch."

Interview Spotlight – The Sparks That Endure

Anonymous Community Advocate (on Freedom and Autonomy)

A peer advocate who had spent years in and out of institutions describes how freedom itself became his spark. He recalls the first time he was trusted with a set of house keys at a group home. "It wasn't just a key—it meant I was trusted to come and go, to live again." For him, recovery was about more than stability. It was about reclaiming choices, whether deciding what to eat, where to walk, or when to rest. "Freedom," he explains, "is the spark that tells you you're alive, not just surviving."

Appendix I:
Glossary of Terms

- **Serious Mental Illness (SMI):** A mental, behavioral, or emotional disorder that causes serious functional impairment and limits major life activities.
- **Sparks:** Persistent passions, drives, or interests—such as music, food, intimacy, rituals, or creativity—that often endure in mental illness and support identity, motivation, and recovery. *(See also: Money, Music, Food, Sex and Intimacy, Spirituality, Creativity, Movement, Rituals, Nature, Humor, Touch, Storytelling, Hope, Freedom.)*
- **Recovery-Oriented Care:** An approach to treatment that emphasizes personal strengths, hope, self-determination, and inclusion in community life, rather than only symptom reduction. *(See also: Hope, Autonomy, Peer Support.)*
- **Peer Support:** Assistance offered by people who have lived through mental health challenges and recovery, providing empathy, role modeling, and shared understanding. *(See also: Lived Experience.)*
- **Trauma-Informed Care:** A care framework that recognizes the widespread impact of trauma and emphasizes safety, trust, empowerment, and collaboration. *(See also: Rituals, Movement, Grounding.)*
- **Polyvagal Theory:** A model developed by Stephen Porges describing how the vagus nerve regulates stress, safety, and social connection, shaping emotional and physiological responses. *(See also: Movement, Rituals, Touch.)*
- **Person-Centered Care:** Treatment that prioritizes the individual's values, preferences, and goals, tailoring interventions around what matters most to them. *(See also: Autonomy, Recovery-Oriented Care.)*
- **Lived Experience:** The knowledge and insights gained from personally experiencing and recovering from mental illness. *(See also: Peer Support, Storytelling.)*
- **Stigma:** Negative stereotypes, prejudice, or discrimination directed at individuals because of mental illness, often leading to shame and isolation. *(See also: Recovery-Oriented Care, Hope.)*

- **Psychosis:** A condition in which a person loses touch with reality, often involving hallucinations, delusions, or disorganized thinking.
- **Hallucinations:** Sensory experiences (hearing, seeing, smelling, or feeling) that seem real but are not based in external reality, such as hearing voices others cannot hear. *(See also: Music, Storytelling.)*
- **Delusions:** Strongly held false beliefs that are not based in reality and are resistant to contrary evidence (e.g., believing one is being persecuted without proof). *(See also: Money, Spirituality.)*
- **Negative Symptoms:** Features of illnesses like schizophrenia that involve reduced motivation, emotional expression, or social engagement (e.g., flat affect, lack of initiative). *(See also: Creativity, Movement.)*
- **Mania:** A state of elevated or irritable mood with increased energy, decreased need for sleep, impulsivity, or rapid speech, often associated with bipolar disorder. *(See also: Creativity, Freedom.)*
- **Depression:** A state of persistent sadness or loss of interest, often accompanied by fatigue, sleep changes, feelings of worthlessness, and impaired concentration. *(See also: Food, Movement, Hope.)*
- **Conservatorship/Guardianship:** A legal arrangement where another person is given authority to make decisions for someone deemed unable to do so safely on their own. *(See also: Autonomy, Money.)*
- **Cognitive Remediation:** A set of therapeutic strategies aimed at improving attention, memory, problem-solving, and other thinking skills affected by serious mental illness. *(See also: Creativity, Storytelling.)*
- **Resilience:** The ability to adapt, recover, and grow stronger in the face of stress, adversity, or illness. *(See also: Hope, Nature.)*
- **Rituals:** Structured, repeated behaviors (such as prayer, routines, or symbolic acts) that provide comfort, predictability, and meaning. *(See also: Sparks, Trauma-Informed Care.)*
- **Hope:** A belief in the possibility of a better future, even in the midst of difficulty; considered a cornerstone of recovery. *(See also: Sparks, Recovery-Oriented Care.)*
- **Autonomy:** The ability to make choices and exercise independence in daily life and treatment. *(See also: Sparks, Freedom, Recovery-Oriented Care.)*
- **Creative Expression:** The use of art, writing, music, or other outlets to process emotions, communicate, and foster healing. *(See also: Sparks, Music, Storytelling.)*

- **Grounding:** Techniques that connect a person to the present moment—often through nature, sensory experiences, or mindfulness—to reduce anxiety or dissociation. *(See also: Sparks, Nature, Touch.)*
- **Narrative Therapy/Storytelling:** A therapeutic approach that encourages people to share personal or cultural stories as a way of making meaning and reclaiming identity. *(See also: Sparks, Lived Experience.)*
- **Protective Factors:** Conditions or supports (such as strong relationships, coping skills, or access to care) that reduce the impact of illness and promote recovery. *(See also: Resilience, Hope.)*

Appendix J:
Bibliography

Recovery, Lived Experience & Narrative
- Anthony, W. A. (1993). Recovery from mental illness: The guiding vision of the mental health service system in the 1990s. *Psychosocial Rehabilitation Journal, 16*(4), 11–23. https://doi.org/10.1037/h0095655
- Benson, P. L. (2008). *Sparks: How parents can ignite the hidden strengths of teenagers.* Jossey-Bass.
- Charon, R. (2006). *Narrative medicine: Honoring the stories of illness.* Oxford University Press.
- Deegan, P. E. (1988). Recovery: The lived experience of rehabilitation. *Psychosocial Rehabilitation Journal, 11*(4), 11–19. https://doi.org/10.1037/h0099565
- Lysaker, P. H., & Lysaker, J. T. (2008). *Schizophrenia and the fate of the self: A narrative account.* Oxford University Press.
- Slade, M. (2009). *Personal recovery and mental illness: A guide for mental health professionals.* Cambridge University Press.

Culture, Meaning & Global Psychiatry
- American Psychiatric Association. (2013). *Diagnostic and statistical manual of mental disorders* (5th ed.). American Psychiatric Publishing.
- Good, B. J. (1994). *Medicine, rationality and experience: An anthropological perspective.* Cambridge University Press.
- Kleinman, A. (1988). *The illness narratives: Suffering, healing, and the human condition.* Basic Books.
- Lewis-Fernández, R., Aggarwal, N. K., Hinton, L., Hinton, D. E., & Kirmayer, L. J. (2015). DSM-5® Cultural Formulation Interview: Progress, controversies, and future directions. *Transcultural Psychiatry, 53*(4), 397–406. https://doi.org/10.1177/1363461515617289
- Luhrmann, T. M. (2012). *When God talks back: Understanding the American Evangelical relationship with God.* Alfred A. Knopf.

Spirituality, Religion & Mental Health

- Exline, J. J., Pargament, K. I., Grubbs, J. B., & Yali, A. M. (2014). The Religious and Spiritual Struggles Scale: Development and initial validation. *Psychology of Religion and Spirituality, 6*(3), 208–222. https://doi.org/10.1037/a0036465
- Hodge, D. R. (2006). A template for spiritual assessment: A review of the JCAHO requirements and guidelines for implementation. *Social Work, 51*(4), 317–326. https://doi.org/10.1093/sw/51.4.317
- Huguelet, P., & Mohr, S. (2004). Spirituality and meaning in persons with schizophrenia. *Journal of Nervous and Mental Disease, 192*(8), 559–567. https://doi.org/10.1097/01.nmd.0000135573.48204.6c
- Koenig, H. G., King, D. E., & Carson, V. B. (2012). *Handbook of religion and health* (2nd ed.). Oxford University Press.
- Koenig, H. G. (2009). Research on religion, spirituality, and mental health: A review. *Canadian Journal of Psychiatry, 54*(5), 283–291. https://doi.org/10.1177/070674370905400502
- Pargament, K. I. (2007). *Spiritually integrated psychotherapy: Understanding and addressing the sacred.* Guilford Press.

Trauma, Catatonia & Neurobiology

- Felitti, V. J., Anda, R. F., Nordenberg, D., et al. (1998). Relationship of childhood abuse and household dysfunction to many of the leading causes of death in adults: The ACE Study. *American Journal of Preventive Medicine, 14*(4), 245–258. https://doi.org/10.1016/S0749-3797(98)00017-8
- Fink, M., & Taylor, M. A. (2003). *Catatonia: A clinician's guide to diagnosis and treatment.* Cambridge University Press.
- Northoff, G. (2002). What catatonia can tell us about "top-down modulation": A neuropsychiatric hypothesis. *Behavioral and Brain Sciences, 25*(5), 555–577. https://doi.org/10.1017/S0140525X02000104
- Porges, S. W. (2011). *The polyvagal theory: Neurophysiological foundations of emotions, attachment, communication, and self-regulation.* W. W. Norton.
- van der Kolk, B. A. (2014). *The body keeps the score: Brain, mind, and body in the healing of trauma.* Viking.

Creativity, Art & Music

- Beaty, R. E., Benedek, M., Silvia, P. J., & Schacter, D. L. (2016). Creative cognition and brain network dynamics. *Trends in Cognitive Sciences, 20*(2), 87–95. https://doi.org/10.1016/j.tics.2015.10.004

- Bradt, J., & Dileo, C. (2017). Music interventions for improving psychological and physical outcomes in cancer patients. *Cochrane Database of Systematic Reviews, 2017*(10), CD006911. https://doi.org/10.1002/14651858.CD006911.pub3 *(use as a high-quality exemplar of music therapy evidence; for schizophrenia see Geretsegger et al., 2014)*
- Crawford, M. J., Killaspy, H., Barnes, T. R. E., et al. (2012). Group art therapy as an adjunctive treatment for people with schizophrenia: Multicentre pragmatic RCT (MATISSE). *BMJ, 344*, e846. https://doi.org/10.1136/bmj.e846
- Dietrich, A. (2004). The cognitive neuroscience of creativity. *Psychonomic Bulletin & Review, 11*(6), 1011–1026. https://doi.org/10.3758/BF03196731
- Geretsegger, M., Elefant, C., Mössler, K. A., & Gold, C. (2014). Music therapy for people with schizophrenia and schizophrenia-like disorders. *Cochrane Database of Systematic Reviews, 2014*(6), CD004025. https://doi.org/10.1002/14651858.CD004025.pub4
- Jamison, K. R. (1993). *Touched with fire: Manic-depressive illness and the artistic temperament.* Free Press.
- Kinney, D. K., Richards, R., Lowing, P. A., LeBlanc, D., Zimbalist, M. E., & Harlan, P. (2001). Creativity in offspring of schizophrenic and bipolar disorder probands. *American Journal of Psychiatry, 158*(8), 1288–1292. https://doi.org/10.1176/appi.ajp.158.8.1288
- Stuckey, H. L., & Nobel, J. (2010). The connection between art, healing, and public health: A review of current literature. *American Journal of Public Health, 100*(2), 254–263. https://doi.org/10.2105/AJPH.2008.156497

Movement, Exercise & Embodiment

- Rizzolatti, G., & Craighero, L. (2004). The mirror-neuron system. *Annual Review of Neuroscience, 27*, 169–192. https://doi.org/10.1146/annurev.neuro.27.070203.144230
- Vancampfort, D., Knapen, J., Probst, M., et al. (2012). Physical activity and sedentary behaviour in people with severe mental illness: A systematic review and meta-analysis. *General Hospital Psychiatry, 34*(6), 599–611. https://doi.org/10.1016/j.genhosppsych.2012.06.013

Nature, Environment & Ecotherapy

- Antonelli, M., Barbieri, G., & Donelli, D. (2019). Effects of forest bathing (shinrin-yoku) on levels of cortisol as a stress biomarker: A systematic review and meta-analysis. *International Journal*

- *of Biometeorology, 63*(8), 1117–1134. https://doi.org/10.1007/s00484-019-01717-x
- Bratman, G. N., Hamilton, J. P., Hahn, K. S., Daily, G. C., & Gross, J. J. (2015). Nature experience reduces rumination and subgenual prefrontal cortex activation. *Proceedings of the National Academy of Sciences, 112*(28), 8567–8572. https://doi.org/10.1073/pnas.1510459112
- Bratman, G. N., Anderson, C. B., Berman, M. G., Cochran, B., de Vries, S., et al. (2019). Nature and mental health: An ecosystem service perspective. *Science Advances, 5*(7), eaax0903. https://doi.org/10.1126/sciadv.aax0903
- Kaplan, R., & Kaplan, S. (1989). *The experience of nature: A psychological perspective.* Cambridge University Press.
- Park, B.-J., Tsunetsugu, Y., Kasetani, T., et al. (2010). The physiological effects of Shinrin-yoku (taking in the forest atmosphere): Evidence from field experiments in 24 forests across Japan. *Environmental Health and Preventive Medicine, 15*(1), 18–26. https://doi.org/10.1007/s12199-009-0086-9
- Song, C., Ikei, H., & Miyazaki, Y. (2016). Physiological effects of nature therapy: A review of the research in Japan. *International Journal of Environmental Research and Public Health, 13*(8), 781. https://doi.org/10.3390/ijerph13080781

Humor & Play

- Gelkopf, M., Gonen, B., Kurs, R., Melamed, Y., & Bleich, A. (2006). The use of humor in serious mental illness: A review. *Evidence-Based Complementary and Alternative Medicine, 3*(2), 191–198. https://doi.org/10.1093/ecam/nel014
- Martin, R. A., Puhlik-Doris, P., Larsen, G., Gray, J., & Weir, K. (2003). Individual differences in uses of humor and their relation to psychological well-being: Development of the Humor Styles Questionnaire. *Journal of Research in Personality, 37*(1), 48–75. https://doi.org/10.1016/S0092-6566(02)00534-2

Touch, Sensory Regulation & Co-Regulation

- Field, T. (2010). Touch for socioemotional and physical well-being: A review. *Developmental Review, 30*(4), 367–383. https://doi.org/10.1016/j.dr.2011.01.001
- Gringras, P., Green, D., Wright, B., et al. (2014). Weighted blankets and sleep in autistic children—A randomized controlled trial. *Pediatrics, 134*(2), 298–306. https://doi.org/10.1542/peds.2013-4285

Meaning, Hope, Motivation & Agency

- Frankl, V. E. (2006). *Man's search for meaning.* Beacon Press. (Original work published 1946)
- Miller, W. R., & Rollnick, S. (2013). *Motivational interviewing: Helping people change* (3rd ed.). Guilford Press.
- Seligman, M. E. P. (1992). *Learned optimism.* Knopf.
- Snyder, C. R. (2002). Hope theory: Rainbows in the mind. *Psychological Inquiry, 13*(4), 249–275. https://doi.org/10.1207/S15327965PLI1304_01

Early Intervention, Psychosocial Treatments & Systems of Care

- Bond, G. R., Drake, R. E., & Becker, D. R. (2012). Generalizability of the Individual Placement and Support (IPS) model of supported employment outside the US. *World Psychiatry, 11*(1), 32–39. https://doi.org/10.1016/j.wpsyc.2012.01.005
- Copeland, M. E. (2002). *Wellness Recovery Action Plan.* Peach Press.
- Drake, R. E., & Bond, G. R. (2011). *Individual placement and support: An evidence-based approach to supported employment.* Oxford University Press.
- McFarlane, W. R. (2002). *Multiple family groups in the treatment of severe psychiatric disorders.* Guilford Press.
- McGorry, P. D., Killackey, E., & Yung, A. (2008). Early intervention in psychosis: Concepts, evidence and future directions. *World Psychiatry, 7*(3), 148–156. https://doi.org/10.1002/j.2051-5545.2008.tb00182.x
- Morrison, A. P. (2004). *Cognitive therapy for psychosis: A formulation-based approach.* Brunner-Routledge.
- Wykes, T., Huddy, V., Cellard, C., McGurk, S. R., & Czobor, P. (2011). A meta-analysis of cognitive remediation for schizophrenia: Methodology and effect sizes. *American Journal of Psychiatry, 168*(5), 472–485. https://doi.org/10.1176/appi.ajp.2010.10060855

Mindfulness, Behavioral Activation & Self-Regulation

- Brewer, J. A., Worhunsky, P. D., Gray, J. R., et al. (2011). Meditation experience is associated with differences in default mode network activity and connectivity. *Proceedings of the National Academy of Sciences, 108*(50), 20254–20259. https://doi.org/10.1073/pnas.1112029108
- Goyal, M., Singh, S., Sibinga, E. M. S., et al. (2014). Meditation programs for psychological stress and well-being: A systematic

review and meta-analysis. *JAMA Internal Medicine, 174*(3), 357–368. https://doi.org/10.1001/jamainternmed.2013.13018
- Kabat-Zinn, J. (1990). *Full catastrophe living.* Delacorte.
- Martell, C. R., Dimidjian, S., & Herman-Dunn, R. (2010). *Behavioral activation for depression: A clinician's guide.* Guilford Press.
- Zeidan, F., Johnson, S. K., Diamond, B. J., David, Z., & Goolkasian, P. (2010). Mindfulness meditation improves cognition: Evidence of brief mental training. *Consciousness and Cognition, 19*(2), 597–605. https://doi.org/10.1016/j.concog.2010.03.014

Reward, Negative Symptoms & Brain Networks

- Damasio, A. R. (1999). *The feeling of what happens: Body and emotion in the making of consciousness.* Harcourt Brace.
- Hamilton, J. P., Farmer, M., Fogelman, P., & Gotlib, I. H. (2015). Depressive rumination, the default-mode network, and the dark matter of clinical neuroscience. *Biological Psychiatry, 78*(4), 224–230. https://doi.org/10.1016/j.biopsych.2015.02.020
- Juckel, G., Schlagenhauf, F., Koslowski, M., et al. (2006). Dysfunction of ventral striatal reward prediction in schizophrenia. *NeuroImage, 29*(2), 409–416. https://doi.org/10.1016/j.neuroimage.2005.07.051
- McGilchrist, I. (2009). *The master and his emissary: The divided brain and the making of the Western world.* Yale University Press.

Neuromodulation, VR & Digital Health

- Firth, J., Torous, J., Nicholas, J., Carney, R., Pratap, A., Rosenbaum, S., & Sarris, J. (2017). The efficacy of smartphone-based mental health interventions for depressive symptoms: A meta-analysis of randomized controlled trials. *World Psychiatry, 16*(3), 287–298. https://doi.org/10.1002/wps.20472
- Freeman, D., Reeve, S., Robinson, A., et al. (2017). Virtual reality in the assessment, understanding, and treatment of mental health disorders. *Psychological Medicine, 47*(14), 2393–2400. https://doi.org/10.1017/S003329171700040X
- Nitsche, M. A., & Paulus, W. (2000). Excitability changes induced in the human motor cortex by weak transcranial direct current stimulation. *The Journal of Physiology, 527*(3), 633–639. https://doi.org/10.1111/j.1469-7793.2000.t01-1-00633.x
- O'Reardon, J. P., Solvason, H. B., Janicak, P. G., et al. (2007). Efficacy and safety of transcranial magnetic stimulation in the acute treatment of major depression. *Biological Psychiatry, 62*(11), 1208–1216. https://doi.org/10.1016/j.biopsych.2007.01.018

- Torous, J., & Roberts, L. W. (2017). Needed innovation in digital health and smartphone applications for mental health: Transparency and trust. *JAMA Psychiatry, 74*(5), 437–438. https://doi.org/10.1001/jamapsychiatry.2017.0262

Housing, Employment & Social Determinants

- Repper, J., & Carter, T. (2011). A review of the literature on peer support in mental health services. *Journal of Mental Health, 20*(4), 392–411. https://doi.org/10.3109/09638237.2011.583947
- Soga, M., Gaston, K. J., & Yamaura, Y. (2017). Gardening is beneficial for health: A meta-analysis. *Preventive Medicine Reports, 5*, 92–99. https://doi.org/10.1016/j.pmedr.2016.11.007
- Tsemberis, S. (2010). *Housing First: The Pathways model to end homelessness for people with mental illness and addiction.* Hazelden.

History, Biography & Exemplars (Madness & Brilliance)

- Dickinson, E. (1998). *The poems of Emily Dickinson* (R. W. Franklin, Ed.). Belknap Press of Harvard University Press.
- Kempe, M. (2004). *The book of Margery Kempe* (A. Bale, Ed.). Oxford University Press.
- Nasar, S. (1998). *A beautiful mind.* Simon & Schuster.
- Nijinsky, V. (1999). *The diary of Vaslav Nijinsky* (J. Acocella, Ed.; K. Everett, Trans.). Farrar, Straus and Giroux.
- Plath, S. (2004). *Ariel: The restored edition.* HarperCollins.
- van Gogh, V. (2009). *The letters of Vincent van Gogh* (R. Pickvance, Ed.). Penguin Classics.
- Woolf, V. (2008). *A writer's diary* (L. Woolf, Ed.). Mariner Books. *(Original work published 1953)*
- Woolf, V. (2005). *Mrs Dalloway.* Harcourt. *(Original work published 1925; for literary context)*

Appendix K:
Index

A

- Acceptance — role in recovery, pp. 241–244
- Adverse Childhood Experiences (ACE) — trauma and long-term impact, pp. 28–33
- Agency — personal choice, autonomy, pp. 244–249
- Art Therapy — creativity, emotional expression, pp. 178–184
- Autonomy — decision-making, patient choice (see also Freedom), pp. 244–249

B

- Boundaries, Personal — sexuality, intimacy, consent, pp. 62–68
- Budgeting — financial literacy, supported employment (see also Money), pp. 94–98

C

- Caregivers — support strategies, pp. 403–404
- Case Vignettes — examples of sparks, pp. 67, 121, 182
- Cognitive Remediation — improving attention, memory, problem-solving, pp. 128–130
- Creativity — art, writing, and expression, pp. 175–184

D

- Delusions — money, spirituality, psychosis, pp. 88–92, 231–234
- Depression — loss of interest in sparks, pp. 35–38, 213–215

E

- Empowerment — recovery-oriented care, pp. 236–240
- Exploitation, financial/sexual — risks in SMI, pp. 98–102, 215–216

F

- Food — nourishment, cultural meals, rituals, pp. 107–115
- Freedom — autonomy, conservatorship, patient choice, pp. 244–249

H

- Hallucinations — auditory, visual, and sensory, pp. 224–227
- Hope — cornerstone of recovery, pp. 257–262
- Humor — playfulness, group engagement, pp. 198–203

I

- Identity — role of sparks in sustaining self, pp. 30–34, 165–167
- Intimacy — sexuality, relationships, trust, pp. 59–70

L

- Lived Experience — peer support, recovery narratives, pp. 323–329

M

- Mania — creativity, impulsivity, pp. 179–181
- Medication — side effects on sexuality, food, weight, pp. 75–77, 114–115
- Money — financial independence, exploitation, symbolic meaning, pp. 85–102
- Movement — exercise, dance, yoga, pp. 188–192

N

- Nature — grounding, gardening, connection, pp. 193–197
- Negative Symptoms — loss of motivation, affect, pp. 33–35, 228–230

P

- Peer Support — role in recovery, pp. 323–329
- Person-Centered Care — values-driven treatment, pp. 332–339
- Polyvagal Theory — safety, vagus nerve, regulation, pp. 341–344
- Psychosis — delusions, hallucinations, disorganization, pp. 221–228

R

- Recovery — definition, recovery-oriented care, pp. 235–241
- Resilience — adaptation, strength, pp. 212–216, 259
- Rituals — structure, trauma recovery, pp. 193–197, 205–209

Appendix L:
Endnotes

Supporting Notes

Spark 2: Sex
- Deegan, P. E. (1988). Recovery: The lived experience of rehabilitation. *Psychosocial Rehabilitation Journal, 11*(4), 11–19. https://doi.org/10.1037/h0099565
- McCann, E. (2010). Investigating mental health service user views of sexual and relationship issues. *Journal of Psychiatric and Mental Health Nursing, 17*(3), 251–259. https://doi.org/10.1111/j.1365-2850.2009.01524.x

Spark 3: Money
- Rosen, M. I., & Rosenheck, R. A. (2012). Managing money in supported housing: A manual for mental health practitioners. Yale University Program for Recovery and Community Health.
- Lysaker, P. H., & Buck, K. D. (2008). Addressing financial issues in recovery from serious mental illness. *Psychiatric Rehabilitation Journal, 32*(1), 71–74. https://doi.org/10.2975/32.1.2008.71.74

Spark 4: Food
- Fawzi, W. W., & Rich-Edwards, J. W. (2004). Malnutrition and mental illness. *Lancet, 364*(9449), 2106–2107. https://doi.org/10.1016/S0140-6736(04)17662-0
- Davison, K. M., & Kaplan, B. J. (2012). Food intake and mental health in community-dwelling adults. *Canadian Journal of Psychiatry, 57*(2), 85–92. https://doi.org/10.1177/070674371205700205

Spark 5: Music
- Aldridge, D. (1996). *Music therapy research and practice in medicine: From out of the silence.* Jessica Kingsley Publishers.
- Gold, C., Mössler, K., Grocke, D., Heldal, T. O., Tjemsland, L., et al. (2009). Individual music therapy for mental health care clients with low therapy motivation: Multicentre randomised controlled

trial. *Psychotherapy and Psychosomatics, 78*(5), 319–327. https://doi.org/10.1159/000229768

Spark 6: Spirituality

- Koenig, H. G. (2009). Research on religion, spirituality, and mental health: A review. *Canadian Journal of Psychiatry, 54*(5), 283–291. https://doi.org/10.1177/070674370905400502
- Pargament, K. I. (2007). *Spiritually integrated psychotherapy: Understanding and addressing the sacred.* Guilford Press.

Spark 7: Creativity

- McGilchrist, I. (2009). *The master and his emissary: The divided brain and the making of the Western world.* Yale University Press.
- Forgeard, M. J. C., & Elstein, J. G. (2014). Creative thinking in mental illness: A review. *Psychology of Aesthetics, Creativity, and the Arts, 8*(2), 113–127. https://doi.org/10.1037/a0036480

Spark 8: Movement

- Callaghan, P. (2004). Exercise: A neglected intervention in mental health care? *Journal of Psychiatric and Mental Health Nursing, 11*(4), 476–483. https://doi.org/10.1111/j.1365-2850.2004.00751.x
- Vancampfort, D., Probst, M., Helvik Skjaerven, L., Catalán-Matamoros, D., Lundvik-Gyllensten, A., Gómez-Conesa, A., & De Hert, M. (2012). Systematic review of physical therapy interventions for patients with schizophrenia. *Physical Therapy, 92*(1), 11–23. https://doi.org/10.2522/ptj.20100231

Spark 9: Rituals

- Porges, S. W. (2011). *The polyvagal theory: Neurophysiological foundations of emotions, attachment, communication, and self-regulation.* W. W. Norton.
- Hobson, N. M., Schroeder, J., Risen, J. L., Xygalatas, D., & Inzlicht, M. (2018). The psychology of rituals: An integrative review and process-based framework. *Personality and Social Psychology Review, 22*(3), 260–284. https://doi.org/10.1177/1088868317734944

Spark 10: Nature

- Bratman, G. N., Anderson, C. B., Berman, M. G., Cochran, B., de Vries, S., et al. (2019). Nature and mental health: An ecosystem service perspective. *Science Advances, 5*(7), eaax0903. https://doi.org/10.1126/sciadv.aax0903
- Berman, M. G., Jonides, J., & Kaplan, S. (2008). The cognitive benefits of interacting with nature. *Psychological Science, 19*(12), 1207–1212. https://doi.org/10.1111/j.1467-9280.2008.02225.x

Spark 11: Humor
- Klein, A., & Kuiper, N. A. (2006). Humor styles, peer relationships, and bullying in middle childhood. *Humor, 19*(4), 383–404. https://doi.org/10.1515/HUMOR.2006.019
- Martin, R. A. (2007). *The psychology of humor: An integrative approach.* Elsevier Academic Press.

Spark 12: Touch
- Field, T. (2010). Touch for socioemotional and physical well-being: A review. *Developmental Review, 30*(4), 367–383. https://doi.org/10.1016/j.dr.2011.01.001
- Hertenstein, M. J., Verkamp, J. M., Kerestes, A. M., & Holmes, R. M. (2006). The communicative functions of touch in humans. *Developmental Review, 26*(2), 69–88. https://doi.org/10.1016/j.dr.2005.09.001

Spark 13: Storytelling
- Charon, R. (2006). *Narrative medicine: Honoring the stories of illness.* Oxford University Press.
- Lysaker, P. H., & Lysaker, J. T. (2008). *Schizophrenia and the fate of the self: A narrative account.* Oxford University Press.

Spark 14: Hope
- Snyder, C. R. (2002). Hope theory: Rainbows in the mind. *Psychological Inquiry, 13*(4), 249–275. https://doi.org/10.1207/S15327965PLI1304_01
- Schrank, B., Stanghellini, G., & Slade, M. (2008). Hope in psychiatry: A review of the literature. *Acta Psychiatrica Scandinavica, 118*(6), 421–433. https://doi.org/10.1111/j.1600-0447.2008.01271.x

Spark 15: Freedom
- Deci, E. L., & Ryan, R. M. (2000). The "what" and "why" of goal pursuits: Human needs and the self-determination of behavior. *Psychological Inquiry, 11*(4), 227–268. https://doi.org/10.1207/S15327965PLI1104_01
- Davidson, L., O'Connell, M. J., Tondora, J., Styron, T., & Kangas, K. (2006). The top ten concerns about recovery encountered in mental health system transformation. *Psychiatric Services, 57*(5), 640–645. https://doi.org/10.1176/ps.2006.57.5.640

Appendix M
Peer-Reviewed Articles

Core Psychiatry & Recovery

- Anthony, W. A. (1993). Recovery from mental illness: The guiding vision of the mental health service system in the 1990s. *Psychosocial Rehabilitation Journal, 16*(4), 11–23.
- Deegan, P. E. (1988). Recovery: The lived experience of rehabilitation. *Psychosocial Rehabilitation Journal, 11*(4), 11–19.
- Insel, T. R. (2010). Rethinking schizophrenia. *Nature, 468*(7321), 187–193.
- Keshavan, M. S., Nasrallah, H. A., & Tandon, R. (2008). Schizophrenia, "Just the facts": What we know in 2008. *Schizophrenia Research, 100*(1–3), 4–19.
- Davidson, L., O'Connell, M., Tondora, J., Styron, T., & Kangas, K. (2005). Recovery in serious mental illness: A new wine or just a new bottle? *Professional Psychology: Research and Practice, 36*(5), 480–487.
- Farkas, M. (2007). The vision of recovery today: What it is and what it means for services. *World Psychiatry, 6*(2), 68–74.
- Leamy, M., Bird, V., Le Boutillier, C., Williams, J., & Slade, M. (2011). Conceptual framework for personal recovery in mental health: Systematic review and narrative synthesis. *The British Journal of Psychiatry, 199*(6), 445–452.

Sparks in Psychiatry

- Sex/Intimacy
  - McCann, E. (2010). Investigating mental health service user views regarding sexual and relationship issues. *Journal of Psychiatric and Mental Health Nursing, 17*(3), 251–259.
  - Quinn, C., & Happell, B. (2012). Talking about sex: Exploring the views of consumers living with mental illness. *International Journal of Mental Health Nursing, 21*(1), 21–29.
- Money/Security

- Lund, C., et al. (2011). Poverty and mental disorders: Breaking the cycle in low-income and middle-income countries. *The Lancet, 378*(9801), 1502–1514.
- Rosenheck, R., Leslie, D., Keefe, R., McEvoy, J., Swartz, M., Perkins, D., ... & Lieberman, J. (2006). Barriers to employment for people with schizophrenia. *American Journal of Psychiatry, 163*(3), 411–417.

- Food/Nourishment
  - Jacka, F. N., et al. (2017). A randomised controlled trial of dietary improvement for adults with major depression (the "SMILES" trial). *BMC Medicine, 15*(1), 23.
  - Rahe, C., Unrath, M., & Berger, K. (2014). Dietary patterns and the risk of depression in adults: A systematic review of observational studies. *European Journal of Nutrition, 53*(4), 997–1013.
- Music/Resonance
  - Aldridge, D. (1996). *Music therapy research and practice in medicine: From out of the silence.* Jessica Kingsley Publishers.
  - Gold, C., Solli, H. P., Krüger, V., & Lie, S. A. (2009). Dose–response relationship in music therapy for people with serious mental disorders: Systematic review and meta-analysis. *Clinical Psychology Review, 29*(3), 193–207.
- Spirituality/Meaning
  - Koenig, H. G. (2009). Research on religion, spirituality, and mental health: A review. *Canadian Journal of Psychiatry, 54*(5), 283–291.
  - Mohr, S., Brandt, P. Y., Borras, L., Gillieron, C., & Huguelet, P. (2006). Toward an integration of spirituality and religiousness into the psychosocial dimension of schizophrenia. *American Journal of Psychiatry, 163*(11), 1952–1959.
- Creativity/Expression
  - Johnson, J. (2008). The therapeutic role of creative arts in mental health recovery: A systematic review. *Journal of Psychiatric and Mental Health Nursing, 15*(8), 725–736.
  - Kaimal, G., Ray, K., & Muniz, J. (2016). Reduction of cortisol levels and participants' responses following art making. *Art Therapy, 33*(2), 74–80.
- Movement/Embodiment
  - Stanton, R., & Reaburn, P. (2014). Exercise and the treatment of depression: A review of reviews. *Journal of Science and Medicine in Sport, 17*(2), 177–182.

- Sharma, A., Madaan, V., & Petty, F. D. (2006). Exercise for mental health. *Primary Care Companion to the Journal of Clinical Psychiatry, 8*(2), 106.
- Rituals/Structure
  - Schneider, F. (2024). Symbol, ritual, and the psychotic process. *International Journal of Social Psychiatry, 70*(1), 15–25.
  - Hobson, N. M., Schroeder, J., Risen, J. L., Xygalatas, D., & Inzlicht, M. (2018). The psychology of rituals: An integrative review and process-based framework. *Personality and Social Psychology Review, 22*(3), 260–284.
- Nature/Grounding
  - Kaplan, S. (1995). The restorative benefits of nature: Toward an integrative framework. *Journal of Environmental Psychology, 15*(3), 169–182.
  - Bratman, G. N., Hamilton, J. P., Hahn, K. S., Daily, G. C., & Gross, J. J. (2015). Nature experience reduces rumination and subgenual prefrontal cortex activation. *PNAS, 112*(28), 8567–8572.
- Humor/Playfulness
  - Mobbs, D., Greicius, M. D., Abdel-Aziz, H., Menon, V., & Reiss, A. L. (2003). Humor modulates the mesolimbic reward centers. *Neuron, 40*(5), 1041–1048.
  - Wilkins, J. F., & Eisenbraun, A. J. (2023). Laughter and the brain: Dopamine, stress buffering, and social bonding. *Neuropsychology Review, 33*(2), 137–154.
- Touch/Sensation
  - Field, T. (2010). Touch for socioemotional and physical well-being: A review. *Developmental Review, 30*(4), 367–383.
  - Cascio, C. J., Moore, D., & McGlone, F. (2019). Social touch and human development. *Developmental Cognitive Neuroscience, 35*, 5–11.
- Storytelling/Meaning-Making
  - White, M., & Epston, D. (1990). *Narrative means to therapeutic ends*. Norton.
  - Lysaker, P. H., & Buck, K. D. (2007). Narrative enhancement and cognitive therapy: A new approach to addressing metacognitive deficits and promoting recovery in schizophrenia. *Journal of Clinical Psychology, 63*(2), 166–178.
- Hope/Possibility
  - Slade, M. (2009). *Personal recovery and mental illness: A guide for mental health professionals*. Cambridge University Press.

- o Schrank, B., & Slade, M. (2007). Recovery in psychiatry. *Psychiatric Bulletin, 31*(9), 321–325.
- Freedom/Autonomy
  - o Priebe, S., & McCabe, R. (2008). Therapeutic relationships in psychiatry: The basis of autonomy and recovery. *Psychotherapy and Psychosomatics, 77*(4), 241–249.
  - o O'Donnell, M., et al. (2003). Patient autonomy and choice in mental health services: A review of the literature. *Psychiatric Services, 54*(9), 1181–1185.

Further Reading for Clinicians and Caregivers

- Copeland, M. E. (2001). *The Depression Workbook: A guide for living with depression and manic depression.* New Harbinger Publications.
- Goodwin, F. K., & Jamison, K. R. (2007). *Manic-Depressive Illness: Bipolar Disorders and Recurrent Depression.* Oxford University Press.
- Repper, J., & Carter, T. (2011). A review of the literature on peer support in mental health services. *Journal of Mental Health, 20*(4), 392–411.
- Herman, J. L. (1992). *Trauma and recovery: The aftermath of violence.* Basic Books.
- van der Kolk, B. (2014). *The body keeps the score: Brain, mind, and body in the healing of trauma.* Viking.
- Frankl, V. E. (1959). *Man's search for meaning.* Beacon Press.
- Jamison, K. R. (1995). *An unquiet mind: A memoir of moods and madness.* Knopf.
- Deegan, P. (1997). *Recovery as a journey of the heart.* Psychiatric Rehabilitation Journal, 19(3), 91–97.
- NAMI (National Alliance on Mental Illness). (2023). Family guide to mental health recovery. www.nami.org.

Appendix N:
Online Resources by Spark

General Mental Health & Recovery
- National Alliance on Mental Illness (NAMI): https://www.nami.org
- Mental Health America (MHA): https://www.mhanational.org
- Substance Abuse and Mental Health Services Administration (SAMHSA): https://www.samhsa.gov
- National Institute of Mental Health (NIMH): https://www.nimh.nih.gov

1. Sex & Intimacy
- American Association of Sexuality Educators, Counselors, and Therapists (AASECT): https://www.aasect.org

2. Money & Security
- Consumer Financial Protection Bureau (Financial Wellness Resources): https://www.consumerfinance.gov
- National Disability Institute (Financial Wellness and Disability Resources): https://www.nationaldisabilityinstitute.org

3. Food & Nourishment
- National Eating Disorders Association (NEDA): https://www.nationaleatingdisorders.org
- Academy of Nutrition and Dietetics (Eat Right): https://www.eatright.org

4. Music & Resonance
- American Music Therapy Association (AMTA): https://www.musictherapy.org

5. Spirituality & Meaning
- Association for Clinical Pastoral Education (ACPE): https://www.acpe.edu
- Faith Communities and Mental Health Resources (NAMI): https://www.nami.org/faithnet

6. Creativity & Expression
- National Coalition of Creative Arts Therapies Associations (NCCATA): https://www.nccata.org

7. Movement & Embodiment
- National Center on Health, Physical Activity, and Disability (NCHPAD): https://www.nchpad.org

8. Rituals & Structure
- ACPE (also listed under Spirituality): https://www.acpe.edu
- Daily structure tools: SAMHSA Wellness Planning: https://store.samhsa.gov/product/Creating-a-Healthier-Life-A-Step-by-Step-Guide/PEP12-VIPPPTX

9. Nature & Grounding
- Association of Nature and Forest Therapy Guides: https://www.natureandforesttherapy.earth
- Children & Nature Network: https://www.childrenandnature.org

10. Humor & Playfulness
- Association for Applied and Therapeutic Humor (AATH): https://www.aath.org

11. Touch & Sensation
- STAR Institute for Sensory Processing: https://www.spdstar.org

12. Storytelling & Meaning-Making
- National Storytelling Network: https://storynet.org
- Narrative Therapy Centre (Toronto): https://www.narrativetherapy-centre.com

13. Hope & Possibility
- Depression and Bipolar Support Alliance (DBSA): https://www.dbsalliance.org
- Schizophrenia and Related Disorders Alliance of America (SARDAA): https://www.sardaa.org

14. Freedom & Autonomy
- Center for Excellence in Supported Decision Making: https://www.cesdm.org
- Bazelon Center for Mental Health Law: https://www.bazelon.org

Crisis & Peer Support
- 988 Suicide & Crisis Lifeline (U.S.): Dial or text **988** (24/7)
- Veterans Crisis Line: Dial **988**, then press 1
- Crisis Text Line: Text **HOME** to 741741 (24/7)
- Hearing Voices Network USA: https://www.hearingvoicesusa.org

Appendix O:
The Fourteen Sparks Assessment Tool

Introduction

Throughout this book, we have explored the enduring sparks—the core human drives that often survive and persist even in the presence of serious mental illness. These sparks include: sex, money, food, music, spirituality, creativity, movement, rituals, nature, humor, touch, storytelling, hope, and freedom.

The **Fourteen Sparks Assessment Tool** is designed to help clinicians, caregivers, and patients collaboratively explore and engage these sparks in everyday psychiatric care. It offers a structured yet flexible way to understand what still matters, what still brings meaning, and how to build from those points of light.

Purpose

This assessment is not diagnostic. It is a **relational guide**—a conversation starter, a bridge between symptom-focused care and person-centered engagement.

In clinical settings, it can:
- Guide intake and recovery planning
- Uncover protective factors or hidden motivators
- Create language around meaning and values
- Provide a way to track engagement over time

It can be adapted for inpatients, outpatients, peer specialists, and family members alike.

How to Use the Tool

Each spark is presented as a short section with:
- **Exploratory Questions** (to prompt conversation)
- **Observational Cues** (what to notice in behavior/affect)
- **Rating Scale (0–5)** (patient/clinician rating of spark strength)
- **Personal Goal Prompt** (small next step)
- **Notes Space** (for quotes, observations, or plans)

The tool can be completed over one or several sessions and revisited periodically to track change and recovery.

Sparks Assessment Worksheet

1. Sex and Intimacy
- **Exploratory Question:** "What does closeness mean to you right now?"
- **Observational Cues:** Comfort/discomfort when discussing intimacy, references to trust or relationships.
- **Rating (0–5):** ____
- **Personal Goal Prompt:** "One step I'd like to take toward intimacy is…"
- **Notes:** _____

2. Money and Security
- **Exploratory Question:** "What role does money play in your sense of control or independence?"
- **Observational Cues:** Talk of independence, exploitation, anxiety, budgeting struggles.
- **Rating (0–5):** ____
- **Personal Goal Prompt:** "One small way I'd like to feel more secure is…"
- **Notes:** _____

3. Food and Nourishment
- **Exploratory Question:** "Are there foods or meals that bring you comfort or memories?"
- **Observational Cues:** Appetite, meal rituals, cultural foods, relationship with eating.
- **Rating (0–5):** ____
- **Personal Goal Prompt:** "One meal or food ritual I'd like to bring back is…"
- **Notes:** _____

4. Music and Resonance
- **Exploratory Question:** "Is there a song or type of music that helps shift your mood?"
- **Observational Cues:** Engagement when talking about music, tapping, humming, or recalling favorites.
- **Rating (0–5):** ____
- **Personal Goal Prompt:** "A piece of music I'd like to use for healing is…"
- **Notes:** _____

5. **Spirituality and Belief**
   - **Exploratory Question:** "Where do you find comfort or strength when things are hard?"
   - **Observational Cues:** References to prayer, rituals, values, or faith community.
   - **Rating (0–5):** _____
   - **Personal Goal Prompt:** "A spiritual practice I'd like to explore is…"
   - **Notes:** _____

6. **Creativity and Expression**
   - **Exploratory Question:** "Have you ever enjoyed making, writing, or imagining something?"
   - **Observational Cues:** References to past hobbies, current interests, openness to art/creative activities.
   - **Rating (0–5):** _____
   - **Personal Goal Prompt:** "One way I'd like to express myself creatively is…"
   - **Notes:** _____

7. **Movement and the Body**
   - **Exploratory Question:** "How do you feel when your body is active or still?"
   - **Observational Cues:** Posture, energy, enthusiasm about walking, dancing, stretching.
   - **Rating (0–5):** _____
   - **Personal Goal Prompt:** "One movement activity I'd like to try is…"
   - **Notes:** _____

8. **Rituals and Structure**
   - **Exploratory Question:** "Are there routines or habits that help you feel grounded?"
   - **Observational Cues:** Daily habits, organization, bedtime rituals, comfort from repetition.
   - **Rating (0–5):** _____
   - **Personal Goal Prompt:** "One ritual or routine I'd like to add is…"
   - **Notes:** _____

9. **Nature and Grounding**
   - **Exploratory Question:** "What role does the outdoors or nature play in your life?"
   - **Observational Cues:** Interest in walking, gardening, or outdoor spaces; calming effect.
   - **Rating (0–5):** _____

- **Personal Goal Prompt:** "One way I'd like to spend more time in nature is…"
- **Notes:** _____

10. Humor and Playfulness
- **Exploratory Question:** "When was the last time you really laughed?"
- **Observational Cues:** Smile, laughter, enjoyment in playful recall.
- **Rating (0–5):** _____
- **Personal Goal Prompt:** "One way I'd like to bring more humor into my life is…"
- **Notes:** _____

11. Touch and Sensation
- **Exploratory Question:** "What kinds of touch or sensory experiences feel safe and comforting?"
- **Observational Cues:** Comfort with weighted blankets, hugs, textures, or sensory tools.
- **Rating (0–5):** _____
- **Personal Goal Prompt:** "One sensory experience that soothes me is…"
- **Notes:** _____

12. Storytelling and Meaning-Making
- **Exploratory Question:** "Are there personal or cultural stories that help explain who you are?"
- **Observational Cues:** Ability to share life narrative, cultural continuity, coherence in story.
- **Rating (0–5):** _____
- **Personal Goal Prompt:** "A story I want to tell or pass on is…"
- **Notes:** _____

13. Hope and Possibility
- **Exploratory Question:** "What are you looking forward to, even in small ways?"
- **Observational Cues:** Future orientation, optimism, connection to goals.
- **Rating (0–5):** _____
- **Personal Goal Prompt:** "Something I feel hopeful about is…"
- **Notes:** _____

14. Freedom and Autonomy
- **Exploratory Question:** "What choices or freedoms matter most to you right now?"

- **Observational Cues:** Desire for independence, references to control or self-direction.
- **Rating (0–5):** ____
- **Personal Goal Prompt:** "One decision I'd like to have more control over is..."
- **Notes:** _____

Using the Results

This tool is **not about scoring or comparison**. It is about noticing: what is present, what is missing, and what might be possible again.

- **Strong sparks** → integrate them into treatment and recovery planning.
- **Weaker sparks** → explore gently, considering trauma, stigma, or systemic barriers.
- **Over time** → revisit to track changes and progress, always grounding in person-centered care.

Conclusion

Recovery is not a checklist. It is a reengagement with life. This tool is one small invitation toward that reengagement—a way to see patients not just as collections of symptoms, but as people living with hidden sparks waiting to be seen, heard, and honored.

By asking these questions, and listening for the answers, we help sparks not only survive, but grow.

APPENDIX

Fourteen Sparks Wheel Assessment

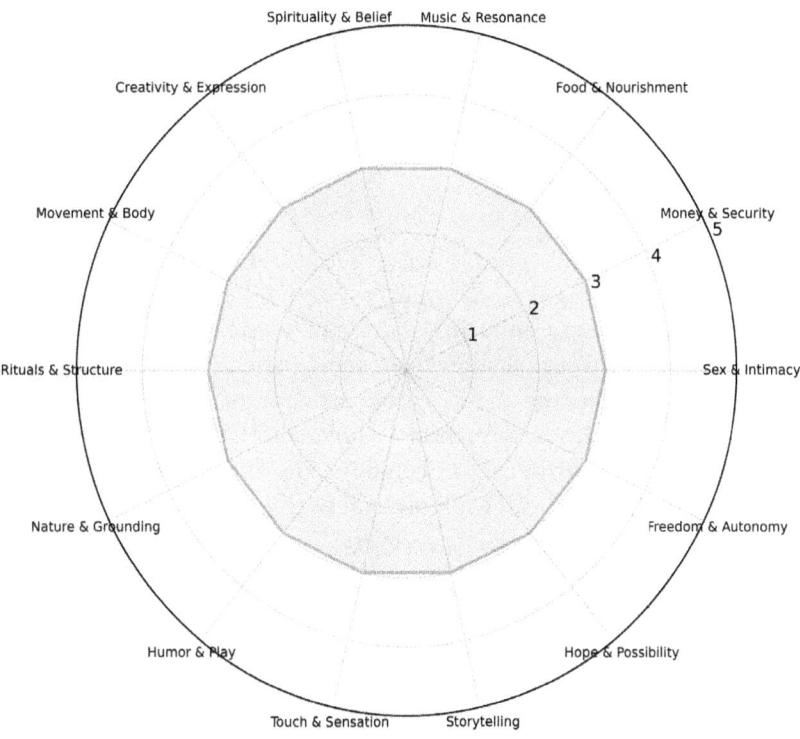

Appendix P:
Clinical Tools — How to Engage the Shadow Sparks

Introduction

While sparks represent enduring sources of passion, identity, and resilience, they can also cast shadows. For some patients, sparks appear distorted, over-amplified, or tied to symptoms in ways that complicate care. For example, sexuality may manifest as hypersexual behavior, money as financial delusions, or rituals as compulsions. Rather than suppressing these sparks, clinicians can explore them with nuance, recognizing both their risks and their potential for recovery.

What Are Shadow Sparks?

- **Sexuality** → hypersexuality, boundary violations, or shame
- **Money** → spending sprees, hoarding, or delusional beliefs about wealth
- **Food** → binge eating, anorexia, or food refusal tied to psychosis
- **Music** → obsessive listening, triggering content, or song-based delusions
- **Spirituality** → religious delusions, rigid dogma, or spiritual despair
- **Creativity** → pressured, chaotic output during mania; withdrawal from creative outlets during depression
- **Movement** → psychomotor agitation, stereotyped behavior, or avoidance of embodiment after trauma
- **Rituals** → compulsions, rigidity, or rituals rooted in paranoia
- **Nature** → isolation in wilderness, avoidance of people
- **Humor** → sarcasm, self-deprecation, or humor used as a defense mechanism
- **Touch** → unsafe or intrusive touch, sensory defensiveness
- **Storytelling** → fragmented narratives, confabulations, or persecutory plots
- **Hope** → unrealistic optimism, denial of illness
- **Freedom** → impulsivity, refusal of treatment, disregard for safety

Clinical Tools for Engagement

1. **Normalize the Spark**
   - Frame the spark as a *drive for connection or meaning,* not only as pathology.
   - Example: "I hear that money feels really important to you. Let's look at what role it plays in your life."
2. **Differentiate Spark vs. Symptom**
   - Distinguish between healthy expression and distorted expression.
   - Example: enjoying spiritual practices vs. persecutory religious delusions.
3. **Channel Safely**
   - Identify safer ways to express the spark (e.g., budgeting groups for money, art therapy for creativity, walking groups for movement).
4. **Contain, Don't Extinguish**
   - Instead of suppressing, create boundaries.
   - Example: setting spending limits rather than forbidding money conversations.
5. **Leverage Peer Narratives**
   - Use lived experience accounts to model how sparks can be reclaimed.
6. **Use Trauma-Informed Lenses**
   - Recognize that shadow sparks often trace back to trauma, neglect, or institutionalization.
7. **Revisit Periodically**
   - A spark in shadow form today may reemerge as a strength tomorrow.

> **Clinical Insight Box**
>
> Engaging shadow sparks requires curiosity and balance, validating the spark's presence while gently shaping its expression toward safety and growth.

Appendix Q:
How Sparks Are Shaped by Culture

Introduction
Sparks are universal, but their **expression, value, and meaning** are shaped by cultural, regional, and historical context. What brings hope, intimacy, or meaning in one community may carry stigma or symbolic weight in another. For clinicians, understanding cultural shaping is essential to avoid imposing one-size-fits-all models of care.

Examples of Cultural Shaping
- **Sex and Intimacy**
  o In Western settings, open discussion of sexuality is increasingly normalized, while in more conservative cultures, it remains taboo.
  o Gender roles and family expectations influence how intimacy is expressed.
- **Money and Security**
  o In immigrant communities, money may symbolize survival, migration success, or family honor.
  o In collectivist societies, financial resources may be shared across extended family, reshaping individual notions of autonomy.
- **Food and Nourishment**
  o Food rituals carry deep cultural meaning (e.g., Sabbath meals, Ramadan fasting, Thanksgiving).
  o Illness can disrupt access to cultural foods, intensifying isolation.
- **Music and Resonance**
  o Spiritual chants, gospel, hip-hop, and folk traditions each resonate differently depending on heritage.
  o Music may carry political or historical identity (e.g., protest songs, cultural preservation).

- **Spirituality and Belief**
  - Religious affiliation often determines acceptable expressions of illness and healing.
  - In some cultures, spiritual explanations of psychosis (ancestral voices, possession) shape care pathways.
- **Creativity and Expression**
  - Art, storytelling, and crafts often serve as cultural survival tools.
  - In some traditions, creative work is sacred rather than recreational.
- **Movement and the Body**
  - Dance as healing ritual (e.g., Haitian rara, Native American powwow).
  - Cultural attitudes toward exercise or rest vary (e.g., yoga in South Asia vs. aerobics in the West).
- **Rituals and Structure**
  - Religious, seasonal, and family rituals define belonging.
  - Institutional rituals (hospitals, prisons) may clash with cultural ones.
- **Nature and Grounding**
  - Land, farming, and ecological ties are central in Indigenous traditions.
  - Access to natural spaces is inequitable across urban vs. rural communities.
- **Humor and Playfulness**
  - Humor can be culturally bound; irony, satire, or slapstick may resonate differently across groups.
  - Humor can be resistance (e.g., jokes under oppression).
- **Touch and Sensation**
  - Cultures differ in comfort with physical affection, greetings, and caregiving touch.
  - Some communities rely more on touch rituals (anointing, healing touch, hugs).
- **Storytelling and Meaning-Making**
  - Oral traditions, myth, and folklore shape identity.
  - Storytelling may be intergenerational, sustaining resilience under oppression.
- **Hope and Possibility**
  - Hope may be framed in religious salvation, collective liberation, or personal success.
  - Cultures facing systemic barriers may cultivate "radical hope" as survival.

- **Freedom and Autonomy**
  - Individualist societies value independence; collectivist ones value harmony.
  - Patients' autonomy is mediated by family structures, gender roles, and legal norms.

Clinical Applications

- Cultural humility: Approach sparks with openness. Ask; don't assume.
- Community integration: Involve families, faith leaders, and cultural healers.
- Language matters: Use culturally resonant terms (e.g., "ritual" vs. "tradition").
- Equity lens: Recognize structural inequities in access to sparks (e.g., safe outdoor spaces, financial stability).

> **Clinical Insight Box**
>
> Sparks may be universal, but they are never neutral. To honor them fully, we must honor the cultural soil in which they grow.

Appendix R:
The Spark Self-Assessment & Reflective Journal Tool

Section 1: Spark Identification Checklist
Instructions: For each spark, reflect and complete the items.
- Is this spark important to you? (Yes/No)
- How strongly do you feel this spark right now? (1–5)
- Has it changed due to illness or care? (Yes/No)
- Describe how it appears—or has disappeared—in your life.

The Fourteen Sparks
1. Sex and Intimacy
2. Money and Security
3. Food and Nourishment
4. Music and Resonance
5. Spirituality and Belief
6. Creativity and Expression
7. Movement and the Body
8. Rituals and Structure
9. Nature and Grounding
10. Humor and Playfulness
11. Touch and Sensation
12. Storytelling and Meaning-Making
13. Hope and Possibility
14. Freedom and Autonomy

Section 2: Spark Reflection Questions
Choose one or two sparks and reflect in writing or conversation.
1. When did you first realize this spark was important to you?
2. How does this spark show up during difficult times?
3. Has anyone ever misunderstood or pathologized this spark in you?
4. What role does culture, identity, or belief play in this spark?
5. What would it mean to reclaim or nurture this spark more fully?

Section 3: Spark-Specific Reflection Prompts

Use these questions to deepen your reflection on each spark.
- Sex and Intimacy: How do you balance closeness and independence?
- Money and Security: What does financial independence mean to you?
- Food and Nourishment: What food connects you to your family or culture?
- Music and Resonance: Is there a song that carries you through hard times?
- Spirituality and Belief: When have you felt connected to something bigger than yourself?
- Creativity and Expression: What have you made that you are most proud of?
- Movement and the Body: What activity makes your body feel alive?
- Rituals and Structure: Which routine gives you stability?
- Nature and Grounding: Where outdoors do you feel most at peace?
- Humor and Playfulness: What always makes you laugh?
- Touch and Sensation: What textures, hugs, or sensory experiences comfort you?
- Storytelling and Meaning-Making: What story do you want others to remember about you?
- Hope and Possibility: What do you look forward to?
- Freedom and Autonomy: What choice feels most important to you right now?

Section 4: Spark Journaling Templates

Weekly Spark Journal
- Date: _____
- Spark I noticed most this week: _____
- How it showed up (thoughts, behaviors, desires): _____
- What helped it grow or shrink?: _____
- How did my environment support or silence it?: _____
- What do I want to carry forward?: _____

Monthly Spark Progress Tracker
Instructions: Rate each spark from 0–5 at the end of each month.
- 0 = Absent
- 1 = Very weak
- 2 = Slight presence

- 3 = Moderate presence
- 4 = Strong presence
- 5 = Very strong, life-shaping presence

Spark	Month 1	Month 2	Month 3	Notes
Sex & Intimacy				
Money & Security				
Food & Nourishment				
Music & Resonance				
Spirituality & Belief				
Creativity & Expression				
Movement & Body				
Rituals & Structure				
Nature & Grounding				
Humor & Playfulness				
Touch & Sensation				
Storytelling & Meaning-Making				
Hope & Possibility				
Freedom & Autonomy				

Section 5: Clinician and Caregiver Integration

For Clinicians
- Use the self-assessment to initiate strength-based conversations.
- Validate the patient's self-identified sparks, even if they conflict with clinical goals.
- Integrate strong sparks into care planning, therapy, or group activities.
- Revisit the tool periodically to track recovery and meaning, not just symptoms.

For Caregivers
- Ask directly: "What still brings you joy or meaning?"
- Watch for sparks in behavior: humming music, repeating stories, choosing foods.
- Support small rituals or pleasures, even if they seem insignificant.
- Encourage sparks by joining in (listening to music together, taking a walk outdoors).
- Celebrate progress when sparks reappear after times of silence.

Closing Note

This tool is not about measuring deficits. It is about noticing sparks, honoring them, and letting them guide recovery. By journaling, reflecting, and sharing, patients and caregivers alike can help sparks not only survive, but flourish.

www.ingramcontent.com/pod-product-compliance
Lightning Source LLC
Chambersburg PA
CBHW070608030426
42337CB00020B/3716